THE GREENWOOD ENCYCLOPEDIA OF LOVE, COURTSHIP, & *Sexuality* THROUGH HISTORY

THE GREENWOOD ENCYCLOPEDIA OF LOVE, COURTSHIP, AND SEXUALITY THROUGH HISTORY

The Ancient World, Volume 1
James W. Howell

The Medieval Era, Volume 2
William E. Burns

The Early Modern Period, Volume 3
Victoria L. Mondelli and Cherrie A. Gottsleben, with the assistance of Kristen Pederson Chew

The Colonial and Revolutionary Age, Volume 4
Merril D. Smith

The Nineteenth Century, Volume 5
Susan Mumm

The Modern World, Volume 6
James T. Sears

THE GREENWOOD ENCYCLOPEDIA OF
LOVE, COURTSHIP, *& Sexuality* THROUGH HISTORY

THE MEDIEVAL ERA
Volume 2

Edited by
WILLIAM E. BURNS

GREENWOOD PRESS
Westport, Connecticut • London

Dedicated to
Robert Sargent Jr. and Janie Sargent

Library of Congress Cataloging-in-Publication Data

The Greenwood encyclopedia of love, courtship, and sexuality through history / volume editors, James W. Howell ... [et al.].
    p. cm.
  Includes bibliographical references and index.
    Contents: v. 1. The ancient world / James W. Howell, editor—v. 2. The medieval era / William E. Burns, editor—v. 3. The early modern period / Victoria L. Mondelli and Cherrie A. Gottsleben, editors—v. 4. The colonial and revolutionary age / Merril D. Smith, editor—v. 5. The nineteenth century / Susan Mumm, editor—v. 6. The modern world / James T. Sears, editor.
  ISBN-13: 978–0–313–33359–0 (set : alk. paper)—ISBN-13: 978–0–313–33583–9 (vol. 1 : alk. paper)—ISBN-13: 978–0–313–33519–8 (vol. 2 : alk. paper)—ISBN-13: 978–0–313–33653–9 (vol. 3 : alk. paper)—ISBN-13: 978–0–313–33360–6 (vol. 4 : alk. paper)—ISBN-13: 978–0–313–33405–4 (vol. 5 : alk. paper)—ISBN-13: 978–0–313–33646–1 (vol. 6 : alk. paper)
  1. Sex—History—Encyclopedias. 2. Love—History—Encyclopedias. 3. Courtship—History—Encyclopedias. I. Howell, James W. II. Title.
  HQ21.G67125 2008
  306.703–dc22   2007023728

British Library Cataloguing in Publication Data is available.

Copyright © 2008 by William E. Burns

All rights reserved. No portion of this book may be reproduced, by any process or technique, without the express written consent of the publisher.

Library of Congress Catalog Card Number: 2007023728
ISBN-13: 978–0–313–33359–0 (set code)
          978–0–313–33583–9 (Vol. 1)
          978–0–313–33519–8 (Vol. 2)
          978–0–313–33653–9 (Vol. 3)
          978–0–313–33360–6 (Vol. 4)
          978–0–313–33405–4 (Vol. 5)
          978–0–313–33646–1 (Vol. 6)

First published in 2008

Greenwood Press, 88 Post Road West, Westport, CT 06881
An imprint of Greenwood Publishing Group, Inc.
www.greenwood.com

Printed in the United States of America

The paper used in this book complies with the Permanent Paper Standard issued by the National Information Standards Organization (Z39.48–1984).

10 9 8 7 6 5 4 3 2 1

Contents

List of Entries   vii

Set Preface   xi

Preface   xiii

Introduction   xv

Guide to Related Topics   xix

Chronology of Selected Events   xxiii

The Encyclopedia   1

Bibiliography   255

Index   273

About the Editor and Contributors   277

List of Entries

'Abbas ben al-Ahnaf, al-
  (c. 750–808)
Abelard, Peter (1079–1142), and
  Heloise (c. 1098–1164)
Abortion
Abu Nuwas (750–810)
Adab Literature
Adultery
Africa
Alain of Lille (c. 1120–1202)
Albas
Albertus Magnus (c. 1206–1280)
Anal and Intercrural Sex
Ananga Ranga
Andreas Capellanus
Aphrodisiacs
Aquinas, Thomas (1224/5–1274)
Aristotle and the Phyllis Legend
Arthurian Legend
Aucassin and Nicolette (c. 1250)
Augustine (354–430)
Averroes. *See* Ibn Rushd
Avicenna. *See* Ibn Sina

Bastardy. *See* Illegitimacy
Bernard of Clairvaux (1090–1153)
Bernardino of Siena (1380–1444)
Bestiality
Bestiary
Bhakti
Bieris de Romans
Bigamy
Bisexuality
Bo Xingjian (776–826)
Boccaccio, Giovanni (1313–1375)
Buddhism
Byzantine Empire. *See* Byzantium
Byzantium

Cakrasamvara Tantra
Canon Law
Cantigas de Santa Maria
Castration
Cathars. *See* Manicheans and
  Cathars
Catholic Europe
Catholicism
Celibacy
Central Asia
Chastity in Marriage
Chaucer, Geoffrey
  (c. 1343–1400)
Childbirth
China
Chinese Paintings of Elite Women
  (*Shinü hua*)
Christine de Pisan (1363–1430)
Chrysostom, John (349–407)
Circumcision
Clitoridectomy
*Collatio Legum Mosaicarum et
  Romanarum* (392/395)
Concubinage
Confession
Consanguinity
Contraception
Courtly Love
Cross-Dressing. *See*
  Transgenderism and
  Cross-Dressing

Dante Alighieri (1265–1321)
Daoism
Devadasis
Divorce
Domestic Violence
Droit du Seigneur

Edward II, King of England
  (1284–1327)
Ejaculation. *See* Orgasm, Male
Ermengaud, Matfre
Eunuchs

Ferrer, Vicente (1350–1419)
Fifteen Joys of Marriage
Footbinding. *See* China
Freya/Frigg

Genital Contact in Islamic Law
Gershom ben Judah
  (c. 960–c. 1040)
Ghazal
Giles of Rome (c. 1243/7–1316)
Goliard Poets
Gonorrhea. *See* Sexually
  Transmitted Diseases
Gower, John (d. 1408)

Hafiz (1327–1391)
Hafsa Bint al-Hadjdj
  (c. 1135–1190)
Halevi, Judah (c. 1075–1141)
Harem
Heloise. *See* Abelard, Peter and
  Heloise
Hermaphrodites
Hijras
Hildegard of Bingen (c. 1098–1179)
Hindu Literature
Hinduism
Homosexuality, Female
Homosexuality, Male
Houris

Ibn Dawud al-Zahir, Muhammad
  (d. 909)

LIST OF ENTRIES

Ibn Gabirol, Solomon (c. 1022–c. 1070)
Ibn Hazm, Abu Muhammad Ali (994–1064)
Ibn Qayyim al-Jawziyya (1292–1350)
Ibn Rushd (Averroes) (1126–1198)
Ibn Sina (Avicenna) (980–1037)
Illegitimacy
Impotence
Incest
India
Interconfessional Sex and Love
Intercrural Sex. *See* Anal and Intercrural Sex
Islam
Islamic Society

Jahiz, Abu Uthman Amr b. Bahr al- (c. 776–868)
Jainism
Japan
Jayadeva (1147–1170)
Jeanne d'Arc. *See* Joan of Arc
Jerome, Eusebius Hieronymus (347–420)
Jews
Joan, Pope. *See* Pope Joan
Joan of Arc (Jeanne d'Arc) (1412–1431)
Judaism

Kailasanath Temple at Ellora
Kalidasa
Kama Sutra
Khajuraho Temple Complex
Kiss of Infamy
Krishna
Kyteler, Alice (1280–c. 1325)

Lent
Lesbianism. *See* Homosexuality, Female
Lust

Magic
Maimonides, Moses (1135–1204)
Manicheans and Cathars
Marcabru (fl. 1130–1150)
Margaret of Henneberg (1254–1276)
Marianism

Marie de France (fl. 1165–1215)
Marriage
Mary Magdalene, Cult of
Masturbation
Medb (fl. first century BCE)
Medicine
Meistersinger
Menstruation
Mesoamerica
Midwives
Minnesinger (Minnesänger)
Misogyny in Latin Christendom
Monasticism, Female
Monasticism, Male
Monophysite Churches
Murasaki Shikibu (c. 970–c. 1031)
Mut'a Marriage

Nestorian Churches
New Songs from a Jade Terrace
Nizami (1141–1203)

Orgasm, Female
Orgasm, Male
Orthodox Christianity
Orthodox Europe
Osculum Infame. *See* Kiss of Infamy
Ovidianism

Pagan Europe
Pederasty
Penitentials
Peter Damian (1007–1072)
Peter of Abano (fl. late thirteenth/early fourteenth centuries)
Petrarch (or Petrarca), Francesco (1304–1374)
Phallic Worship
Philip II Augustus, King of France (1165–1223)
Phyllis Legend. *See* Aristotle and the Phyllis Legend
Physiognomics
Polygamy
Pope Joan
Pornography
Prithviraj III (r. 1178–1192)
Prostitution

Qiyan. *See* Singing Girls

Rape
Razi, Abu Bakr Muhammad ibn Zakariya al- (Rhazes) (865–925)

Remarriage
Rhazes. *See* al-Razi, Abu Bakr Muhammad ibn Zakariya
Roman Law
Romance
Romance of the Rose
Ruiz, Juan
Rumi, Jalaluddin (1207–1273)

Saga Literature
Sakthism
Scholastic Philosophy
Seclusion of Women
Secrets of Women (De Secretis Mulierum)
Sex Manuals
Sexual Differences. *See* Theories of Sexual Difference
Sexually Transmitted Diseases
Shajarat ad-Durr (fl. thirteenth century)
Sharia
Sheela-na-Gig
Shinü hua. See Chinese Paintings of Elite Women
Shonagon, Sei (fl. tenth–eleventh century)
Singing Girls (*Qayna,* sing./ *Qiyan,* pl.)
Slavery
Sodomy
Sorel, Agnes (c. 1422–1450)
Sufism
Sukayna bint al-Husayn (fl. seventh century)
Sun Simiao (581–682)

Tachikawa-ryu
Tantric Buddhism
Templars, Trial of. *See* Trial of the Templars
Theodora (c. 500–548)
Theophylactus of Ochrid (c. 1050–c. 1110)
Theories of Sexual Difference
Thousand and One Nights
Tibet
Transgenderism and Cross-Dressing
Trial of the Templars (1307–1308)
Tristan
Trobairitz
Trotula (c. 1097–?)
Troubadours

LIST OF ENTRIES

Udhrite Love
Umar Ibn Abi Rabia (644–712/721)

Veil
Virgin Martyrs
Virgin Mary. *See* Marianism
Virginity

Wallada bint al-Mustakfi
 (1011–1091)
Wedding Rituals
Wilgefortis, Saint
William IX, Duke of Aquitaine
 and Gascony, Count of Poitiers
 (1071–1126)

Witches and Witch-Hunting
Wu Zetian (627–705)

Yang Guifei (719–756)

Zhang Boduan (983–1082)
Zhang Zhuo (c. 660–740)

Set Preface

Sex and love are part of the very fabric of daily life—universal concepts that permeate every human society and are central to how each society views and understands itself. However, the way sex and love are expressed or perceived varies from culture to culture, and, within a particular society, attitudes toward sex and love evolve over time alongside the culture from which they arose. To capture the multicultural and chronological dimensions of these vital concepts, the six-volume *The Greenwood Encyclopedia of Love, Courtship, and Sexuality through History* explores the array of ideas, attitudes, and practices that have constituted sex and love around the world and across the centuries.

Each volume of alphabetically arranged entries was edited by an expert in the field who has drawn upon the expertise of contributors from many related disciplines to carefully analyze views toward sex and love among many cultures within a specified time period. Students and interested general readers will find in this work a host of current, informative, and engaging entries to help them compare and contrast different perceptions and practices across time and space. Entries cover such topics as customs and practices; institutions; legislation; religious beliefs; art and literature; and important ideas, innovations, and individuals. Users of this encyclopedia will, for instance, be able to learn how marriage in ancient Rome differed from marriage in Victorian England or in colonial America; how prostitution was viewed in medieval Europe and in the contemporaneous Islamic societies of Africa and the Middle East; and how or even if celibacy was practiced in eighteenth-century India, ancient Greece, or early modern Europe.

Edited by James W. Howell, Volume 1, *The Ancient World*, explores love and sexuality in the great societies of Europe, Africa, and Asia in the period before around 300 CE. Entries include Marriage, Homosexuality, Temple Prostitution, and Sex in Art. Volume 2, *The Medieval Era*, by William E. Burns examines sex and love in Europe, East Asia, India, the Middle East, Africa, and pre-Columbian Mesoamerica in the period between around 300 and 1400. Entries in this volume include Arthurian Legend, Concubinage, Eunuchs, Krishna, Seclusion of Women, *Thousand and One Nights*, and Virginity.

Volume 3, *The Early Modern Period*, edited by Victoria L. Mondelli and Cherrie Ann Gottsleben, with the assistance of Kristen Pederson Chew, focuses on sex and love in Europe, India, China, the Middle East, Africa, and the Americas in the fifteenth and sixteenth centuries. Some important entries in this volume are Bastardy, Confucianism, Dowries, Sex Toys, Suttee, and William Shakespeare. Edited by Merril D. Smith,

SET PREFACE

Volume 4, *The Colonial and Revolutionary Age*, looks at love and sexuality in western Europe, eastern Asia, India, the Middle East, Africa, and the Americas in the seventeenth and eighteenth centuries. The volume offers entries such as Bestiality, Castration, Berdache, Harems, Pueblo Indians, and Yoshiwara.

Volume 5, *The Nineteenth Century*, edited by Susan Mumm, explores sex and love in the Victorian period, primarily in Europe and the United States, but also in India, Asia, and the Middle East. Entries in this volume include Birth Control, Courtship, Fetishism, Native Americans, and Ottoman Women. Edited by James T. Sears, Volume 6, *The Modern World*, explores major topics in sex and sexuality from around the world in the twentieth and twenty-first centuries. Entries include AIDS/HIV, Domestic and Relationship Violence, Internet Pornography, Politics and Sex, Premarital Sex, Television, and the Women's Movement.

Each volume is illustrated and several cross-references to entries are provided. The entries conclude with a list of additional information resources, including the most useful books, journal articles, and Web sites currently available. Other important features of the encyclopedia include chronologies of important dates and events; guides to related topics that allow readers to trace broad themes across the entries; bibliographies of important general and standard works; and useful appendices, such as lists of Chinese dynasties and selections of important films and Web sites. Finally, detailed subject indexes help users gain easy access to the wealth of information on sex, love, and culture provided by this encyclopedia.

Preface

The Medieval Era is the second book in the six-volume *The Greenwood Encyclopedia of Love, Courtship, and Sexuality through History*, which covers its topic from antiquity to the present. This volume contains more than 200 entries on various topics relating to love, sex, and culture in the medieval world, defined roughly as the period from 300 to 1400 CE. Topics range from specific individuals and documents to surveys of regions and civilizations to examinations of phenomena across cultures. There is a particular focus on areas of Europe that followed the Catholic Church in the period, but there are numerous articles on other civilizations as well, including East Asia, India, the Middle East, and even Africa and Mesoamerica. This volume is intended as a reference work for the general public and for students at various levels from high school through college who want to learn about the topic of sex and culture in the medieval period.

The entries are arranged alphabetically. Each entry begins by describing or defining its topic and its importance to the general themes of medieval sex and culture, before proceeding to a general overview of the subject. Since almost sixty authors have contributed to this volume, they sometimes have different perspectives or disagreeing interpretations. Each entry concludes with a bibliography of further information sources, including books, articles, and Web sites. Cross-references to other entries in the volume are in **bold**, and a Guide to Related Topics helps users to quickly and easily trace broad themes and concepts across the entries. The volume also includes an introduction providing overall context for the entries, a chronology of significant events of the period, and a general bibliography.

Introduction

The history of love and sex in the medieval period, like love and sex in other periods and cultures, combines elements that are familiar to us in the twenty-first century with concepts that are far different and in some ways even shocking. (For the purposes of this book, the "medieval period" is defined roughly as the period from 300 to 1400 CE.) Although arranged marriage is far from unknown in our own time, few readers of this book will expect to have their marriages arranged by their parents, nor will brides expect to move into the house of their husband's parents, as has been the case for millions of newly married women in India and China during the medieval period and long after.

The medieval period in the history of sex and love, like the medieval period in general, can be defined in terms of the expansion of several religions, philosophies, and legal systems across Eurasia and Africa. The most important religions in this regard are Christianity and Islam, but Confucianism, Hinduism, Mahayana and Tantric Buddhism, and Rabbinical Judaism have also played a major role in shaping love and sexuality to the present day. Ideas less embodied in institutions, such as romantic love, also spread during this period.

PATRIARCHY AND RELIGION IN THE CHRISTIAN AND ISLAMIC LANDS

Among the most remarkable phenomena of the medieval period is the dramatic expansion of the religious and cultural systems of Christianity and Islam. After the adoption of Christianity by the Roman emperor Constantine in the fourth century, the institutions and practices of the Christian churches spread to the population of the Mediterranean basin and Europe. The rise of Islam was even more striking, beginning with its unification of the Arabian peninsula in the seventh century and the rapid conquest of the Persian and much of the Byzantine empire thereafter—Islam grew through both conquest and peaceful expansion throughout the medieval period. These religions, which dominated western Eurasia and North Africa, had common roots within Judaism, and both Christian and Islamic societies included Jewish populations. Although Judaism in the medieval period did not seek converts, its geographic spread was wide, and it underwent important transformations with the rise of rabbinic authority and the creation and spread of the Talmud.

Despite the hostility they often displayed toward one another, these three religions had many similarities in their approaches to the problems of love and sex. All three religions endorsed male supremacy, Christianity placing the most emphasis on characterizing God as "Father." In many areas, conversion to Islam or Christianity was followed by a decline in the autonomy, including the sexual autonomy, of women.

All three asserted that sexual expression should be limited by divine law. The Sharia law of Islam, the Christian penitentials, and the Talmud along with its rabbinic commentaries handled sexual issues, like other issues, with unprecedented range and subtlety. The expansion of Christianity and Islam forced societies from Ireland to India to remake their sexual customs and practices to conform to the dictates of their new faith, although this process was often incomplete.

CHRISTIANITY AND SEXUAL LIFE

As the Christian centuries continued in Europe and the eastern Mediterranean, there was a steadily increasing involvement of religious authority with key sexual institutions such as marriage. From being an arrangement between two families, marriage became a sacrament of the church. An example of this growing importance of church regulation can be seen in the doctrine of consanguinity. Through the selective enforcement of the bar on relatives marrying, the church was able to control much of aristocratic marital life.

The most striking difference between Christianity and its Western monotheistic rivals, Judaism and Islam, in the sexual realm was the high value Christianity placed on celibacy, and its corresponding suspicion of sex. While Judaism and Islam viewed marriage as the highest spiritual state, something appropriate for the holiest saints and prophets, Christianity in its Catholic, Orthodox, and Monophysite variations viewed virginity and celibacy as spiritually superior to married life. Its founder, Jesus, and his apostles were portrayed as celibate men, with Jesus enjoying the unique status of not even having been conceived through intercourse. His mother, Mary, who rivaled him as an object of devotion for much of the Middle Ages, was portrayed as a virgin mother, pure from the stain of sex. Monks, priests, and nuns emulated these sacred role models in the sphere of sexuality; married and sexually experienced men and women did not.

This meant that not only was sex of any kind barred to priests, monks, nuns, and unmarried people, but it was also viewed ambiguously even between married partners. This was a subject of debate, but some viewed lust as problematic even within marriage. This was one reason that medieval Christian societies never developed sex manuals oriented to and celebrating sexual pleasure, as did Islamic, Indian, and East Asian civilizations. Another unique characteristic of the Christian approach to married life was its extreme emphasis on monogamy, which distinguished it from East Asian, Islamic, Indian, and African societies, all of which had a place for polygamy. European Jews, on the other hand, followed their Christian neighbors to a religiously enforced monogamy. Christianity also drew a strong distinction between children born to married partners and "illegitimate" children born of other kinds of relationships.

On a deeper level, Catholic Christianity and, to a lesser degree, Orthodox and Monophysite Christianity created a system in which celibate men were treated as the authorities on matters sexual. As confessors, theologians, canon lawyers, and professors, men vowed to celibacy (whether or not they actually practiced it), defined the limits of permissible sexual behavior in thought and deed, and established and enforced the penalties for their violation.

ISLAM

By the late Middle Ages, Islam spread from central Asia to West Africa, from Indonesia to southern Spain. Unlike Jesus and the Buddha, Muhammad, the founder of Islam, was portrayed as a multiply married man with a vigorous sexual life. Islam followed the tradition of Muhammad by generally approving of sex within a defined context, and, except for some Sufis, it did not associate holiness with celibacy. While the

Christian heaven was a place without sex, many depictions of the Islamic heaven had a place for sex, whether literal or metaphorical. However, Islam's Sharia law covered sexuality in as much detail as did the Christian penitential code or the Talmud, and Islam brought with it a body of customs, including male circumcision and the seclusion and veiling of women, which often greatly changed those societies that fell under its sway, whether by force or conversion. In addition to legal commentaries, Islam produced a wide variety of genres discussing sex, from poetry to medical writings to *adab*, or advisory, literature.

Despite its rejection of religious celibacy, Islam did not endorse an "anything goes" sexual ethic. It regarded chastity and the limitation of sex to marriage as a religious duty for both men and women, although men were allowed up to four wives, and women's chastity (as in the Christian world and elsewhere) was far more ferociously policed than men's. Followers were also told to associate sex, just like many other activities, with ritual cleansing.

SOUTH ASIA

One of the areas that Islam affected, particularly in the later medieval period, was South Asia, which had its own sexual culture strongly influenced by the religions grouped together as "Hinduism." Hinduism went considerably farther than Islam or any Western religious tradition in linking the sexual and the divine, ascribing sexual activity to its gods, conceptualizing the relationships of devotees and their deities as erotic, and even including depictions of people having sex in its religious art. The close association of the erotic and the divine also influenced Buddhism, leading to the formation of Tantric Buddhism, a religious tradition that began in India and later spread to China and Tibet. Medieval India also produced voluminous literature advising people on the proper ways and occasions to have sex, the most famous example being the *Kama Sutra*.

Despite its overall sex-positive culture, which included a recognized position in society for "third-gender" individuals, India also placed a high value on female chastity and virginity and exercised tight control over the sexuality of married women, practicing seclusion and strictly forbidding widow remarriage.

SEX AND LOVE IN EAST ASIA

Analogous to the spread of Christianity and Islam in western and central Eurasia was the spread of Buddhism and Confucianism in the East. Many forms of Buddhism had one thing in common with Christianity—its suspicion of sex and desire. Although legend portrayed the Buddha as having been married, it also portrayed him as having renounced his wife and family to seek enlightenment. Both Buddhism and Christianity promoted the spread of celibate religious institutions. (The indigenous Chinese religion of Daoism was influenced by Buddhism to found its own monastic institutions as well.) However, Buddhism was never able to establish itself in the dominant hegemonic position that Christianity and Islam had, nor did it create and impose an elaborate sexual code in the manner of the Western religions.

The philosophy that became dominant in many aspects of day-to-day life in East Asia was not Buddhism (marginalized in China from around the middle of the Tang dynasty) but Confucianism, which both secured a dominant position in China during the Song dynasty and spread to Korea and Japan. Confucianists had a healthy respect for the power of sex—Confucius himself was alleged to have claimed that he had never met a man who loved virtue as much as he loved sex—and took a generally positive view of sex within the context of the family, which was the individual's highest obligation to carry on and support. However, Confucianists in authority lacked either the legalism or the obsession with categorizing and forbidding sexual acts of their Christian and Muslim contemporaries. Confucianism did parallel the Western monotheisms, though, in its support for male authority. Indeed, Confucianism grew more repressive over time owing to its opposition to widow remarriage and its support for the seclusion of women, among other things. Another aspect of the increasingly authoritarian Chinese sexual culture was the spread of foot binding, a phenomenon that originated in the medieval period.

SEX AND LOVE IN LITERATURE

During the medieval period, love was central to the development of many national literatures. Some of the most marked examples can be found in Islamic and Catholic European literature. The Persian poet Nizami's *Layla and Majnun* and the romances of medieval France shaped approaches to love and sex in their literatures for centuries following the end of the Middle Ages. In Hindu India, the works of Kalidasa played a similar role, while the long-lived Chinese genre of the "scholar-and-beauty romance" was inaugurated by Zhang Zhuo's *The Dwelling of Playful Goddesses*, which was even more influential in Japan and Korea than in China.

The period also saw in many societies the beginnings of the literary exploration of love and sex by women. Before the medieval period, women who wrote of these things, like women writers in general, were few and far between, the most notable being Sappho. Although still vastly outnumbered by male writers, the female company of the Middle Ages included Murasaki and Sei Shonagon from Heian Japan, Hafsa Bint-al Hajj and Wallada from Muslim Andalusia, Marie de France and Christine de Pisan from the courts of late medieval western Europe, and the Catholic nun Hildegard of Bingen.

One of the most important developments in literature, if not necessarily in practice, was the development of forms of romantic love not oriented to physical consummation. This development occurred in Christian and Islamic cultures. Udhrite love was associated with tribal Bedouin Arabs, while "courtly love" emerged in the royal and noble courts of high medieval Europe. The two cultures met in medieval Spain.

SCIENCE AND MEDICINE

Drawing on ancient roots, the treatment of sex in science and medicine continued to develop throughout the Middle Ages as did these disciplines themselves. The ancient medicine of Galen and Hippocrates was further developed in the Arab world by philosopher-physicians such as Ibn Sina, Ibn Rushd, and al-Razi and then in the universities of the Latin West. Chinese medicine was carried forward by Sun Simiao. With the flourishing of these medical traditions came a growing awareness of sexual medicine as a distinct field.

Medicine did not challenge religion for authority on sexual matters during the Middle Ages, as it would do in subsequent centuries. However, medicine did provide an alternative way of categorizing sexual behavior as a natural and healthy function. Physicians in several medical traditions regarded sex as necessary for health for both men and women to purge matter that would otherwise build up in the body.

It is important to remember, however, that medical theory did not always determine medical practice. One important difference is that while learned medicine as practiced by physicians like Ibn Sina and Simiao was, like other learned disciplines, a near monopoly of men, medicine as practiced was, especially in some areas such as delivery, dominated by women. Much of what was practiced in contraception, the care of menstruating or pregnant women, and childbirth cannot be recovered because it was not written down, but transmitted orally or by example.

Guide to Related Topics

CULTURAL AND REGIONAL GROUPINGS

REGIONAL AND ETHNIC SURVEYS
Africa
Byzantium
Catholic Europe
Central Asia
China
India
Islamic Society
Japan
Jews
Mesoamerica
Orthodox Europe
Pagan Europe
Tibet

EAST ASIA
Bo Xingjian
Buddhism
Cakrasamvara Tantra
China
Chinese Paintings of Elite
 Women
Daoism
Japan
Murasaki Shikibu
New Songs from a Jade Terrace
Shonagon, Sei
Sun Simiao
Tachikawa-ryu
Tibet
Wu Zetian
Yang Guifei
Zhang Boduan
Zhang Zhuo

INDIA
Ananga Ranga
Bhakti
Buddhism
Devadasis
Hijras
Hindu Literature
Hinduism
India
Jainism
Jayadeva
Kailasanath Temple at Ellora
Kalidasa
Kama Sutra
Khajuraho Temple Complex
Krishna
Prithviraj III
Sakthism
Tantric Buddhism

ISLAMIC WORLD
'Abbas ben al-Ahnaf, al-
Abu Nuwas
Adab Literature
Africa
Central Asia
Genital Contact in Islamic Law
Ghazal
Hafiz
Hafsa Bint al-Hadjdj
Harem
Houris
Ibn Dawud al-Zahir, Muhammad
Ibn Hazm, Abu Muhammad Ali
Ibn Qayyim al-Jawziyya
Ibn Rushd (Averroes)
Ibn Sina (Avicenna)
Islam

Islamic Society
Jahiz, Abu Uthman Amr b.
 Bahr al-
Mut'a Marriage
Nizami
Physiognomics
Razi, Abu Bakr Muhammad
 ibn Zakariya al-
Rumi, Jalaluddin
Shajarat ad-Durr
Sharia
Singing Girls (*Qayna*)
Sufism
Sukayna bint al-Husayn
Thousand and One Nights
Udhrite Love
Umar Ibn Abi Rabia
Veil
Wallada bint al-Mustakfi

JEWISH WORLD
Gershom ben Judah
Halevi, Judah
Ibn Gabirol, Solomon
Jews
Judaism
Maimonides, Moses

LATIN CHRISTENDOM
Abelard, Peter, and Heloise
Alain of Lille
Albas
Albertus Magnus
Andreas Capellanus
Aquinas, Thomas
Aristotle and the Phyllis legend
Arthurian Legend
Aucassin and Nicolette

GUIDE TO RELATED TOPICS

Augustine
Bernard of Clairvaux
Bernardino of Siena
Bestiary
Bieris de Romans
Bigamy
Boccaccio, Giovanni
Canon Law
Cantigas de Santa Maria
Catholic Europe
Catholicism
Chastity in Marriage
Chaucer, Geoffrey
Christine de Pisan
Collatio Legum Mosaicarum et Romanarum
Confession
Courtly Love
Dante Alighieri
Droit du Seigneur
Edward II, King of England
Ermengaud, Matfre
Ferrer, Vicente
Fifteen Joys of Marriage
Giles of Rome
Goliard Poets
Gower, John
Hildegard of Bingen
Jerome, Eusebius Hieronymus
Joan of Arc
Kiss of Infamy
Kyteler, Alice
Lent
Lust
Marcabru
Margaret of Henneberg
Marianism
Marie de France
Mary Magdalene, Cult of
Meistersinger
Minnesinger
Misogyny in Latin Christendom
Monasticism, Female
Monasticism, Male
Ovidianism
Penitentials
Peter Damian
Peter of Abano
Petrarch, Francesco
Philip II Augustus, King of France
Pope Joan
Romance
Romance of the Rose

Ruiz, Juan
Saga Literature
Scholastic Philosophy
Secrets of Women
Sheela-na-Gig
Sodomy
Sorel, Agnes
Trial of the Templars
Tristan
Trobairitz
Trotula
Troubadours
Virgin Martyrs
Wilgefortis, Saint
William IX, Duke of Aquitaine and Gascony, Count of Poitiers
Witches and Witch-Hunting

Orthodox Christendom
Byzantium
Chrysostom, John
Orthodox Christianity
Orthodox Europe
Theodora
Theophylactus of Ochrid

Pagan Europe
Freya/Frigg
Medb
Pagan Europe

THEMATIC GROUPINGS

Art, Music, and Literature
'Abbas ben al-Ahnaf, al-
Abu Nuwas
Adab literature
Albas
Arthurian Legend
Aucassin and Nicolette
Bieris de Romans
Bo Xingjian
Boccaccio
Cantigas de Santa Maria
Chaucer, Geoffrey
Chinese Paintings of Elite Women
Christine de Pisan
Dante Alighieri
Ermengaud, Matfre
Fifteen Joys of Marriage
Ghazal
Goliard Poets
Gower, John

Hafiz
Hafsa Bint al-Hadjdj
Halevi, Judah
Hindu Literature
Ibn Hazm, Abu Muhammad Ali
Ibn Gabirol, Solomon
Ibn Qayyim al-Jawziyya
Jahiz, Abu Uthman Amr b. Bahr al-
Jayadeva
Kailasanath Temple, Ellora
Kalidasa
Khajuraho Temple Complex
Marcabru
Marie de France
Meistersinger
Minnesinger
Murasaki Shikibu
New Songs from a Jade Terrace
Nizami
Ovidianism
Petrarch, Francesco
Romance
Romance of the Rose
Ruiz, Juan
Rumi, Jalaluddin
Saga Literature
Sheela-na-Gig
Shonagon, Sei
Singing Girls (*Qayna*)
Thousand and One Nights
Tristan
Trobairitz
Troubadours
Wallada bint al-Mustakfi
William IX, Duke of Aquitaine and Gascony, Count of Poitiers
Zhang Zhuo

The Body
Abortion
Castration
Childbirth
Circumcision
Clitoridectomy
Contraception
Impotence
Menstruation
Virginity

Individuals
'Abbas ben al-Ahnaf, al-
Abelard, Peter, and Heloise

Abu Nuwas
Alain of Lille
Albertus Magnus
Aquinas, Thomas
Aristotle and the Phyllis Legend
Augustine
Bernard of Clairvaux
Bernardino of Siena
Bo Xingjian
Boccaccio, Giovanni
Chaucer, Geoffrey
Christine de Pisan
Chrysostom, John
Dante Alighieri
Edward II, King of England
Ermengaud Matfre
Ferrer, Vicente
Gershom ben Judah
Giles of Rome
Gower, John
Hafiz
Hafsa Bint al-Hadjdj
Halevi, Judah
Hildegard of Bingen
Ibn Dawud al-Zahir, Muhammad
Ibn Gabirol, Solomon
Ibn Hazm, Abu Muhammad Ali
Ibn Qayyim al-Jawziyya
Ibn Rushd (Averroes)
Ibn Sina (Avicenna)
Jahiz, Abu Uthman Amr b. Bahr al-
Jayadeva
Jerome, Eusebius Hieronymus
Joan of Arc (Jeanne d'Arc)
Kyteler, Alice
Maimonides, Moses
Marcabru
Margaret of Henneberg
Marie de France
Medb
Murasaki Shikibu
Nizami
Peter Damian
Peter of Abano
Petrarch, Francesco
Philip II Augustus, King of France
Prithviraj III
Razi, Abu Bakr Muhammad ibn Zakariya al-
Ruiz, Juan
Rumi, Jalaluddin
Shajarat ad-Durr

Shonagon, Sei
Sorel, Agnes
Sukayna bint al-Husayn
Sun Simiao
Theodora
Theophylactus of Ochrid
Trotula
Umar Ibn Abi Rabia
Wallada bint al-Mustakfi
William IX, Duke of Aquitaine and Gascony, Count of Poitiers
Wu Zetian
Yang Guifei
Zhang Boduan
Zhang Zhuo

LAWS AND INSTITUTIONS
Bigamy
Canon Law
Collatio Legum Mosaicarum et Romanarum
Concubinage
Consanguinity
Divorce
Domestic Violence
Genital Contact in Islamic Law
Illegitimacy
Marriage
Polygamy
Roman Law
Seclusion of Women
Sharia
Slavery
Trial of the Templars
Wedding Rituals
Witches and Witch-Hunting

PHILOSOPHY, SCIENCE, AND MEDICINE
Alain of Lille
Albertus Magnus
Aquinas, Thomas
Augustine
Giles of Rome
Hildegard of Bingen
Ibn Rushd (Averroes)
Ibn Sina (Avicenna)
Magic
Maimonides, Moses
Medicine
Peter of Abano
Physiognomics
Razi, Abu Bakr Muhammad ibn Zakariya al-

Scholastic Philosophy
Secrets of Women
Sexually Transmitted Diseases
Sun Simiao
Theories of Sexual Difference
Trotula
Zhang Boduan

POPULATIONS
Devadasis
Eunuchs
Hermaphrodites
Hijras
Midwives
Singing Girls (*Qayna*)

RELIGIONS, SECTS, AND DEVOTIONAL PRACTICES
Bhakti
Buddhism
Catholicism
Daoism
Hinduism
Islam
Jainism
Krishna
Manicheans and Cathars
Monophysite Churches
Nestorian Churches
Orthodox Christianity
Phallic Worship
Sakthism
Sufism
Tachikawa-ryu
Tantric Buddhism

SEX
Adultery
Anal and Intercrural Sex
Aphrodisiacs
Bestiality
Bisexuality
Celibacy
Chastity in Marriage
Courtly Love
Homosexuality, Female
Homosexuality, Male
Incest
Interconfessional Sex and Love
Masturbation
Orgasm, Female
Orgasm, Male
Pederasty

Pornography
Prostitution
Rape
Remarriage
Sex Manuals
Transgenderism and Cross-Dressing
Udhrite Love

WOMEN
Abelard, Peter, and Heloise
Abortion
Childbirth
Chinese Paintings of Elite Women
Christine de Pisan
Clitoridectomy
Concubinage
Contraception
Divorce
Domestic Violence
Droit du Seigneur
Freya/Frigg
Hildegard of Bingen
Homosexuality, Female
Joan of Arc (Jeanne d'Arc)
Kyteler, Alice
Margaret of Henneberg
Marianism
Marie de France
Marriage
Mary Magdalene, Cult of
Medb
Menstruation
Midwives
Misogyny in Latin Christendom
Monasticism, Female
Orgasm, Female
Pope Joan
Prostitution
Rape
Remarriage
Seclusion of Women
Shajarat ad-Durr
Shonagon, Sei
Singing Girls
Sorel, Agnes
Sukayna bint al-Husayn
Theodora
Veil
Virgin Martyrs
Wedding Rituals
Witches and Witch-Hunting
Wu Zetian
Yang Guifei

Chronology of Selected Events

206 BCE–220 CE	Reign of the Han dynasty in China.
312	Constantine, one of the contenders for the throne of the Roman empire, converts to Christianity.
325	Council of Nicea forbids human castration.
330	Founding of Constantinople as the new capital of the Roman empire. It will remain the capital of the East Roman and Byzantine empires until 1453.
431	Council of Ephesus proclaims the doctrine of the perpetual virginity of Mary.
524	Justinian, nephew of the Eastern Roman emperor Justin, spearheads a change in the law allowing former actresses to marry patricians. The next year he marries the former actress Theodora, and they succeed to the imperial crown in 527.
533	Emperor Justinian declares sodomy subject to civil sanctions.
545	Xu Ling compiles the first anthology in Chinese devoted entirely to love poems, titled *New Songs from a Jade Terrace*.
581–617	Rule of the Sui dynasty in China.
622	Muhammad's flight from Mecca to Medina, the Hegira, later recognized as the starting date for the Islamic calendar.
636–751	Islamic empire established, extending from Spain to the borders of China.
652	Publication of Sun Simiao's *Prescriptions Worth a Thousand Pieces of Gold for Every Emergency*, containing the foundations of the Chinese tradition of gynecological medicine.
618–907	Rule of the Tang dynasty in China.
721	Pope Gregory II forbids marriage between a parent and a godparent of the same child.
732	Pope Gregory III extends the forbidden degrees of kinship to those sharing a common ancestry in the last seven generations.
736	Yang Guifei selected to be the wife of the eighteenth son of the Chinese emperor Xuanzong.
745	Yang Guifei becomes the "Precious Consort" of Xuanzong.
756	Rebels force Yang Guifei to commit suicide, but her love will be celebrated in Chinese literature for centuries.
907–960	The Five Dynasties period in China.
960–1127	Period of the Northern Song dynasty in China.
1000	Approximate date of Rabbi Gershom ben Judah's decree against polygamy.
1008	Murasaki Shikubu begins writing *The Tale of Genji*.
1115–1234	Jin dynasty rules North China.
1049	Appearance of Peter Damian's work denouncing male homosexuality, *Liber Gomorrhianus*.

CHRONOLOGY OF SELECTED EVENTS

1116	Beginning of the love affair between Heloise and Peter Abelard.
1127–1279	Reign of the Southern Song dynasty in China.
1152	Eleanor of Aquitaine's marriage to Henry II of England helps spread southern French courtly love culture to the north and to England.
1163	The long love affair between the Spanish poets Hafsa Bint Al Hajj and Abu Ja'afar Ibn Said ends when Said is executed for plotting against the government.
1175	Composition of Nizami's *Khusrau u Shirin*, an influential Persian love story.
	Traditional date for the elopement of Prithviraj and Sanjukta.
1184	Philip Augustus of France demands a divorce from his fourteen-year-old wife Isabella of Hainault. She successfully resists this demand.
1188	Appearance of Nizami's *Laila u Majnun*.
1193	Philip Augustus of France, now a widower, marries Ingeborg of Denmark, but a few hours after the wedding demands an annulment on the grounds of consanguinity.
1196	French clergy grant Philip Augustus an annulment. He marries Agnes of Meuran.
1198	In his letter *Universis Christifidelibus*, Pope Innocent III exhorts all Christians to promote the redemption of prostitutes.
1200	Enraged at Philip Augustus's bigamy, Innocent III lays France under interdict.
1201	Death of Agnes of Meuran followed by reconciliation between Philip Augustus and Innocent III, with Philip recognizing papal supremacy in marital issues.
1215	Fourth Lateran Council defines marriage as a sacrament and establishes many aspects of marriage in canon law.
1233	Pope Gregory IX's bull, *Vox in Rama*, charges heretics with the kiss of infamy and bisexual orgies.
1236–1240	Reign of Sultana Razziya of the Delhi sultanate, who cross-dresses as a way of playing the traditionally male role of ruler.
1237	Guillame de Lorris begins the *Romance of the Rose* around this date.
1250	Shajarat ad-Durr rises from the harem to briefly rule as Sultan of Egypt.
1274	First meeting of Dante and Beatrice.
1277	The bishop of Paris, Etienne Tempier, condemns many texts, including Andreas Capellanus's *On Love*.
1279–1368	Yuan (Mongol) dynasty rules China.
1298	Boniface VIII's bull, *Periculoso*, mandates stricter seclusion of nuns.
1307	Philip IV the Fair of France begins his attack on the knightly Order of the Temple, in which charges of sodomy will play a central role.
1308	Coronation of Edward II of England. The prominent role of the Gascon nobleman Piers Gaveston at the ceremony will arouse concern about his relationship with the king, and Gaveston will be forced into exile later in the year.
1312	Under French pressure, Pope Clement V dissolves the Order of the Temple.
	Piers Gaveston captured and killed by English nobles.
1318	Edward II appoints Hugh Despenser his lord chamberlain.
1324	Trial of Alice Kyteler in Ireland links magical powers and human women having sex with demons.
1326	Edward II and Hugh Despenser defeated by forces of Edward's wife, Queen Isabella, and her lover, Roger Mortimer. Despenser is executed, and Edward deposed and executed the following year.
1347	First appearance of the Black Death in Europe, often interpreted as a punishment for the sins of the people.
1368–1644	Ming dynasty in China.
1390	Probable date of completion of John Gower's poem *Confessio Amantis*.
1399	Christine de Pisan writes *L'Epistre au Dieu d'Amours*, a response to the *Romance of the Rose*.

1432	Italian city-state of Florence establishes the Office of the Night, the first institution devoted solely to suppressing sex between men.	**1443**	Agnes Sorel meets Charles VII of France. She will bear him several children and become the first mistress of a European king with a quasi-official status.

The Encyclopedia

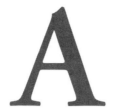

'ABBAS BEN AL-AHNAF, AL- (c. 750–c. 808). Al-'Abbas ben al-Ahnaf of the Arab tribe Hanifa, named Abu al-Fadl (Father of Excellence), was a famous love poet under the Abbasid caliph Harun al-Rashid. He began his career at an early age at Baghdad and soon entered the court, where he became a protégé of Harun who, at least in his younger days, preferred the **harem** to the world of politics. Al-'Abbas died between 803 and 808 while on a pilgrimage, and was buried in Basra.

The love poems (**ghazal**) of al-'Abbas, seemingly the only genre he cultivated, continue the tradition of Umayyad love poetry, especially in its elegiac (udhri) forms. They were in vogue among the women of the caliphal harem, and were often set to music and performed by the most famous singers of the time. They were also highly esteemed by contemporary colleagues, scholars, and critics. As a traditional Arab love poet, al-'Abbas would have alluded to his personal emotions in his poetry. However, reports about his life contain no details of his own love affairs. Speculations on the identity of his beloved Fawz (luck), whom he meaningfully also calls Zalum (evil), have been in vain. On the contrary, even prose commentaries to some of his verses add nothing new to the poetry itself.

The poetry of al-'Abbas has been named "courtly," which makes him a precursor of courtly poetry in medieval France, Italy, and Germany. Although there are affinities between the traditions, in particular the inaccessibility of the lady, the humbleness of the lover, and the connection of love and religion, medieval Arab and European love poetry are not the same. "Love for love's sake," a claim by which the aristocracy justified and defended its cultural hegemony in Europe, went beyond any equivalent in the Arab setting. Love poetry in Arab society never denied having its roots in the desert, and therefore never developed an equivalent to the courtly "joy." Love for love's sake, in the context of city and court no less, connoted loss more than benefit and consequently maintained the elegiac mood.

The poetry of al-'Abbas represents the summit of profane love poetry in Arabic literature. His verses inspired mystical poets, who from then on turned most of their attention to God as the ultimate object of desire, longing, and union. Al-'Abbas, like many poets from the Arab East, may have had an influence on Andalusian poets, too, and from there on courtly poetry in Europe. *See also* Udhrite Love.

Further Reading: Enderwitz, Susanne. *Liebe als Beruf: al-'Abbas ibn al-Ahnaf und das Ghazal*. Stuttgart: Franz Steiner Verlag. 1995; Torrey, C. C. "The History of al-'Abbas b. al-Ahnaf and His Fortunate Verses." *Journal of the American Oriental Society* 15 (1894): 43–70;

Vadet, Jean Claude. *L'Esprit courtois en Orient dans les cinq premiers siècles de l'Hègire*. Paris: G. P. Maisonneuve et Larose, 1968.

Susanne Enderwitz

ABELARD, PETER (1079–1142), **AND HELOISE** (c. 1098–1164). Peter Abelard and Heloise had one of the most famous and tragic love relationships in history. Every aspect of that relationship, from Abelard's fame to their deaths and burials, has excited the imagination of scholars and writers for centuries.

Abelard, a renowned teacher and philosopher specializing in dialectic (logic), was an instructor at the cathedral school of Notre Dame in Paris when he met Heloise. The niece of Fulbert, one of the subdeacons of the cathedral school, Heloise had a deserved reputation for intellectual brilliance. She was about one-half Abelard's age, by most accounts still in her teens, when they became lovers in 1116. By his own admission in his *Historia calamitatum* (*The History of His Misfortunes*), Abelard set out to seduce her. He entered into an agreement with Fulbert to move into the home that Fulbert shared with his niece in order to tutor her.

Abelard's stratagem worked, and teacher and pupil were soon involved in a passionate affair. When Heloise became pregnant, Abelard sent her disguised as a nun to stay with his sister in Brittany, where she gave birth to their son, Astralabe. Abelard then came to an agreement with Fulbert that included **marriage** and the uncle keeping their relationship a secret. Heloise strongly resisted marriage, convinced that it would hurt Abelard's reputation and that true love could exist only when freely given, but finally acquiesced.

After Fulbert began to speak publicly of the marriage, Abelard took Heloise to the convent at Argenteuil north of Paris, where she had been educated as a child. Assuming Abelard was trying to dispose of Heloise by making her a nun, Fulbert sought revenge. Some of Fulbert's men entered Abelard's lodgings by bribing one of his servants and then castrated him. The resulting shame and confusion led Abelard to take refuge at the Abbey of St. Denis and persuade Heloise also to accept a monastic life.

The two lovers spent the rest of their lives within the church, Heloise ultimately becoming abbess of a monastery called the Paraclete, which had been built for Abelard. A copy of *Historia calamitatum* coming into Heloise's hands precipitated the passionate, tormented letters she sent to Abelard that inspired many of the later writings about the lovers, including Alexander Pope's eighteenth-century poem *Eloisa to Abelard*. In later years, communication between the two primarily involved the proper functioning of Heloise's religious community.

After Abelard's death in 1142, his body was interred at the Paraclete. Heloise died in 1164 and was buried beside Abelard in the abbey church, not, as has often been asserted, in the same tomb. After several reburials, they now share a sarcophagus in the Père Lachaise cemetery in Paris.

Further Reading: Mews, Constant J. *Abelard and Heloise*. New York: Oxford University Press, 2005; Mews, Constant J. *The Lost Love Letters of Heloise and Abelard*. New York: St. Martin's Press, 1999.

Edward J. Rielly

ABORTION. Medieval society generally condemned abortion, though the knowledge of abortion and how it was carried out was very different from today's. Injunctions against abortion were common in medieval law codes, even from the earliest part of the period. Penalties could be fairly extreme, ranging from fines to corporal punishment to death. However, in practice, these penalties do not seem to have been rigorously enforced. **Islamic society** adopted the most lenient attitude toward abortion, and was largely responsible for the medical knowledge about abortion available in Western universities of the later medieval period.

In their attempts to define abortion, both the modern and medieval ages have grappled with the question "when does life begin"; both eras, however, have come up with very different responses. What we today consider abortion—generally the ejection or extraction of a fetus from the womb before the twentieth week of gestation—would have been understood in the medieval Christian world only as **contraception**, a sinful act that was generally disregarded. In discussing abortion, the medieval church, following in the footsteps of St. **Augustine** of Hippo, focused on two pivotal moments: First, the physical formation of the fetus (roughly fifteen weeks), which was significant because only after this moment could a fetus be said to "have been endowed with its senses." Second, and perhaps most important, was the quickening, meaning the earliest observance of fetal movement (around eighteen weeks); the medieval church believed that it was at this moment that a fetus acquired its soul. Interfering with a fetus after these two events was considered abortion, and was subject to harsh penalties under the law.

The medieval world also had much different expectations as to how an abortion might be carried out. Rather than surgery, a *maleficium* or abortifacient, herbs or other agents imbibed with the purpose of producing an abortion, was usually employed. In secular law, however, the definition was sometimes extended even further. English common law argued that anyone who struck a woman with the intention of killing the child in her womb was also guilty of abortion.

References to abortion can be found in the earliest law codes of the founding European peoples. The Merovingians, Bavarians, and Ostrogoths of the sixth and seventh centuries all included injunctions against abortion in their law codes. At times, their laws even suggested a sophisticated understanding of abortion. For example, the Allemanian law of the late sixth century imposed a sliding scale of fines that increased with the stage of fetal development. The usual punishment seems to have been a fine, although hardening attitudes toward abortion over time are reflected in the harsher penalties toward the High and late Middle Ages. In continental Europe, an abortionist might expect a fine, accompanied by a jail term or time spent in the pillories. In England, abortion was considered a form of homicide; as such, it was subject to death penalty. It is significant, however, that cases of abortion in the courts were exceedingly rare. In general, the secular and ecclesiastical courts seem to have been content to overlook cases of abortion. This attitude may be best explained by the handbooks of penance surviving from the early Middle Ages. Burchard of Worms's *Decretum* (c. 1008–1012) notes that the sin was less for a woman who committed abortion because she could not afford to have another child.

Islamic law took a much more lax approach toward the prosecution of abortion. In large part, this attitude results from their unique interpretation of abortion. Muhammad recognized three stages of fetal development, but he believed that it was only in the final stage that ensoulment occurred. Such a late date for the definition of abortion, coupled with a largely tolerant attitude toward **contraception**, probably made actual abortion unnecessary. Even still, abortion was treated leniently under the law, and it was thought that a woman could abort even without her husband's permission, providing she had a good reason for wanting the abortion. It is significant that Islamic **medicine**, especially the writings of Ibn Sina (known in the West as Avicenna, 980–1037), transmitted to the West during the period of the Crusades, significantly increased the knowledge about birth control and abortion in Western universities. There is reason to believe, however, that the Christian church's negative attitude toward abortion may have had an impact on the teaching of these texts at the universities, and certainly impeded any widespread transmission of this information in Western society.

Further Reading: Noonan, John T., Jr. *Contraception: A History of Its Treatment by the Catholic Theologians and Canonists.* Cambridge, MA: Belknap Press, 1965; Riddle, John M. *Eve's Herbs: A History of Contraception and Abortion in the West.* Cambridge, MA: Harvard University Press, 1997.

Sara M. Butler

ABU NUWAS (750–810). Abu Nuwas al-Hasan ibn Hani al-Hakam, one of the earliest poets of male homosexuality in Arabic, was an iconoclast who became famous for his poems on *mudhakkarat* (the love of boys), *khamriyyat* (wine), and *majouniyyat* (ribaldry). He wrote with superb technical fineness and without inhibition. Born at Ahwaz in Persia, Abu Nuwas was sold by his mother, Golban, at a young age. He came to the seaport of Basrah and became the lover and student of a poet, Waliba ibn al-Hubab (d. 786). Afterward, Abu Nuwas came into contact with Harun al-Rashid (764–809), the Abbasid caliph, and became a court poet. Although a patron of arts and literature, the caliph found Abu Nuwas's bold poetry too much. The poet was imprisoned many times. When the powerful Barmakis family lost favor with Harun in 798, Abu Nuwas wrote an elegy as a reaction, as he was close with the family. He went on a pilgrimage to Mecca and then traveled to Egypt to escape Harun's anger. He returned to Baghdad at the time of the new caliph, Al-Amin (809–813), who had a similar taste for boys. However, he jailed the poet for excessive drinking. The next caliph, Abdullah al-Mamun (813–833), was a patron of scholars, but was against deviants like Abu Nuwas. There is no definite information on the last part of his life. He either met a violent death in prison or was poisoned.

Abu Nuwas threw a gauntlet against the conventional mores of the society and was steadfast in his convictions. In a couplet he mentioned that he had left girls and clear water for boys and wine respectively. In another place he claimed that he was delighted in the things that were forbidden by Holy texts and eschewed God and gold. Unabashedly, the poet in many of his verses described in detail his lovemaking with handsome boys. His poetry has survived after twelve centuries, much to the wrath of fundamentalists. His ribald character and outrageous exploits appeared many times in the **Thousand and One Nights**. He was not only imprisoned and derided while alive, but remains controversial even today. In January 2001, the Ministry of Culture of Egypt burned 6,000 copies of his books. *See also* Pederasty.

Further Reading: Bey, Hakim. *O Tribe That Loves Boys.* Amsterdam: Entimos Press, 1993; Colville, Jim. *Poems of Wine and Revelry: The Khamriyyat of Abu Nuwas.* London: Kegan Paul, 2004; Kennedy, Philip F. *The Wine Song in Classical Arabic Poetry: Abu Nuwas and the Literary Tradition.* Oxford: Clarendon Press, 1997.

Patit Paban Mishra

ADAB LITERATURE. *Adab* is an important term in Arabic, used since the Middle Ages. It has a long history that follows the evolution of Arab-Islamic culture, from the pre-Islamic period until today. If in modern times *adab* simply means "literature" in the specific sense of the word, in the pre-Islamic period it was a synonym for "tradition" in the sense of "custom, or hereditary norm of conduct," derived from the forefathers and enshrined in proverbs, anecdotes, and poetry. It therefore assumed a twofold connotation, being both praiseworthy and an heritage from the ancestors. The concept underwent an evolution and in later times came to refer to "good upbringing, or urbanity," both in the sense of refining of bedouin customs and contact with foreign cultures. In the eighth century it was a synonym for the Latin *urbanitas*, and was also for the first time mentioned in relation to literature. The ethical and social meaning continued to exist during medieval **Islam**, covering in specific cases the meaning of etiquette (e.g., of drinking, of dressing). Another important meaning of intellectual nature was soon added to the social and ethical one: in this sense *adab* referred to the sum of knowledge the well-educated person had to acquire. Following the expansion of Islam, the range of interests of the cultured person progressively broadened to the Indian, Iranian, and Hellenistic worlds, thus including epic, gnomic, and narrative traditions from these cultures. In a narrower acception, already present in the Abbasid period, the complexity of *adab* as "culture" was reduced to "specific knowledge for a given office."

All the meanings of the term are reflected in what has been defined as *adab* literature, that is, books that aim to describe or transmit *adab*. The expression *adab* literature thus does not identify a specific literary genre in the technical sense of the word; it mostly refers to works that are usually miscellaneous and encyclopedic and have a didactic aim, and to works of diverse character and with diverse formal traits, monographs or anthologies. Most of these books are compilations more than original productions, thus stressing the social nature of *adab*: the reluctance that the authors show in producing original works points to the consciousness that *adab* is something inherited that must be transmitted. The writers could nevertheless bring a personal contribution through the criteria of selection and arrangement of the materials. They were also able to give old materials a new significance simply by changing the context of quotation or slightly altering the wording of narratives.

Canonical features of *adab* literature are the blending of prose and poetry, of anecdotes and poems, and the wide range of subjects—political, ethical, and religious themes as well as philological and rhetoric ones. Among these, love is often treated under different aspects, both physical and psychological: specific chapters or monographs dwell on the rules of courtesy between lovers, the phenomenology of passion, unhappy love stories, and even homosexual intercourse. A typical trait of *adab* literature is the combination of joke and earnest: *adab* literature has to educate without being boring. Therefore, entertaining passages and funny stories are included in the treatment of serious themes to relieve the reader, even though in cases of extremely important subjects this practice is disregarded to make room for a thorough treatment.

Further Reading: Bonebakker, Seeger Adrianus. "Adab and the Concept of Belles-Lettres." In '*Abbasid Belles-Lettres*, edited by Julia Ashtiany et al., 16–30. The Cambridge History of Arabic Literature series. Cambridge: Cambridge University Press, 1990; Nallino, Carlo Alfonso. *La litterature arabe des origines a l' epoque de la dynastie umayyade*. Paris: G. P. Maisonneuve et Larose, 1950.

Antonella Ghersetti

ADULTERY. As a social and religious concept, adultery (from the Latin *adulterium*) developed many different manifestations between 300 and 1400 CE. In late antiquity, adultery was often confused with fornication, since both acts could be characterized as illicit love outside the bonds of **marriage**, culminating in the couple's consummation of their passions. By the Middle Ages, however, adultery had multiple definitions. In European societies, the term could refer, as it did in late antiquity, to extramarital relations, but it also encompassed the marriage of a man or a woman who had taken a vow of chastity, as well as the marriage between people of different faiths. Within Arabic, Islamic, and Jewish cultures, the legal concept was broadly understood as a married woman's sexual congress with a man other than her husband. It was not until after the twelfth century that the Western definition of adultery was refined to include only extramarital relations and the marriage of one bound by an oath of chastity.

JURISDICTION. At the beginning of the fourth century, **Roman law** considered adultery a domestic matter. It was only when the affair came to the notice of the general public that cases of adultery would be prosecuted in legal courts. In Arabic and Islamic societies, authority over instances of adultery was placed in the hands of male family members through Shari'a law, from a combination of religious and judicial influences in Qur'anic and legal commentaries. Within **Judaism**, jurisdiction over such cases fell to the Sanhedrin, the state religious court, after a local priest was informed of the transgression.

Through Constantine's reforms in 318, church laws could be enforced by the state, leading to religiously regimented control over what was previously a familial matter within European society. As ecclesiastical courts gained power, jurisdiction began to change from secular to religious provenance. From Charlemagne at the turn of the ninth century until the fourteenth century, the church had almost sole jurisdiction over any crimes of a sexual nature, including, but not limited to, adultery. It was not unheard of for such cases to be judged in secular courts, due to the decretists' argument that the consequences of adultery were both religious and social. However, if the crime never came to the attention of the spouse of the adulterer, it was considered to be a private religious affair to be settled in the confessional rather than in the courtroom.

PUNISHMENT. In both late antiquity and the Middle Ages, adultery was most often seen as a female crime. In late antiquity, Roman common law gave a husband the right to kill his wife if she and her consort were caught in the act, but overall, punishment for an adulteress was considered a matter for the *paterfamilias* (the eldest ranking male of the family), who had a variety of methods of discipline available. The first-century Roman writer Tacitus claimed that according to Germanic custom, an adulteress could be sentenced to death, a fate that could also come up on her paramour unless the injured husband was willing to accept monetary compensation. Furthermore, Roman legislation held that an adulteress could lose the right of control over her dowry, as was also true in Qur'anic law. Because of the ideas of **Augustine** and other patristic writers in the fourth century, there was a legal change that made adultery a crime for both sexes, but the severity of punishment remained much greater for females than for males. By the time of Justinian's sixth-century *Corpus Iurus Civilis*, adultery laws were still biased against women, but severe penalties also became a reality for men. If a woman formally prosecuted her husband in court, the adulterer could lose his rights to his wife's dowry, as well as to any wedding gifts. In addition, by 589, a Western husband was required to give three legally recorded warnings before he was allowed to lawfully kill his wife if she was caught in the act. At this time, Germanic law stated that a woman could be killed by her husband, father, or brother for her extramarital affair. If either spouse knowingly failed to prosecute the other's dalliance, they would receive a large fine, and possibly lose a great deal of property. Similarly, Sharia law allowed an Islamic adulteress to be killed by her father and brother, and her adulterous partner by her husband.

In the Middle Ages, many of the same punishments were still applicable, especially those in the Germanic tradition. However, the influence of penitential Christian writers upon the conclusions reached in the *Summa Theologica* allowed the religious ideals of forgiveness and repentance to surface in cases of adultery. A husband was exhorted by church law to forgive his adulterous wife, provided that she completed the penance prescribed by the ecumenical court. Correspondingly, Islamic tradition held that reconciliation, mediated by both families, was more desirable socially and religiously than **divorce**. Jewish culture, however, saw divorce as the main solution to adultery after ending the archaic punishment of stoning. The Christian church also forbade a husband to kill his adulterous wife, and ecclesiastical authorities were prepared to prosecute the husband for murder. Conversely, the Qur'anic tradition continued to permit men to use violence against their wives. Other possible punishments for a Christian adulteress were excommunication or exile. According to ecclesiastical law, both adulterous males and females were forbidden from marrying their paramour even after their offended spouse was dead. An adulteress's marriage to her lover was also unlawful in Judaic society, while it was not encouraged, but could be allowed, in the Islamic tradition.

Further Reading: Brundage, James A. *Law, Sex, and Christian Society in Medieval Europe.* Chicago: University of Chicago Press, 1987; Epstein, Lewis M. *Sex Laws and Customs in Judaism.* New York: Ktav Publishing House, 1967; Sayyid-Marsot, Afaf Lutfi, ed. *Society and the Sexes in Medieval Islam.* Malibu, CA: Undena Publications, 1979.

Bethany Hope Allen and T. Brice Pearce

AFRICA. Much of the medieval history of Africa outside the Mediterranean littoral and Ethiopia is difficult to recover due to the lack of literacy and record keeping. The coming of **Islam** to many African regions helped create a written record, but much of medieval African history has been reconstructed from archeological records and oral traditions. African societies, Islamic and traditional, were extraordinarily diverse, and generalizing about them is difficult.

Celibacy had little place in African cultures except in those areas that had been affected by Christianity, such as Ethiopia and Nubia, which had **Monophysite churches** and flourishing monastic communities. Under most circumstances, people were expected to be married. Africa's high land-to-population ratio made children especially valuable, and most African societies placed childbirth at the center of family life. **Polygamy** was very common in traditional and Islamic communities alike, usually in the form of multiple wives, although societies in which one woman married more than one man were not unknown. In many cultures, polygamy was not practiced only by the social elite, as was often the case outside Africa, but extended farther down the social hierarchy. **Concubinage** was also practiced. Sex and fertility outside institutional arrangements were generally frowned upon, and unmarried adults were viewed with suspicion. There were some exceptions, though—among some West African groups, a chieftain's eldest daughter was expected to stay home and take care of her mother rather than marry, and was encouraged to have nonmarital sexual relationships to bear children for the family.

Men in many traditional African societies married for the first time when they were ready to work a farm and support a family economically, around the age of twenty-one. Women married younger, when they became fully fertile, around the age of sixteen. Islam had the effect of lowering the age of first **marriage**. Courtship played a role in marriage, but often marriages involved go-betweens and negotiations between families.

The custom of "bride-price," in which the groom's family pays money or goods to the bride's, was found in many African societies, although some practiced the custom of dowry, in which the transfer was from the bride's family to the new couple.

In some societies, married women refrained from sex with their husbands throughout pregnancy and for a three-year period afterward while nursing their children. Women were also secluded during **menstruation** in many African cultures, as menstrual blood was believed to have sacred power that made it highly dangerous and potentially contaminating.

Many African cultures practiced **circumcision**, even before the coming of Islam made it a religious requirement, and female genital mutilation, including **clitoridectomy**, and in some cultures the sewing shut of the labia. The age at which these procedures were carried out varied. Among some peoples, it was performed soon after birth, while others used it as a rite of passage to adulthood before marriage.

Traditional religion varied widely over the length and breadth of sub-Saharan Africa. Some societies incorporated sex into their religious rituals and artwork. Naked figures were associated with sexuality and fertility. Heterosexual intercourse, both vaginal and anal, has been depicted in West African metalwork—often in contexts suggesting ritual acts. Fertility rituals associated with sexuality have a long history in Africa, having seemingly been depicted in rock art from both Algeria in Africa's far north to Botswana in the south. Barrenness for women and impotence for men were often seen as being caused by magic or cursing, and specific deities could be prayed to for the lifting of the curse.

Much of the sexual culture of North, West, and East Africa during the Middle Ages was transformed by the encounter with Islam, although conversion did not mean the immediate extinction of indigenous African traditions. Muslim travelers from the Middle East or North Africa claimed to be shocked by the amount of freedom permitted to sub-Saharan African Muslim women. Islam was also often associated with increased trade and urbanization, which had an independent effect on African societies. Households tended to be smaller in urban areas, which also developed prostitution. This was particularly true during trading seasons, when a city might temporarily play host to hundreds of young male traders, away from their wives and families.

The heterosexual family dominated African sexual life. However, the presence of all-male and all-female "homosocial" institutions permitted same-sex sex play and emotional bonding. Herd boys, who spent long months isolated from society looking after the cattle in their charge, were particularly associated with same-sex relationships.

Further Reading: Conner, Randy P. "Sexuality and Gender in African Spiritual Traditions." In *Sexuality and the World's Religions*, edited by David W. Machacek and Melissa M. Wilcox, 3–30. Santa Barbara, CA: ABC-Clio, 2003; Mvuyekure, Pierre-Damien. *West African Kingdoms, 500–1590*. Detroit, MI: Gale Group, 2004.

William E. Burns

ALAIN OF LILLE (c. 1120–1202). Alain of Lille, a leading French theologian and philosopher, was born in the town of Lille around 1120. Little is known about his life. Many referred to him as Alain the Great or Universal Doctor. Once he moved to Paris, he studied under philosopher Gilbert de la Porree at a school in Chartres. He later taught at universities in Paris and Montpellier. In perhaps his most famous work, *De Planctu Naturae* (*On the Lamentation of Nature*), which was written during 1160–1175, Alain attempts to reconcile the role of nature with that of God and humans. Not long after this manuscript was published, he wrote his poem *Anticlaudianus* in 1182.

In this epic poem, Alain continues expanding his ideas about the role of nature and attempts to explain how human beings could achieve perfection. *Anticlaudianus* is essentially a treatise on society's morals.

Alain's discussion of nature and the ways in which humans challenged her rightful sovereignty included condemnation of many sexual expressions, particularly those involving male homosexuality, that Alain deemed unnatural. In *De Planctu*, Alain avoids specifically Christian arguments and evidence to focus on "universal" laws of morality, those that could be agreed upon by Christians and pagans. Alain particularly condemns homosexual prostitution and anal intercourse. He also discusses male sexuality in grammatical terms in *On the Catholic Faith against the Heretics*, dividing men into masculine (homosexual), feminine (heterosexual), and neuter (bisexual) categories.

In addition to being a poet and theologian, Alain was a mystic and a philosopher, who followed the theories of Neo-Platonism and Pythagoras. After teaching in Paris, he eventually joined the Cistercian order of monks at the Monastery of Citeaux. He remained in Citeaux until his death in 1202.

Further Reading: Boswell, John. *Christianity, Social Tolerance, and Homosexuality: Gay People in Western Europe from the Beginning of the Christian Era to the Fourteenth Century*. Chicago: University of Chicago Press, 1980.

Nicole Mitchell

ALBAS. The Old Occitan *alba* or "dawn-song" (Old French *aube*, Middle High German *tageliet*) is a genre of love lyric depicting adulterous lovers forced to separate at the arrival of the dawn (*alba*). Its origins remain debatable, but the *alba* certainly attained notable expression among the **troubadours** of southern France during the twelfth century, and eventually appeared in many of the major European vernacular languages, including French, German, Galician, Italian, and English. Thematically, the *alba* contrasts the joy of lovers brought together under the cover of night with the sorrow of their separation at the break of day. Also characteristic of the genre is the appearance of a third party, the *gaita* or watchman, whose task it is to warn the lovers of the approaching dawn so that they may part without drawing the unwanted suspicion of, among others, the *gelos*, the jealous husband of the female beloved.

The song itself can assume a variety of forms. Many are monologues delivered by the male or female lover or the watchman. The earliest surviving Occitan *alba*, "Reis glorios, verais lums e clardatz" ("Glorious King, true light and splendor") by the twelfth-century troubadour Giraut de Bornelh, offers such a monologue by the watchman, whose growing anxiety is juxtaposed with the imperturbable ecstasy of the lovers seemingly deaf to his warnings. The lament of Giraut's watchman is further punctuated by a refrain at the conclusion of each stanza, another common marker of the genre. Dialogues between the lovers or between one of the lovers and the watchman also survive and are especially common in German dawn-songs. Several particularly accomplished examples can be found in the works of Heinrich von Morungen (d. 1222) and Wolfram von Eschenbach (d. c. 1220).

Although the *alba* initially flourished among professional and amateur minstrels in France and Germany during the twelfth through fourteenth centuries, its popularity was enduring. English readers can discover an *alba* embedded in **Geoffrey Chaucer**'s *Troilus and Criseyde*, while the setting and themes are unmistakable in the sweet sorrow with which Shakespeare's Romeo and Juliet famously part.

Further Reading: Hatto, Arthur T., ed. *Eos: An Enquiry into the Theme of Lovers' Meetings and Partings at Dawn in Poetry.* London: Mouton, 1965; Sigal, Gale. *Erotic Dawn-Songs of the Middle Ages: Voicing the Lyric Lady.* Gainesville: University Press of Florida, 1996.

John T. Sebastian

ALBERTUS MAGNUS (c. 1206–1280). Albertus Magnus, also known as Albert of Cologne, Albert the Great, and Doctor *Universalis*, was a philosopher, theologian, and scientist who advocated the study of Aristotle and helped to legitimize the study of nature by medieval Christians. Albertus was born around 1206 in Lauingen on the Danube River near Ulm, Swabia (now Germany). He attended the University of Padua. In the summer of 1223 he joined the Dominican order. After further study at Bologna and in Germany, he taught at several convents in Germany. Around 1241 Albert went to the Dominican convent of Saint-Jacques at the University of Paris. There he studied the works of Aristotle, recently translated from the Greek and Arabic, along with commentaries on Aristotle by **Ibn Rushd (Averroes)**. Eventually, he wrote his own commentaries in which he expressed his own observations, experiments, and speculations.

For Albertus "experiment" denoted a careful process of observing, describing, and classifying. Through his study of Aristotle, Albertus acquired an advanced knowledge of the science of his time. He was invested as the bishop of Regensburg in 1259. He died on November 15, 1280, at Cologne.

Albertus took part in the medieval discussion on the nature of sex. He rejected the idea that prelapsarian sex in the Garden of Eden was radically different from postlapsarian coitus after the Fall of Man. Rather, sex was a natural part of human biology fashioned in the original creation. Sex was not a result of the curse of original sin. This meant that desire, arousal, and procreation were the same both before and after the Fall. Albertus's view of sex in **marriage** was that it was inherently good and could be spiritually meritorious if approached in the spirit of love and with procreative intentions. If the couple merely endured the pleasure of the coitus because it was unavoidable, their lovemaking was not sinful and might even be meritorious. Albertus interpreted marital sex as a conjugal debt that had been contracted. Husbands and wives could pay the conjugal debt even in penitential seasons, but the one who initiated the payment committed a venial sin. Marital sexual intercourse could be sinful if the intentions of the partners were wrongly motivated. Albertus held that marital coitus initiated by **lust** was sinful, but the sin was not mortal, especially if the intention was to conceive a child. In that case, lust made the act merely venially sinful. He thought that sex during pregnancy was acceptable

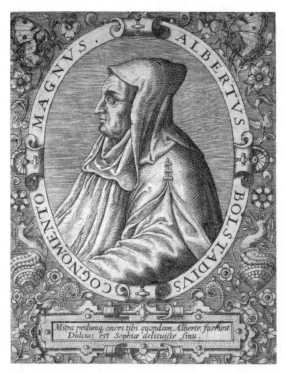

Albertus Magnus. Courtesy of the Library of Congress.

because the fetus stimulated the woman. Intercourse was a kind of **medicine** for her sexual hunger.

Albertus described five coital positions: missionary, side-by-side, seated, standing, and *a tergo*. He held that the missionary position was the least sinful. However, the other positions were acceptable in certain circumstances. Pregnancy would warrant the side-by-side position; obesity could warrant other positions. Nonmissionary positions were sinful only if they were used merely to increase sexual pleasure. He believed that excessive sexual intercourse could produce debilitating symptoms such as trembling, nervousness, ringing in the ears, and abdominal pain. He opposed premarital sex and homosexuality.

There are a number of pseudonymous treatises falsely ascribed to Albertus, such as *De secretis mulierum* (**Secrets of Women**), a manual for marital coitus. *See also* Scholastic Philosophy.

Further Reading: Albertus Magnus. *Man and the Beasts* (*De animalibus*, books 22–26). Translated by James J. Scanlan. Binghampton, NY: Medieval & Renaissance Texts & Studies, 1987; Clifford, John J. "The Ethics of Conjugal Intimacy according to St. Albert the Great." *Theological Studies* 3 (1942): 1–26.

Andrew J. Waskey

ANAL AND INTERCRURAL SEX. During the Middle Ages, anal and intercrural sex were considered unacceptable by the church because they could not lead to procreation, which for purists was the only acceptable excuse for sexual interaction, pleasure being a sin in itself. The vast majority of theologians viewed anal intercourse as the most sinful position, but early on, from the sixth until the early seventh century, anal sex, even between men, was not treated any more harshly than any other form of sex that was not meant for procreation.

Information about anal and intercrural sex during the Middle Ages is relatively scarce. For the early period, until the eleventh century, the richest and the most candid sources are the **penitentials** that the clergy used as confessional handbooks. From mid-eleventh century on, the documentation becomes more varied and includes poems, **romance**s, philosophical works, medical treatises, historical chronicles, and the updated version of the penitential handbook, the *summa confessorum*. The most specific and extensive texts to deal with these practices are probably **Peter Damian**'s *Liber Gomorrhianus* (Book of Gomorrah, 1049) and **Alain of Lille**'s *Complaint of Nature* (1165).

Damiani, who was beatified, coined the word "sodomy" in the eleventh century. He classified the sexual sins in ascending order of sinfulness: first **masturbation**, then mutual masturbation, followed by intercrural sex, and finally **sodomy**. Sodomy, which had grown synonymous with anal sex (*coitus in ano*), became a legal crime by the end of the thirteenth century, and governments and courts attended to its monitoring and prosecution. The Inquisition tribunals even linked it to heresy, making it a capital crime. Later on, under the influence of St. Paul's writings about the Romans (1:26–27), all forms of same-sex intercourse, including intercrural sex, were included in the "sodomy" category. This eventually led to the exclusion from this group of heterosexual anal intercourse, which was seen as a minor irregularity.

The seventh-century Frankish Cummean Penitential prescribed two degrees of penance for intercrural sex. The first was one hundred days for the first offence and one year for the second, and was meant probably for those below twenty years of age or for laymen. The second degree of penance was two years, and probably meant for those above twenty or for the clergy. For anal intercourse the penance was seven years.

A Visigothic law from the same century prescribed **castration** for both the *inferens* (inserter) and the *patiens* (passive). The term for "inserter" varied later on among *agens*, *activus*, and *faciens* (doing), and *patiens* was occasionally substituted by *receptivus*.

Intercrural sex, also known as interfemoral connection, had been the acceptable form of male homosexual intercourse in ancient Greece, and the approved technique, abundantly illustrated visually, consisted in the mature man leaning over the boy, who was always in an upright position, and rubbing his penis between the boy's thighs. The practice was common in many parts of the world during the Middle Ages. It was very popular throughout the Muslim world, as illustrated in literary texts such as the poetry of the eighth-century Baghdadi poet **Abu Nuwas** and in the ***Thousand and One Nights***, and even in **Japan**, where the documented practice of *shudo* ("the way of the young") was the equivalent of Western **pederasty**. In Europe there was considerable reference to intercrural sex in late medieval romance, in which pederasty seems still as popular as it had been in the classical, Greco-Roman age. *Altercatio Ganimedis et Helene*, written in France during the late twelfth or early thirteenth century, is probably the most relevant example of the very popular debate-on-pederasty genre. The debate is between Ganymede and Helen, on the merits of boy love versus woman love. Young Ganymede speaks in favor of pederasty, and unapologetically praises both the sensual and financial gratification that boys derive from this practice. Along these lines, he describes the predominant sexual practice of those times, intercrural frottage, as the most desirable and sought after by the wealthy adult male, who discharges "Venus's tear" (semen) by rubbing his penis against the "slippery thighs of boys" who sell their *crura* (thighs). *See also* Homosexuality, Male.

Further Reading: Boswell, John. *Christianity, Social Tolerance, and Homosexuality: Gay People in Western Europe from the Beginning of the Christian Era to the Fourteenth Century*. Chicago: University of Chicago Press, 1980; Boswell, John. *Rediscovering Gay History: Archetypes of Gay Love in Christian History*. London: Gay Christian Movement, 1982; Farmer, Sharon A., and Carol Braun Pasternack. *Gender and Difference in the Middle Ages*. Minneapolis: University of Minnesota Press, 2003; Jordan, Mark D. *The Invention of Sodomy in Christian Theology*. Chicago: University of Chicago Press, 1997.

Georgia Tres

ANANGA RANGA. The fifteenth-century work *Ananga Ranga* is an updated version of the ***Kama Sutra***, written in far more accessible Sanskrit than its predecessor. As a result, for many centuries the *Ananga Ranga* actually superseded the *Kama Sutra* as the text of choice for knowledge about sexual pleasure. The writing of the *Ananga Ranga* was commissioned by the nobleman Ladakhana for one of the Lodi dynasty monarchs. The Lodis were part of the powerful Delhi Sultanate that ruled northern **India** before the Mughal dynasty took its place. Kalyanamalla, the author of the *Ananga Ranga*, was a Hindu poet, who drew heavily upon the *Kama Sutra* in preparing his text. Kalyanamalla wrote in an accessible Sanskrit style, and its royal Muslim patronage assured that the text enjoyed a wide circulation among the medieval Muslim empires. Versions of the *Ananga Ranga* also appeared in Arabic, Persian, and Urdu.

Opening with a dedication to Ladakhana, the text's patron, the book contains prescriptive advice for married couples, and for their conduct both social and sexual. Body types are classified according to their mutual compatibility, and advice given for sexual satisfaction. The goal of the text is to promote happiness within **marriage** by teaching married couples to bring variety to their sexual practices, along with mutual enjoyment. The title of the book has been variously translated as "Stage of the Bodiless

One," "The Hindu Art of Love," and "Theatre of the Love God," among others. Some scholars see this text as less woman-centered than the earlier *Kama Sutra*, perhaps reflective of a more sexist social environment, and note places where the author neglects to provide normative advice for producing women's pleasure, such as the use of fingers.

As part of the romanticism of colonial rule, Europeans sought out Eastern texts to bring ancient wisdom to the modern world. However, the Orientalist engagement in the *Ananga Ranga* ironically led to the text's decreased relevance and the prominence of the earlier *Kama Sutra*. Sir Richard Francis Burton's experiences living in India as a part of the British military and his fascination with the sexual practices of Oriental societies, coupled with his desire to bring this knowledge to the attention of his cocitizens of the British metropole, made him interested in the canon of sexual knowledge preserved in Sanskrit texts. Because of the relative popularity of the *Ananga Ranga* among Sanskrit specialists, it was natural that it should be the text of choice for Burton's purposes. When reviewing their translations, however, Burton made note of the many references made to an earlier compilation by Vatsyayana. Burton believed that this earlier text, the *Kama Sutra*, was a far more foundational work, and requested that the Pandits locate a copy. Because of centuries of relative neglect, the *Kama Sutra* at this stage only existed in parts. The text had to be recompiled from Sanskrit manuscript library collections across India and in the princely states. Once the text was translated into English, its popularity grew, and Indian scholars set aside the *Ananga Ranga* with a renewed interest in its predecessor. *See also* Sex Manuals.

Further Reading: Burton, Sir Richard Francis, trans. *The Kama Sutra and Ananga Ranga*. New York: Barnes and Noble, 2006.

Anne Hardgrove

ANDREAS CAPELLANUS. The name Andreas Capellanus (Andrew the Chaplain) is associated with the late twelfth- or early thirteenth-century Latin prose treatise *De amore*, or *On Love*, a guidebook written for the edification of the otherwise anonymous figure "Walter." The treatise is modeled on the writings on love by the Roman poet Ovid (43 BCE–17 CE), especially his *Art of Love* and *Remedies of Love*.

On Love is divided into three books. The first book opens with a definition of love, which for Andreas is an internal suffering prompted by the sense of sight and characterized by a deep reflection on the beauty of the beloved and a longing for her embraces. Because of this emphasis on sight as the main conduit for desire, the blind are prohibited from participation in the pleasures of love, as are the elderly, the too young, and those whose passions are so uncontrollable that they merely **lust** indiscriminately after any woman they encounter. More than half of the first book is devoted to a series of dialogues between men and women of various social classes (e.g., a non-noble man addresses a noblewoman, or a member of the higher nobility addresses one equal in station). These dialogues illustrate the means by which love can and should be pursued. Book 1 also briefly instructs Walter on the love of nuns, peasants, and prostitutes. In the much briefer second book, Andreas attends to the means by which love may be nourished and maintained or, alternately, diminished and even ended. Book 2 concludes with a list of thirty-one rules of love. Book 3, however, turns in a very different direction. Here Andreas takes pains to convince Walter that he should not read the previous chapters as a guide to pursuing love but rather as an instruction on how to avoid love altogether with an eye toward pleasing God. This sudden and striking departure has led scholars to speculate variously on the degree of irony or seriousness with which Andreas approaches each of the books of *On Love*.

The name Andreas Capellanus has traditionally been linked to the court of Marie, the twelfth-century Countess of Champagne, who most famously patronized the **romance**-writer Chrétien de Troyes and who is mentioned by name in *On Love*. Recently, however, scholars have questioned the association of Andreas with Champagne, with the twelfth century, and even with any historical figure called Andreas Capellanus at all. What little is known about Andreas comes from *On Love* itself, where he is identified not only as the chaplain of the royal court (presumably that in Paris) but also as a lover himself. Regardless of the identity of Andreas Capellanus, real or assumed, the influence of *On Love* was certainly immense in the Latin West, if its official condemnation in 1277 by the bishop of Paris, Etienne Tempier, is any measure. *See also* Courtly Love; Ovidianism.

Further Reading: Andreas Capellanus. *On Love*. Translated by P. G. Walsh. London: Duckworth, 1982; Dronke, Peter. "Andreas Capellanus." *Journal of Medieval Latin* 4 (1994): 51–63.

John T. Sebastian

APHRODISIACS. Use of and preoccupation with aphrodisiacs have existed since the earliest times and continued through the Middle Ages, when Arab and Asian products and practices were incorporated into the local and Greco-Roman traditions of Europe.

A wide range of foods and beverages were regarded as sexual enhancers, and many still are. However, some aphrodisiacs were nonedible. The most prestigious from the animal kingdom was the Spanish fly, not actually a fly but a beetle from the Cantharidae genus. Probably the most popular and commonly used vegetal aphrodisiac was the mandrake, whose presumed effectiveness was attributed to its phallic appearance. Another well-known aphrodisiac was the root of orchid, believed to induce fertility, also based on its appearance, in this case resembling testicles. However, it was considered important to ingest the hard part of the root because the soft one had the opposite effect, which, however, was considered beneficial by nuns, who ate lily root to ensure chastity.

Magical preparations were also added to the age-old food- and drug-based recipes. They contained such fantastic ingredients as human excrement; body parts, including the putrefied flesh of a corpse; and wormwood. Increasing love and becoming one would be induced, for example, by drinking each other's blood. Eating a dead spouse's heart would ensure the endurance of the surviving spouse's love.

A remarkable list of recipes for aphrodisiacs meant to enhance a man's sexual prowess and pleasure appears at the end of *De coitu* (*On Coitus*), a treatise written by the eleventh-century monk Constantine the African. This work deals with topics like sexual pleasure and conception without ever mentioning women. The French alchemist Nicolas Flamel (1330–1418), supposedly the most accomplished of all European alchemists, was a very innovative creator of love recipes. The ingredients for one of his potions were thistle, the left-side testicle of a three-year-old goat, ashes of hair from the backside of a completely white dog (cut on the first day of the new moon and burned on the seventh), brandy, and the sperm of a crocodile.

The use of aphrodisiacs is abundantly documented in the **sex manuals** circulated in the medieval Arab world, the most well known being *Al-Raudh al-'Atir fí Nouzhat al-Khawátir* (*The Perfumed Garden for the Delectation of Souls*) by Shaykh al-Imám Abú 'Abd-Allah al-Nefzawí and *Kitáb Rujú'a al-Shaykh ila Sabáh fí 'l-Kuwwat al-Báh* (*The Book of Age-Rejuvenescence in the Power of Concupiscence*) by Ahmad bin Sulayman, surnamed Ibn Kamál Pasha. One aspect of aphrodisiacs discussed in almost all Arab sex manuals was their role in increasing penis size. It is remarkable that this topic was rarely mentioned in European handbooks.

Further Reading: Hull Walton, Alan. *Love Recipes Old and New: A Study of Aphrodisiacs throughout the Ages, with Sections on Suitable Food, Glandular Extracts, Hormone Stimulation and Rejuvenation.* London: Torchstream Books, 1956.

Georgia Tres

AQUINAS, THOMAS (1224/5–1274). Thomas Aquinas was an Italian Dominican and one of the most important and influential Christian thinkers of the Middle Ages. His teaching on sexuality is a synthesis of Greek philosophical notions and Christian ideals.

Like Aristotle, Aquinas possessed a teleological understanding of human nature. Human action and desire are for the sake of an end or purpose, which in turn has the character of a good. Aquinas distinguishes three levels of goods naturally desired by human beings, namely, self-preservation, the sexual union of male and female and the raising of offspring, and knowledge of truth and life in society. Sexual activity is both natural and intrinsically good; nevertheless, since reason is the rule and measure of human acts, sexual activity must be governed by reason if it is to be an authentically human good. For human beings to live rightly, they must acquire and cultivate the virtues. Aquinas identifies chastity as the virtue that regulates sexual activity. It involves the chastising of sensual desire by reason. Aquinas holds that sexual intercourse has as its purpose procreation, and it is to be confined within the limits of **marriage**. The vice opposed to chastity is **lust** (*luxuria*), which Aquinas defines as the excessive and irrational pursuit of sexual pleasure. Lust brings disorder to reason and will. It blinds the mind's ability to apprehend an end as good; it impairs its ability to deliberate about what ought to be done; and it renders the mind indecisive and unable to abide by its decisions. Since lust impels human beings to desire inordinately carnal pleasures, it encourages love of self and hatred of God, who prohibits the enjoyment of such pleasures. Aquinas distinguishes six kinds of lust: simple fornication (sexual intercourse with an unmarried woman), **adultery**, **incest**, seduction (sexual intercourse with a virgin), **rape**, and vice against nature. The last one is regarded as the worst form of lust, since it violates the purpose of sex by pursuing intercourse that cannot result in procreation. Aquinas distinguishes four kinds of vice against nature: **masturbation**; **bestiality** (sexual intercourse with a member of a different species); sodomitic vice (homosexual intercourse); and engaging in sex in unnatural ways, either by using an improper organ or by using monstrous or bestial means of intercourse.

Although marriage is intrinsically good, a more excellent state of life is **virginity**, whereby one abstains from sexual activity in order to devote oneself to divine contemplation. Aquinas rejects the claim that virginity is contrary to the teaching of Genesis 1:28 ("Be fruitful and multiply, and fill the earth"), since this command is issued not to any one individual but to the multitude. Thus it is sufficient that some individuals live in a married state, while others maintain their virginity. *See also* Scholastic Philosophy.

Further Reading: Aquinas, Thomas. *Summa Theologiae.* Translated by the Fathers of the English Dominican Province. Westminster, MD: Christian Classics, 1981; Jordan, Mark D. *The Invention of Sodomy in Christian Theology.* Chicago: University of Chicago Press, 1997.

Mark D. Gossiaux

ARABIAN NIGHTS. See Thousand and One Nights

ARISTOTLE AND THE PHYLLIS LEGEND. Around the beginning of the thirteenth century, a legend concerning the ancient Greek philosopher Aristotle began to circulate in Latin Europe. In it, Aristotle rebuked his pupil Alexander the Great for giving excessive attention to his lover, referred to in some versions of the legend as Phyllis. In retaliation, the lady appeared outside the philosopher's window in a sexually provocative manner. So powerful were her displays that Aristotle implored her to have sex with him. She agreed, but only on the condition that he first allow her to ride him like a horse. Rather than carrying out her part of the bargain, she arranged for Alexander to witness his tutor's humiliation. The legend also occurred in Arabic and Indian story collections, which were probably the sources for the Latin versions, although without the connection to Aristotle specifically.

This legend of Aristotle and Phyllis has been defined in various contexts. In collections of *exempla*—anecdotes for preachers to use in their sermons—it was an example of how **lust** could cause the wisest man to fall. The fact that Aristotle assumed the position of a horse made his fall a particularly degrading example of how lust can reduce men to beasts. In verse narratives, the anecdote was used to illustrate the power of love. Aristotle and Phyllis were also frequently represented in art and sculpture.

Further Reading: Smith, Susan L. *The Power of Women: A Topos in Medieval Art and Literature.* Philadelphia: University of Pennsylvania Press, 1995.

William E. Burns

ARTHURIAN LEGEND. The Arthurian legend begins with the poorly documented exploits of an obscure and anonymous military leader who led the resistance against Germanic invaders in Britain during the fifth and sixth centuries. Despite, or perhaps because of, the paucity and unreliability of contemporary sources, the legend of Arthur, king of the Britons, has since flowered into a vast and colorful tradition.

The earliest sources for fifth-century British history are scarce and come primarily in the form of Latin chronicles, chiefly *On the Ruin and Conquest of Britain* by the sixth-century monk Gildas. It was not until the composition of Nennius's *History of the Britons* at the beginning of the ninth century, however, that the name Arthur became first associated with historical events, although an even earlier literary reference appears in the Welsh poem *The Gododdin*. As moralizing castigations of the iniquities of the Britons (in the case of the Latin chronicles), or as heroic elegies for fallen heroes (in the case of *The Gododdin* and similar Welsh poems), these early sources are hardly concerned with the amorous exploits so famously central to the later legend.

The first noteworthy gesture in that direction arrived in the 1130s in the form of Geoffrey of Monmouth's Latin work *History of the Kings of Britain*, which would become world famous almost instantaneously. Like his predecessors, Geoffrey presents Arthur primarily as a great military leader, but he also introduces Arthur's beautiful Roman wife, Guinevere. She appears most notably at the conclusion of Geoffrey's account of Arthur's defeat of the Roman Lucius, where she is depicted as living adulterously with Arthur's nephew and regent-turned-traitor, Mordred, during the king's absence from Britain.

Geoffrey expresses a reluctance to narrate Guinevere's infidelity in any detail, a reluctance that seems only to have inspired his successors to develop the story of Arthur in new directions. Most important among this next generation of innovators was Chrétien de Troyes (late twelfth century), who transferred the legend from Latin to the vernacular and from historical chronicle to **romance**—the chief narrative vehicle of **courtly love**. One of Chrétien's most enduring contributions to Arthurian literature is his elaboration of the adulterous love between Guinevere and the title character of his *Lancelot, or The Knight of the Cart*. For Chrétien, the queen's **adultery** is a given and is presented in a conspicuously unproblematic fashion. Chrétien's chief preoccupation is not sexual indiscretion, but rather Lancelot's performance as a lover in the course of rescuing Guinevere from her kidnapper, the wicked Meleagant.

If the moral failings of Lancelot and Guinevere seem to pass all but unnoticed by Chrétien, they nevertheless become the primary force behind the collapse of Camelot in the sprawling prose "Vulgate Cycle," so called because it was written in

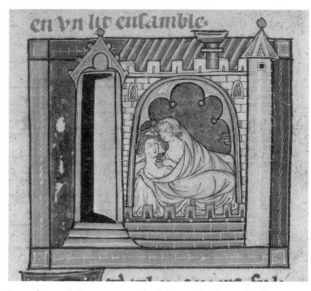

Lancelot and Guinevere in bed. From the Lancelot Romance, ca. 1300–1310. © HIP/Art Resource, NY.

French rather than Latin and compiled during the first half of the thirteenth century, quite possibly under the auspices of Cistercian monks. This massive compilation in five parts expands the career of Lancelot as it simultaneously complicates the relationship between the chivalric values prized by Arthur and the spiritual imperatives of Christianity. Nowhere is this more evident than in the adventure of the Holy Grail, in which Lancelot's failure to achieve the quest is figured explicitly as punishment for his dalliance with Guinevere. Indeed, of the three knights to complete the quest, Galahad (Lancelot's illegitimate son) and Perceval are virgins while Bors is chaste. The adulterous, and ultimately traitorous, relationship of Lancelot and Guinevere results in the deaths of Arthur and many of his knights as well as the destruction of the court. A comparable tension between the competing codes of chivalry and courtly love is similarly explored under the guise of a quest in the fourteenth-century English alliterative poem *Sir Gawain and the Green Knight*. There, Gawain must choose between his feudal duty to his lord and to his host and his amorous duty to the host's wife. The poem's ambivalent conclusion suggests that the two obligations may not have been compatible in the minds of Chrétien's successors.

The medieval Arthurian tradition culminates in the English prose masterpiece *Le Morte d'Arthur* by Thomas Malory (d. 1471). Malory draws heavily on the Vulgate Cycle in his presentation of the Arthurian legend, and so it is again Lancelot's unquenchable passion for Guinevere that leads to the ruin of Camelot. Yet Malory's re-creation of the Arthurian world is tinged with nostalgia, particularly when it comes to matters of the heart. More than once Malory compares the love of his own day, which he finds immoderate and fickle, to the idealized vision of love, adulterous as it may be, that infuses his imagined past. *See also* Tristan.

Further Reading: Pearsall, Derek. *Arthurian Romance: A Short Introduction*. Malden, MA: Blackwell Publishing, 2003; Wilhelm, James J., ed. *The Romance of Arthur: An Anthology of Medieval Texts in Translation*. Exp. ed. New York: Garland Publishing, 1994.

John T. Sebastian

AUCASSIN AND NICOLETTE (c. 1250).   *Aucassin and Nicolette* is one of the best-known medieval love stories. Composed in the south of France, it narrates the forbidden love affair between the two protagonists. The text survives in only one manuscript (Paris B.N.F. fr. 2168) and is unique in that it contains sections written in both prose and verse.

Aucassin, a Christian youth (who bears a Saracen name), is the son of the Count of Beaucaire. Nicolette (who surprisingly has a Christian name) is a Saracen slave, brought to France by the viscount of Beaucaire. Nicolette and Aucassin fall in love, but Aucassin's parents oppose their **marriage**. To prevent the lovers from seeing one another, they are imprisoned. Nicolette escapes, and as soon as Aucassin is released, he joins her in the forest. When the couple arranges to flee by sea, their vessel is pushed off course during a storm and lands in the strange kingdom of Torelore. The lovers are then captured by pirates and taken to separate ships. During a second storm, Aucassin's ship is driven back to Beaucaire, where he learns of the death of his father and becomes ruler of the city. Nicolette's ship, meanwhile, lands in Carthage (Spanish Cartagena), where she is recognized as the long-lost daughter of the king. Throughout her journey, Nicolette does not forget Aucassin. To avoid an arranged marriage to another man, she dresses as a minstrel and abandons her family to travel back to Beaucaire, where she reunites with her lover. Aucassin and Nicolette are finally married and live happily together.

Aucassin and Nicolette is a satirical work that plays with the traditional paradigms of medieval love stories. As the tale unfolds, love and sexuality transcend and transgress political and social norms. Thus, Aucassin, although Christian, declares that he would rather have the Saracen Nicolette as his wife than go to heaven. Hell, he suggests, is a much livelier place full of handsome knights, beautiful ladies with their lovers and husbands, authors, kings, and entertainers. Unlike the heroines of most medieval Christian stories about love affairs between Muslim women and Christian men, Nicolette does not convert to Christianity for her lover. Yet from the very beginning we learn that, as a child, she was forcibly baptized by the viscount of Beaucaire.

Gender roles and expectations are also reversed, especially during the visit to the strange kingdom of Torelore. There, the queen leads her troops in battle shortly after giving birth and makes war by flinging rotten crab-apples, cheese, mushrooms, and eggs on the enemy. Meanwhile, her king recovers from the strains of labor by lying in bed. Aucassin promptly declares the king a fool and beats him with a stick. Yet, throughout the tale Aucassin is content to follow Nicolette, whose decisions drive the narrative. It is she who initiates the couple's escape to the forest and arranges the sailing from France. At the end of the story she seeks out Aucassin, who, as Count of Beaucaire, has made no attempt to use the resources at his disposal to locate his lost love. *See also* Interconfessional Sex and Love.

Further Reading: Gilbert, Jane. "The Practice of Gender in *Aucassin and Nicolette*." *Forum for Modern Language Studies* 33, no. 3 (1977): 217–28; Matarasso, P. *Aucassin and Nicolette and Other Tales*. Harmondsworth, UK: Penguin, 1971.

K. Sarah-Jane Murray

AUGUSTINE (354–430).   Augustine, philosopher and bishop of Hippo, was one of the fathers of the church and a prolific writer who left a deep mark in Western thought. He was born in Tagaste, a little city in Numidia, in 354, the son of Patrick, a pagan, and his wife Monica, a Christian. He first received instruction in his native town and also in nearby Madaura. He continued his studies in Carthage, where he started a long-lasting relationship with a woman, with whom he had a son, Adeodato, meaning "gift of God."

During this time, Augustine read the *Hortensius* of Cicero, which introduced him to philosophy—which soon became his passion. After joining the Manichean sect, in 374 he returned to Tagaste to teach grammar and then again to Carthage to teach eloquence. Increasingly detached from manicheism, he went to Rome, where, from 383 to 386, he taught rhetoric and afterward retired in Cassiciaco, in the vicinity of Milan. In 387, Ambrose, bishop of Milan, baptized Augustine and his son. Subsequently, he came back to Tagaste, where Adeodato died. After that, Augustine established his home in Hippo, becoming first priest and then bishop of the city in 395. He died there in 430.

Augustine wrote many works (about 117 can be attributed to him), some considered masterpieces of Western thought, including *Confessions*, *The City of God*, *On the Trinity*, and *Retractions*. Among the numerous themes he discussed, sexuality has an important place, partly because of his troubled personal experience before his conversion to the faith. The thoughts of Augustine on sexuality are organized around the concepts of **lust**, continence, and **virginity**. Lust is an exaggerated love for sensual pleasures, a frenetic desire that has its center in sexuality and subjects the soul to the body in an irrational way, depriving it in some manner even of its liberty. It is a consequence of original sin. The spiritual man must contain lust as much as possible within the correct limits in the soul and in the body. For Augustine, **marriage** is the remedy for lust. This does not mean that lust becomes right, but it is directed to an honest function: procreation. Marriage also includes the duty of continence, a limit imposed by the faithfulness of the couple and their responsibility to follow the Christian virtues. Continence is not only an inhibition of sexual compulsions, but also an obligation of the whole soul to move toward God. However, those who wish to be perfect must aim toward virginity as a still better condition to reach holiness. Virginity, above and beyond the literal sense, is seen by Augustine as being available and open to God. Christ, in that sense, is the model and source of virginity, and the church is described as a virgin and mother, the same way that Augustine recognizes Mary: both virgin and then devoted to God, and for this, brides and mothers respectively of believers and of Christ.Augustine

Augustine perceives male predominance in nature because everything is submitted to this model. As in the soul of man there is a part that deliberates and dominates and another part that must obey, women must spiritually and physically obey men. Women possess the same rational nature but must submit sexually and in other ways to men. The commonly held opinion that sex is perceived in western European thought as linked to sin is often attributed to Augustine. He considered it the consequence and mode of transmission of original sin, resulting in evil in the world. Augustine's conflicted relationship with sexuality is evident. Strongly sensual, he did not see relations with women as a way to satisfy the sentimental, psychic, and physical needs of both sexes. He saw women as nothing more than simple physical toys, with inferior qualities of sentiment and friendship. For Augustine, the only reason that God created women is for procreation. Any other relationship women can provide is worse than that offered by friendship among men. *See also* Catholicism; Manicheans and Cathars.

Further Reading: Pincherle, Alberto. *Vita di Sant'Agostino*. Bari: Laterza, 1980.

Elvio Ciferri

AVERROES. *See* Ibn Rushd

AVICENNA. *See* Ibn Sina

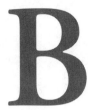

BASTARDY. *See* Illegitimacy

BERNARD OF CLAIRVAUX (1090–1153). Bernard of Clairvaux was one of the most influential religious and political figures of the twelfth century. His theological writings, which include the sermons on the *Song of Songs* and the treatise *On Loving God*, profoundly influenced Western concepts of physical and spiritual love.

Bernard was born at Fontaine-lès-Dijon (Burgundy, France) to a noble family in 1090, and at an early age became a student at Chalons. Renowned for his piety, he entered the abbey of Cîteaux in 1113. Soon Bernard was sent with twelve companions to found a new abbey at Vallée d'Absinthe (Valley of Bitterness) in the Champagne region. Bernard named the new house, of which he was appointed abbot, Clairvaux (Clear Valley). Due to Bernard's saintly reputation and effectiveness as a preacher, Clairvaux grew into a popular pilgrimage destination and, although officially dependent on Cîteaux, became the most influential abbey of the new Cistercian order.

Bernard's mystical theology contributed to the development of a deeply personal Christian faith in medieval Europe. He argued against any dualism between the body and the spirit. By according sensuality a place in the soul's spiritual development, Bernard profoundly shaped the medieval conception of love. The eighty-six sermons on the *Song of Songs* exemplify how the soul must achieve complete and harmonious union with God through love. For Bernard, the human soul (and also the church) resembles the bride of Solomon's Canticle, who passionately yearns for her bridegroom, Christ. Bernard further developed his views in *On Loving God*, a treatise devoted to the four degrees, or ways, in which humankind loves God. Since humans are born of the flesh, explains Bernard, their love must first begin in the flesh. However, when that lust is carefully redirected and guided toward God, human love finds its consummation in the spirit. Thus, humans first love themselves for their own sake. Then, they turn to God and love God, again for their own sake. In the third degree of love, they learn to love God for God's sake. The fourth degree of love—rarely attained during the mortal life—corresponds to the love of self for God's sake. Bernard's influence is particularly evident in **Dante Alighieri**'s *Divine Comedy*, in which the pilgrim, guided by his love for Beatrice, moves through the four degrees of love until he encounters St. Bernard in paradise and beholds, with the abbot's help, the beatific vision.

Bernard was also prominently involved in political affairs. He was the most vocal opponent of **Peter Abelard**, advised two popes, and, at the bequest of Eugenius III, traveled throughout Europe to recruit support for the Second Crusade. Bernard was canonized in 1174 and declared a doctor of the church in 1830. His feast day is August 20. *See also* Catholicism.

Further Reading: Evans, G. R. *The Mind of St. Bernard of Clairvaux*. New York: Oxford University Press, 2000; Gilson, Etienne. *The Mystical Theology of Saint Bernard*. Translated by A.H.C. Downes. New York: Sheed and Ward, 1955.

Jason Lewallen and K. Sarah-Jane Murray

BERNARDINO OF SIENA (1380–1444). The Franciscan friar Bernardino of Siena was a star of early-fifteenth-century Italian preaching, addressing crowds numbering in the thousands in cities throughout Italy on numerous occasions. Although he preached on many subjects, sexual issues, especially **sodomy**, were particularly important to him. The celibate virgin Bernardino's detailed and frank discussions of sexual acts, in and outside **marriage**, were unprecedented in medieval preaching.

Sodomy was the subject of many of Bernardino's sermons as well as a Latin treatise. He employed a broad definition of sodomy to cover a range of sexual behaviors "against nature," from male homosexuality to sexual acts between a married man and woman that were not open to the possibility of procreation, such as **anal and intercrural sex**. (Bernardino devoted little attention to other forms of sodomy, such as **bestiality** and female homosexuality.) He encouraged wives to refuse such acts, as well as refuse sex when the husband was drunk. (He even advised wives to consent to intercourse during **menstruation**, if the alternative was being sodomized.) In some passages, Bernardino suggests that wives separate from sodomitical husbands; in others he is more circumspect. Although in his discussions of marital sodomy Bernardino points to the husband's lust as the problem, in other passages he accepts the traditional idea that women are more naturally lustful than men. He suggests that they restrain themselves by a variety of quasi-ascetic techniques, including fasts and cold baths. Bernardino's general approach to married life and love, however, was positive. Love was a religious duty spouses owed each other.

The most ferociously denounced sodomite for Bernardino was the man who had sex with other men. He reveled in describing the particularly painful experiences such sodomites would suffer in hell, and encouraged, with some success, the passage of the antisodomy legislation in the Italian towns he visited. Like his contemporaries, Bernardino conceived of male same-sex relationships as taking place between an older man and a boy or youth. He placed part of the blame for sodomy with mothers who encouraged their sons to be pretty and effeminate, thus attracting the interest of adult sodomites.

Sodomy was not merely a personal sin for Bernardino, but one that corrupted the very foundations of a city, rendering it a fitting object of God's wrath, like Sodom and Gomorrah. It attacked the entire human race in that sodomites failed in the God-given duty to reproduce. All nonclerical men, claimed Bernardino, should marry so as to avoid falling into this horrible vice. (Bernardino paid little attention to heterosexual **prostitution**, a burgeoning industry in fifteenth-century Italy. This may have been because he believed it provided an alternative to sodomy.) A fierce opponent of heretics and **witches**, he also denounced their alleged propensities for sexual orgies and sex with the devil.

Further Reading: Debby, Nirit Ben-Aryeh. *Renaissance Florence in the Rhetoric of Two Popular Preachers: Giovanni Dominici (1356–1419) and Bernardino of Siena (1380–1444)*. Turnhout, Belgium: Brepols, 2001; Mormando, Franco. *The Preacher's Demons: Bernardino of*

Siena and the Social Underworld of Early Renaissance Italy. Chicago: University of Chicago Press, 1999.

William E. Burns

BESTIALITY. Sexual intercourse between humans and animals has a long history. It is particularly characteristic of rural societies, and is especially common among animal herders. It also has a mythological history. Pre- and non-Christian European pagan societies condemned bestiality, but also allotted it a religious role. The amours of the classical gods in animal form were well known, and ridiculed by Christians. Some Germanic and Celtic royal houses traced their lineage to the offspring of humans and animals, associating animal descent with strength. For example, the royal house of Denmark traced its ancestry to a woman and a bear. (Although intercourse between women and animals is relatively common in mythology and literature, legislation was aimed almost entirely at men.) In day-to-day life, bestiality was often treated casually, as a matter not of much consequence. The early secular laws of the Germanic peoples contain no mention of it.

Christians condemned bestiality from the start, a prohibition ultimately going back to the biblical book of Leviticus and its forbidding both men and women "lying with any beast." Unlike many Levitical bans, this was adopted from **Judaism** into Christianity and even intensified. (Bestiality was also forbidden in Islamic **Sharia** law.) The Council of Ancyra in 314 prescribed penance for committing such acts, the penalty increasing with age and marital status. They prescribed fifteen years' penance for a youth under twenty; a married man above fifty must do penance for the rest of his life. However, with the fall of the Roman empire, bestiality in practice was treated as a minor sexual sin on a par with **masturbation** (a tradition that continued throughout the Middle Ages in Eastern Christendom). The early penitential manuals penalized bestiality on the part of young men with only a few months' penance, although penalties were significantly higher for older men and married men. These were much lighter than the penances for **sodomy**.

Beginning in the seventh and eighth centuries, **penitentials** began assigning penances for bestiality that lasted several years, close to those for sodomy. Penitentials also started to take account of differences between animals, although not in any systematic way. Some assigned greater penances for intercourse with "small animals" or with mammals as opposed to birds. In the mid-eighth century, penalties began to be assigned to the animal as well as the human. Leviticus had also prescribed death for the animal, a provision previously ignored. The new willingness to condemn the animal was accompanied by care that its polluted flesh not be consumed by humans, but fed to dogs or otherwise disposed of. The early canon lawyers of the eleventh century repeated this prohibition, adding that the point of killing the animal was not to punish it, as it could not be held responsible, but to erase the memory of the act.

The twelfth and thirteenth centuries were marked by growing concern about bestiality. The belief that offspring were possible from bestial unions seems to have become more widespread, and visions of hell included scenes in which bestialists were repeatedly raped and impregnated with monsters. **Thomas Aquinas** ranked intercourse with animals, which perverted the order of nature at the most fundamental level, as the worst of all sexual sins. Like sodomy, bestiality became a matter for criminal enforcement rather than just religious penance, and by the fifteenth century it was treated as a capital offence in some parts of Europe.

Further Reading: Salisbury, Joyce E. *The Beast Within: Animals in the Middle Ages*. New York: Routledge, 1994.

William E. Burns

BESTIARY. A bestiary is a western European work on the appearance and habits of real or imaginary animals, especially popular during the twelfth and thirteenth centuries. Bestiary manuscripts were commonly illustrated and were usually adaptations from the Latin *Physiologus* text. *Physiologus* continued to be popular throughout the Middle Ages, while the bestiary developed alongside it.

Some bestiaries begin with Genesis and the naming of animals. From there, creatures are listed by kind (four-footed, birds, fish, then reptiles), starting with the lion. Bestiaries derived their authority from the learning of others rather than direct observation. Creatures' relationships with the outside world were explored as a way of explaining humans' relationships with each other and with God. For example, elephants represented Adam and Eve, because it was claimed they did not practice **adultery** and lived in complete chastity unless they ate mandrake. While links between humans and the natural world are important, an equally important part of the teaching in the bestiary is the difference between humans and animals—that humans act from knowledge and reason.

One role the bestiary played in medieval Christian society was as a bridge between theology and the natural world. Another role was linking classical knowledge with Christian interpretation. The moral and religious nature of the bestiary is therefore essential to understand it, as is its explanation of the human condition through animal characteristics. Issues arising when animals are discussed included chastity and modesty, sexuality and **marriage**. These moralized teachings help the reader understand Christian teachings on these and related subjects.

Because a bestiary included the moral characteristics of an animal, some animals from bestiaries have been used as symbols of love or examples to be followed by human beings, and were adopted into heraldic devices and copied into medieval art. One of the most interesting bestiaries is the thirteenth-century Old French *Bestiary of Love* by Richard de Fournival. He used the animals in his bestiary to illustrate his thoughts on male and female relationships, and the anonymous response to his work used the same animals to refute his argument.

Further Reading: Clark, W. B., and M. T. McMunn. *Beasts and Birds of the Middle Ages: The Bestiary and Its Legacy*. Philadelphia: University of Pennsylvania Press, 1989; Yamamoto, Dorothy. *The Boundaries of the Human in Medieval English Literature*. Oxford: Oxford University Press, 2000.

Gillian Polack

BHAKTI. The *Bhakti* movements began within **Hinduism** in the early Middle Ages. They exercised great cultural influences and became the most widespread of all forms of Hinduism, ultimately influencing Sufism in **India** and contributing to the rise of Sikhism.

Bhakti comes from a Sanskrit word for "sharing" or "devotion." *Bhakti* practices promoted selfless and passionate love of God as a lover, father, mother, child, or any other aspect of the ultimate Brahma that the devotee desired to use for expression. *Bhakti Marga* was one of the three Hindu paths (*margas*) for achieving the final liberation of the soul (*moksha*). People were encouraged to discard caste, rituals, and philosophical speculation, and cast themselves into giving love to God.

The *Bhakti* path arose in South India among Tamil-speaking people some time during the seventh to ninth centuries. *Bhakti* movements were monotheistic and emotional. They stressed devotion to the ultimate in the universe as a single unity as the ultimate reality. They also suppressed iconographic expressions (*rupas*) of the multiple forms of the Brahma, which outsiders regarded as idolatry. *Bhakti* devotees (*bhaktas*) sought to experience ecstatic emotions in giving themselves in worship to Vishnu, Shiva, or Shakti. The monotheistic challenges of **Islam** may have influenced *Bhakti* movements in northern India. Hinduism takes its starting point from the *Vedas*. *Bhakti* scholars found their roots in the Vedic worship of the *Rig Veda* god Varuna. Others found *Bhakti* in portions of the *Ramayana, Bhagavad Gita*, or the *Mahabharata*. Still others saw its origin in the *Padma Purana*.

Bhakti movements gathered people together from all castes and showed them how sharing love would earn salvation from *karma* in a single lifetime. By sharing love for the God with individuals, family, and groups, those who advanced in devotion became *Bhakti* saints. Around them, communities of good people (*satsang*) would gather. It was believed that the gathering together of goodness would overcome evils in the ages and would also have the power to transform lives.

Bhakti movements combined songs with devotion. The defining characteristic of the movement in South India was its expression of devotion in songs (*bhajans*) sung in vernacular languages. Singing in the languages of the common people was not only egalitarian but also very emotional. The emotions experienced, though personal, were shared among fellow worshippers. Two groups of South Indian singer-saints—the Alvars, devoted to Vishnu, and the Nayanars, devoted to Shiva—preached their message with songs after the seventh century. At times the singing involved chanting that continued for a very long time.

Bhakti schools developed devotional practices based upon the emotions in relationships, such as a woman's love for her beloved. These emotional expressions were interpreted as analogous to those in the relationship of the devotee with God.

Some *Bhakti* devotees produced love poetry. Women were highly involved in these movements, even participating in pilgrimages, which was an important practice. Other *Bhakti* practices included chanting the name of the devotee's God, wearing the God's emblem, and group worship at small shrines or large temples rather than individual meditation. *See also* Krishna.

Further Reading: Hardy, Friedhelm. *Viraha Bhakti: The Early Development of Krsna Devotion in South India*. Oxford: Oxford University Press, 1981; Pande, Susmita. *Medieval Bhakti Movement, Its History and Philosophy*. Meerut, India: Kusumanjali Prakashan, 1989; Shobha, Savitri Chandra. *Medieval India and Hindi Bhakti Poetry: A Socio-Cultural Study*. New Delhi: Har-Anand Publications, 1996.

Andrew J. Waskey

BIERIS DE ROMANS. Bieris de Romans (thirteenth century) is commonly identified as a **trobairitz**, or a female troubadour. Virtually nothing is known about her with any certainty. She is the presumed author of a *canso*, or love song, referred to as "Na Maria, pretz e fina valors" ("Lady Maria, merit and pure worth"). She has garnered considerable attention on account of the song's apparent expression of female homosexual desire, which makes "Na Maria" unique among surviving compositions by trobairitz. Besides her association with the composition of "Na Maria" in a single manuscript, Bieris is not mentioned in any other medieval source.

The claims for Bieris's lesbianism derive from the text of the song itself, in which the lyric speaker addresses the otherwise anonymous Lady Maria in terms typical of the conventions of contemporary love songs written by male **troubadours** for women. Bieris praises Maria's physical beauty, her moral virtue, and her courteous manner. The speaker also locates all of her sorrow in Maria's failure to requite her love and all of her joy in the abiding hope that she may yet grant her favors. This is the same rhetoric troubadours routinely used to express heterosexual desire.

Various attempts have been made to explain away the apparent lesbianism in Bieris's song. Some critics have argued for male authorship of the poem, while others have seen in its striking imitation of the troubadours' preferred themes and lexicon no more than the expected language of courtesy and praise customarily traded between women of equal social rank during the thirteenth century. The question of Bieris de Romans's putative homosexuality has yet to be resolved to the satisfaction of all. In the meantime, her sole-surviving song remains a unique specimen among the poetic and musical remains of the trobairitz of southern France. *See also* Homosexuality, Female.

Further Reading: Bruckner, Matilda Tomaryn, Laurie Shepard, and Sarah White, eds. *Songs of the Women Troubadours*. New York: Garland Publishing, 1995; Rieger, Angelica. "Was Bieiris de Romans Lesbian? Women's Relations with Each Other in the World of the Troubadours." In *The Voice of the Trobairitz: Perspectives on the Women Troubadours*, edited by William D. Paden, 73–94. Philadelphia: University of Pennsylvania Press, 1989.

John T. Sebastian

BIGAMY.   Bigamy refers to an individual's **marriage** to two or more people in a society where only monogamy is legally permitted. It differs from **polygamy**, which is a recognized custom in many societies, in that it is a criminal act. Bigamy played a prominent role in a society that strongly emphasized monogamous marriage, that of Christian Europe.

Male bigamy was particularly characteristic of a young and mobile population, and was associated with areas where people moved in and out and often had histories not generally known, such as ports or border areas. (Female bigamy, in which a woman had two or more husbands, was far less common than male bigamy.) The impossibility of **divorce** encouraged clandestine bigamy as "**remarriage** without divorce." This option was particularly available to the poor and landless, whose histories would not be known in the new area. However, if a bigamous marriage was revealed, the second marriage was legally considered no marriage at all, and bigamy was grounds for annulment. The most celebrated case of male bigamy in the Middle Ages was that of King **Philip II Augustus** of France, who married Agnes of Meuran after securing an annulment of his marriage to Ingeborg of Denmark on grounds of consanguinity. Since the annulment was secured from the French clergy rather than the pope, Pope Innocent III denied its validity, and eventually succeeded in securing Philip Augustus's concession of papal supremacy in marital affairs.

The Catholic Church treated bigamy as a religious offence against the sacrament of marriage, and it was usually under the jurisdiction of church courts, like much else in marriage and family law. The technical meaning of "bigamy" in **canon law** extended to other situations (besides a person with two spouses) such as a person previously obligated by religious vows taking a previously married spouse, or a person's second marriage. (In the latter case, bigamy was not considered a crime or an invalidation of the second marriage, but an impediment to the reception of Holy Orders.)

Ashkenazi **Jews** abandoned polygamy in the eleventh century after the *herem* (decree) of Rabbi **Gershom ben Judah**. Jewish law distinguished between female bigamy, in which case the second marriage was invalid and the woman was required to divorce her original husband, and male bigamy, which violated rabbinic law but did not make the second marriage invalid. Jews in Islamic lands continued to allow polygamous relationships.

Further Reading: Gies, Frances, and Joseph Gies. *Marriage and the Family in the Middle Ages.* New York: Harper and Row, 1987.

William E. Burns

BISEXUALITY. In the Middle Ages, bisexuality was not identified or isolated, either legally, medically, or theologically, as a distinct type of sexual behavior. The term itself was coined only around 1809, in the field of botany, to designate plants that have both male and female sexual organs. It is not known when the term was applied to human sexual behavior, but its use continues to be disputed even today. However, medieval records of bisexual behavior do exist, although they overwhelmingly cover male bisexuality, which tends to be ascribed to homosexuality.

Early in the Middle Ages, bisexual behavior and practice were not looked upon as particularly transgressive, as they would be later on, but were tolerated. This attitude reflected the Greek tradition of **pederasty**, seen as a rite of initiation, whereby homosexual relationships between men and boys did not preclude heterosexual **marriage** for the partners, mainly for the purpose of reproduction. This practice endured throughout Europe. The Roman soldier and historian Ammianus Marcellinus (330–395) noticed it among the Taifali, a people who had settled between the Carpathians and the Black Sea but had to withdraw toward the Danube and the Roman territory when the Huns invaded in 375. The Byzantine historian Procopius, in *The Vandalic Wars*, claims that Rome had been captured by the Vandals in 455 because the Vandals, despite their aggressive hypermasculine culture, had sent 300 of their most beautiful boys to serve as house slaves and sexual objects to Roman patricians and then, at a predetermined time, kill their masters and open the gates of Rome.

In time, **penitentials**, the priests' confessional handbooks that prescribed the required atonements for sexual offences, started including references to married sodomites. Lesbian sex, even for married women, was not a major sin and was generally classified under **masturbation**. By the twelfth century, the Christian church became very strict with regard to sexual activity, and severe legislation followed suit to enforce ideal, ascetic heterosexuality. However, due to the strict requirements and prolonged procedures for marriage, young men did resort to the services of prostitutes, and a number of them still pursued sexual satisfaction through intercourse with other men, rather than a prostitute, or both. The Loire poets, a group of poets who lived along the Loire River in the late eleventh and early twelfth centuries, including Marbod of Rennes (c. 1035–1123), Baudri of Bourgueil (1040–1130), and several anonymous clerics, wrote mostly about their love of boys, but some of them also mentioned pursuing both boys and girls or both men and women.

There was even an attempt to establish a diagram of male sexual inclinations. It is attributed to **Alain of Lille** (c. 1128–1202), a French Cistercian theologian and a poet, honored by his contemporaries as the Universal Doctor. In *De fide catholica contra haereticos* (*On Catholic Faith against Heretics*), he used the three grammatical genders of Latin—masculine, feminine, and neuter—to map male desire. The masculine gender described men who were only attracted to and had sex with other men. The feminine gender covered those men who only wanted and had intercourse with women. Alain applied the neuter to those males who equally desired people of either gender and had sex with men in the summer and women in the winter.

In the Arab world, bisexual behavior had remained quite ordinary and acceptable before **Islam** and continued to be so even after its advent. The ninth-century Basra poet al-Jâhiz wrote both about men's passion for the *qayna* (singing slave girls and prostitutes) and about their love of boys. In 1082 Kai Ka'us ibn Iskander, a Persian prince, wrote *Mirror for Princes*, a guide in which he recommends his eldest son not to confine his inclinations to either sex (i.e., women and young men) and suggests that in the summer he might incline toward young men and in the winter toward women. (As for daughters, ibn Iskander wrote that it would be best if they did not come into existence, but if they did, they should be either married or buried, and, by all means, never literate.) In the twelfth century, Samau'al ibn Yahya, a Jewish convert to Islam, wrote that many well-known and powerful men had sought the company of youths because physicians had advised them that intercourse with women would cause gout, hemorrhoids, and premature aging. Beha Ed-Din Zoheir, a thirteenth-century Egyptian poet, wrote that when his mistress rejected him he started pursuing a beautiful boy. *See also* Homosexuality, Male.

Further Reading: Bullough, Vern L., and James A. Brundage, eds. *Handbook of Medieval Sexuality.* New York: Garland Publishing, 1996; Spencer, Colin. *Homosexuality in History.* New York: Harcourt, Brace, 1995.

Georgia Tres

BO XINGJIAN (776–826). Bo Xingjian (courtesy name Tuizhi) was a literati official of Tang **China** (618–907) known for his love stories and poetry. Born to a low-ranking official family, he followed the career path of his older brother, Bo Juyi (772–846), the most prolific literatus of the Tang dynasty. The Bo brothers passed the civil service examinations and obtained the *Jinshi* (advanced scholar) degree, which guaranteed them high-ranking official positions, prominent social status, and great literary reputation. Throughout his life Bo Xingjian's official duties included editor of imperial diary, reminder of the Left in the chancellery, vice director of the Transit Authorization Bureau, and director of the Bureau of Receptions.

He was best known for his "Tale of Li Wa" (*Li Wa zhuan*), a story about a courtesan and a young scholar who fell in love at first sight and got married after enduring many hardships and overcoming many obstacles. Bo Xingjian implied that it was the intense love between the two that guided them to happiness. The "Tale of Li Wa" was long considered a model for the "scholar and beauty" (*caizi jiaren*) romance in Chinese literary history. Another work attributed to Bo Xingjian is "Poetical Essay on the Supreme Joy of the Sexual Union of Yin and Yang and Heaven and Earth" (*Tiandi yinyang jiaohuan dale fu*). The essay explicitly depicts lovemaking acts among men and women of various relations. Bo considered the intimacy of a married couple as the ideal and most pleasant lovemaking situation. A **marriage** was considered formed in the first night of intercourse; along their years together, the excitement of sex reinforced the feelings of love between husband and wife. However, the bluntness of this sex manual probably astounded post-Tang literati, as the work was long considered forged and excluded from most book listings and collectanea. The discovery of the copy among the Dunhuang manuscripts further proved that the Tang dynasty was an unprecedented era of openness and sensuality in Chinese history.

Further Reading: Dudbridge, Glen. *The Tale of Li Wa: Study and Critical Edition of a Chinese Story from the Ninth Century.* London: Oxford University Press, 1983; Van Gulik, Robert Hans, and Paul Rakita Goldin. *Sexual Life in Ancient China: A Preliminary Survey of Chinese Sex and Society from ca. 1500 BC till 1644 AD.* Leiden: Brill Academic Publishers, 2003.

Ping Yao

BOCCACCIO, GIOVANNI (1313–1375).

Giovanni Boccaccio was one of the central figures in the Italian Renaissance. Like his contemporary and friend **Petrarch**, Boccaccio was an avid reader and imitator of the works of ancient Greece and Rome, but he also followed the example of **Dante Alighieri** in developing the Italian vernacular as a literary language. His works are notable for being more realistic, and in some cases much more frankly sexual, than those of his contemporaries.

Boccaccio was born in 1313, probably in Florence. Nothing reliable is known about his mother; his father was a merchant banker, who in the late 1320s was appointed head of the Neopolitan branch of the Compagnia dei Bardi (a prominent Florentine banking concern). Boccaccio went with his father to Naples and was apprenticed to the bank, but he did not do well as a banker and within a few years took up the study of law. Boccaccio was no more a success as a lawyer than he had been as a banker, but he eventually took up both writing and the study of literature, at which he excelled. Naples in the early fourteenth century was a major intellectual center, and Boccaccio profited both from the company of other scholars and writers and his father's connections with the court of Robert of Anjou. Because of political problems, Boccaccio was forced to leave Naples and return to Florence in 1341. Although he was never entirely happy with his native city, he became involved with Florentine politics and was sent on several diplomatic missions by the government, including at least three to the papal court. In 1350 he met Petrarch for the first time and began a friendship that would last until the latter's death in 1374. Although at the time Boccaccio was famous as a writer in Italian, under Petrarch's influence he began to pay more attention to the literature of classical antiquity and write more of his own works in Latin. In 1361, Boccaccio moved from Florence to the nearby town of Certaldo, where he died in 1375.

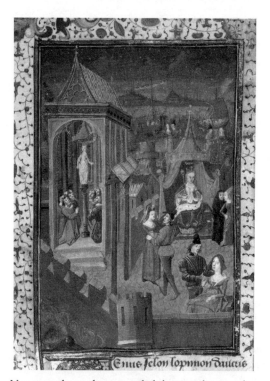

Venus enthroned, surrounded by couples at play; adoration of statue of Venus; and scene with prostitutes. "Des Cleres et Nobles Femmes," by Giovanni Boccaccio, c. 1470. © New York Public Library/Art Resource, NY.

Boccaccio's most famous work is the *Decameron*, a series of one hundred tales, primarily about love and sex, which he wrote around 1350. The tales are written as if told by a group of rich, young Florentine men and women to pass the time while avoiding the plague of 1349 in a secluded villa. The stories range from the serious and tragic to the bawdy and comic and are notable for taking a much more positive view of human sexuality than was common at the time. Boccaccio's other major works include *Filostrato* and *Filocolo* (both from the 1330s), two courtly romances that influenced **Geoffrey Chaucer**; *De mulieribus claris* (*On Famous Women*, written in 1361), which is a series of biographical sketches of famous and infamous women of antiquity; and *Genealogia deorum gentilium* (*The Descent of the Gods of the Pagans*, c. 1360), which was the standard guide to the gods of Greek and Roman myth for several centuries. *See also* Misogyny in Latin Christendom.

Further Reading: Boccaccio, Giovanni. *The Decameron.* Translated by G. H. McWilliam. Harmondsworth, UK: Penguin Books, 1972; Branca, Vittore. *Boccaccio: The Man and His Works.* Translated by Richard Monges and Dennis J. McAuliffe. New York: New York University Press, 1976.

Stephen A. Allen

BUDDHISM. Buddhist traditions, which tend to emphasize the goal of liberation from worldly attachments, generally evaluated sex negatively and valued love in its spiritual form only. Over time, sexuality gained greater acceptance within some Buddhist traditions and achieved the status of a spiritual discipline in **Tantric Buddhism**.

MONASTIC BUDDHISM. Buddhism initially problematized desire and love. A central Buddhist teaching is the four noble truths, the second of which postulates that suffering results from a cause. This cause was commonly identified as thirst or craving, namely, the impulse to appropriate the objects of one's desire. Desire was thought to arise from a deeply conditioned egocentric perspective that in turn derived from ignorance concerning the nature of the self. While Buddhists acknowledge that there are positive forms of desire, it is problematic insofar as it is directed toward sensory objects. They thus argued that those seeking to achieve liberation should renounce worldly attachments and become monks or nuns. The monastic code sought to enforce this renunciant lifestyle, by prohibiting monks and nuns from engaging in worldly behavior. Consciously engaging in sexual acts was one of the gravest violations of the monastic code, resulting in expulsion from the order. The code describes in great detail exactly what sorts of sex acts were prohibited, suggesting that monks and nuns periodically test these boundaries. The monastic code tends to focus on heterosexual sexuality, and largely ignores homosexual sexuality. This may not be coincidental; there have been numerous reports of homosexual love in the monastic context, particularly in East Asia during the medieval and early modern periods.

While inimical to romantic and sexual love, the Buddhist order did not completely condemn love. The *Metta Sutta*, part of the Pali Canon first put into writing around 300 CE, holds that there is a form of love that should be cultivated. It was called *metta*, a term usually translated as "loving kindness," as it designates a spiritual form of love. It is usually compared to the love that a mother has for her child. But unlike motherly love, which is directed toward children, *metta* should be cultivated such that one directs it toward all beings without exception. The idea here is that one should break down the egocentric perspective and give rise to love toward all without discrimination. This text was commonly studied, recited, and used as a basis for meditation in the Theravada tradition during the medieval period.

MAHAYANA BUDDHISM. The ideal of universal love and compassion was emphasized by the Mahayana school of Buddhism, which rose to prominence in **India** during the first millennium of the Common Era. The Mahayana school advanced as its spiritual ideal the *bodhisattvas*, individuals who have dedicated their lives to the attainment of Buddhahood, a goal that can be achieved only through compassionate activity. The Mahayana tradition identified compassion as a form of desire that was free of selfish motivation. It also separated the figure of the *bodhisattva* from the renunciant lifestyle of the monks and nuns.

Several well-known Mahayana Buddhist sutras advanced the notion that the *bodhisattva* could be a layperson, who, out of compassion, engages in actions that appear to be motivated by desire. The *Vimalakirti Sutra*, likely dating back to the fourth century CE, focuses on the lay *bodhisattva* Vimalakirti, who out of compassion would visit brothels and bars. The *Gandhavyuha Sutra*, likely dating back to the fifth century CE, describes a female *bodhisattva* named Vasumitra, who could liberate beings through her glance, wink, kiss, or embrace. As laypeople, these figures were not breaking any Buddhist precepts though their engagement in sexuality.

These developments seem to be influenced by the nondualistic trend in Mahayana philosophy, which eroded confidence in the validity of associating renunciation with liberation, and worldly behavior with bondage. The notion that these actions could be necessary when motivated by compassion constituted a powerful challenge to monasticism. While most Mahayana monks seem to have adhered to their vow of **celibacy**, there are exceptions, such as the Japanese Zen monk Ikkyu Sojun (1394–1481), who visited brothels and recorded his experiences in a celebrated poetry collection.

TANTRIC BUDDHISM. Around the seventh century, Buddhists began composing texts that advanced the proposition that sexual practices could lead to the rapid attainment of Buddhahood. One of the earliest of these, the *Guhyasamaja Tantra*, begins with an extremely unconventional opening verse, which placed the setting of the Buddha's teaching activity within "the vulvae of the adamantine ladies." This text inspired considerable controversy, with critics condemning it as non-Buddhist, and apologists defending it, often by claiming that it represented an exercise of "skillful means," taught in order to bring the lustful into the Buddhist fold.

These Tantras appear to have been influenced by earlier Hindu Tantras that call for the sacramental consumption of sexual fluids. The Buddhist "unexcelled yoga tantras" (*anuttarayogatanta*), which include texts such as the *Guhyasamaja* and the **Cakrasamvara Tantra**, called for sexual acts in the context of their initiation ceremony. This ceremony involved four consecrations (*abhisheka*). The first, the "vase consecration," consisted of a series of initiatory rites derived from earlier strata of Tantric literature. In the second, the "secret consecration," the master would enter into sexual union with his consort, and anoint the disciple with the resulting mixture of sexual fluids. This would be followed by the "wisdom-gnosis consecration," in which the disciple would be instructed in the arts of

The Buddha Vajrasattva with consort, first half of the 13th century. © Réunion des Musées Nationaux/Art Resource, NY.

sexual union or "sexual yogas" with a specially prepared consort. This leads to the mystical "fourth consecration," in which the disciple, through sexual union, realizes the secret gnosis of awakening.

As these Tantras were considered the highest teaching by many Buddhists, they presented a serious challenge to the monastic order, since they called for practices that the monks and nuns could not engage in without violating their vow of celibacy. Some Buddhists thought that this was not a problem, and argued that the "higher" Mahayana and Tantric vows superseded the monastic vows. Other Buddhists, however, saw them as a threat to the foundation of Buddhism, given the fact that Buddhist communities tend to be organized around the institution of the monastery.

These Tantras were transmitted to **Tibet** from the eighth through fourteenth centuries. The Tibetan Buddhist traditions resolved this problem in a novel fashion: The actual practice of sexual acts was eliminated from the public performances of the Tantric rites. Sexual union would be imaginatively visualized rather than actually performed, and disciples would be consecrated with symbolic substitutes. While the sexual yogas could be practiced in secret, it was also possible in some traditions to practice them through visualization only. However, the Tibetan tradition also had religious figures, such as Drukpa Kunley (b. 1455), who openly celebrated sexuality as an integral aspect of the spiritual path. *See also* China; Japan.

Further Reading: Arntzen, Sonja, trans. *Ikkyu and the Crazy Cloud Anthology: A Zen Poet of Medieval Japan*. Tokyo: University of Tokyo Press, 1986; Dowman, Keith, trans. *The Divine Madman: The Sublime Life and Songs of Drukpa Kunley*. Clearlake, CA: Dawnhorse Press, 1980; Faure, Bernard. *The Red Thread: Buddhist Approaches to Sexuality*. Princeton, NJ: Princeton University Press, 1998; Shaw, Miranda. *Passionate Enlightenment: Women in Tantric Buddhism*. Princeton, NJ: Princeton University Press, 1994; Young, Serinity. *Courtesans and Tantric Consorts: Sexualities in Buddhist Narrative, Iconography, and Ritual*. New York: Routledge, 2004.

David B. Gray

BYZANTINE EMPIRE. *See* Byzantium

BYZANTIUM. Byzantium was an old Greek colony founded on the European side of the Bosporus Strait and named after Byzas, the son of the god Neptune. In the first century BCE, the settlement was included in the Roman realm. When the Western Roman empire went into a decline, the emperor Constantine (r. 324–337) decided to move his residence to the east, and selected Byzantium as his new capital. The city was rebuilt under the name Constantinople. In 395 the empire was divided between two sons of Emperor Theodosius I. The eastern part emerged as an independent state and became the cradle of a new civilization that survived for more than a thousand years. During the reign of Emperor Justinian (527–565), Byzantium was the most powerful state in Europe reaching from North **Africa** and Spain to the Balkan peninsula and Caucasus. In the following centuries it faced challenges from the Arabs, who conquered Syria, Egypt, and Palestine in the seventh century; outlived the invasion of the crusaders, who captured Constantinople in 1204; but failed to repulse the Ottoman Turks who subjugated the empire in 1453.

Throughout its history, Byzantine civilization preserved its cultural identity. Since Emperor Constantine officially recognized Christianity as a state religion, the everyday life of the Byzantine commonwealth was heavily influenced by church doctrine. Early Christian theologians formulated certain principles and regulations regarding proper social behavior, **marriage**, and household and monastic life. The famous church fathers Clement of Alexandria, Basil of Caesaria, Gregory of Nyssa, **John Chrysostom**, and

Gregory Nazianzus left a number of accounts on human body, **virginity**, and sexuality. Their teaching finally appeared as a collection of **canon law** (*nomokanon* in Greek). In the eighth century, the Byzantine emperors issued the secular law code, the Ecloga, which also contained rules of conduct for clergy and laypeople.

Both ecclesiastical and secular law considered marriage an important institution that helps to maintain social order. The legitimate marriage required proper religious ceremony and permission from parents of the young couple. Boys were allowed to get married for the first time at the age of fifteen, and girls at the age of twelve. The church also recognized second and third marriages after the death of former spouses, but condemned the fourth one. Orthodox canon law prohibited marriages between close relatives and people with spiritual relationship. A godfather, for example, could not marry his goddaughter.

The church fathers had different perceptions of the nature of sexual relations. John Chrysostom argued that intercourse was meant by God to impel people to increase in number; therefore it is permissible not only for procreation. Most theologians, however, considered sexuality a human's sin and separation from God. Ecclesiastical law attempted to regulate sexual behavior even between married couples. *Nomokanon* forbade marital sex during religious holidays. Many types of sexual intercourse were regarded as unnatural. The only exception was the so-called missionary position with the man on top. Canon law prohibited sexual contacts outside marriage and considered **adultery** a serious crime. The more realistic secular law recognized extramarital sex. The legislation of Emperor Justinian, for example, raised the status of concubines by granting inheritance rights to women who maintained long relations with an unmarried man. Concubine's children might legally inherit their father's property.

In the fifth century, the Byzantine church adopted a policy regarding clerical marriage. Priests and deacons of lower ranks were allowed to marry before ordination, but, if married, could not be elected to higher offices in the church. The sexual behavior of married clergy was strictly regulated by the canon law. A priest, for example, had to refrain from sexual intercourse on days when he served a liturgy. The monastic clergy, who might be promoted to the ranks of bishops and archbishops, on the contrary, had to remain celibate.

The secular law dealt with improper sexual conduct that might disturb public safety. Justinian's code repressed prostitutes and penalized those who owed public houses. Homosexuality was considered a serious offence, as people believed that it might cause famine or earthquake. In general, church and state in the Byzantine empire took active measures to control sexuality by means of legislation and social institutions to avoid its destructive influence on the society. *See also* Eunuchs; Orthodox Christianity; Theophylactus of Ochrid.

Further Reading: Brown, Peter. *The Body and Society: Men, Women, and Sexual Renunciation in Early Christianity*. New York: Columbia University Press, 1988; Brundage, James A. *Law, Sex and Christian Society in Medieval Europe*. Chicago: University of Chicago Press, 1987; Levin, Eve. "Eastern Orthodox Christianity." In *Handbook of Medieval Sexuality*, edited by Vern L. Bullough and James A. Brundage, 329–43. New York: Garland, 1996.

Sergey Lobachev

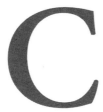

CAKRASAMVARA TANTRA. The *Cakrasamvara Tantra* is an Indian Tantric Buddhist text. While its date of composition is not known, there is evidence suggesting that it was composed between the mid-eighth and early ninth centuries. This scripture was classified as a Yogini Tantra, a goddess-centered genre that highlights eroticism and violence. Many of these texts appear to have been significantly influenced by Hindu Tantric traditions, and their status as genuine Buddhist scriptures are questioned by many Indian Buddhists.

The *Cakrasamvara Tantra* focuses on a class of deities known as *yoginis* or *dakinis*, semidivine, semidemonic female deities who can also manifest as human females. The text proposes that the spiritual development of a male adept depends upon his ability to find and gain the support of a *yogini* or *dakini*. In order to do this, he must first obtain initiation from a qualified master. The initiation process is complex, and involves engagement in sexual practices. According to the text, the master and his consort enter into sexual union, in which they produce sexual fluids. The mixture of these fluids are used to anoint the disciple, who is then instructed in sexual union with a consort.

Following initiation, he needs to discover a woman who belongs to one of the clans of *yoginis* or *dakinis*. The text describes in great detail the distinguishing characteristics of the women of these clans so that the adept can recognize them. It also describes a secret code and sign language that should be used to communicate with them. Once he finds them, he can join them in their Tantric feast, in which they engage in eating, singing, dancing, and sexual union. The text describes in some detail sexual practices, the purpose of which is the production of sexual fluids that are used as sacraments, and giving rise to magical powers such as flight.

Tradition also understands the text to refer obliquely to sexual practices involving the inner subtle body. These involve entering sexual union for the purpose of giving rise to energies that, instead of being released, are diverted upward into the central channel of the subtle body, giving rise to great bliss. The text does not describe these practices explicitly; commentators claim that these practices are secrets of the tradition and hence are not disclosed in the text.

This tradition was disseminated to Nepal and **Tibet**, where it remains popular. The scripture was translated during the medieval period into Tibetan and Mongolian, and has recently been translated into Chinese. Considerable secrecy surrounds its practice. However, in the Tibetan Buddhist traditions, the *Cakrasamvara* initiation rite is performed publicly, with symbolic substitutes for the actual sexual elements. *See also* Buddhism; Tantric Buddhism.

Further Reading: Gray, David B. "Disclosing the Empty Secret: Textuality and Embodiment in the *Cakrasamvara Tantra*." *Numen* 52, no. 4 (2005): 417–44; Gray, David B. *The Cakrasamvara Tantra: A Study and Annotated Translation*. New York: American Institute of Buddhist Studies, 2006.

David B. Gray

CANON LAW. The canon law is the body of legislation that regulates Christian ritual practices and the moral behavior of individual Christians. It thus covers many aspects of sexuality, from individual sexual acts to **marriage** and reproduction. Canon law is derived from a variety of sources, such as the Bible, the decisions of church councils, and papal letters. During the early Middle Ages, canon law was often a matter of local practice, but after the twelfth century the papacy increasingly took over the responsibility for issuing and enforcing it.

The best evidence for the early medieval canon law of sex and sexuality comes from a group of texts called the **penitentials**, which were popular from the sixth to the eleventh centuries. Penitentials were written to provide guidance for priests hearing **confession**s and generally consisted of lists of sins with the appropriate penances to assign to each one. While the penitentials do not provide detailed explanations of why certain acts were considered sinful, they do show the limits placed on sexual activity in early medieval Europe. While there were some collections of canon law circulating in this society, they were frequently unreliable and often did not contain materials addressing sexual matters.

The penitentials, and the other scattered sources of early medieval canon law that discuss sex, reveal a certain uniformity of opinion. Taking its lead from Christian writings of late antiquity (especially those of Saint **Augustine** of Hippo), early canon law viewed **celibacy** as the best possible state of human sexual affairs. If a person did not remain celibate, he or she was required to marry and engage in sexual activity only within the bounds of marriage. Premarital sex, **adultery**, homosexuality, and **masturbation** were forbidden. Even sex between individuals married to each other was highly restricted: couples were supposed to refrain from sex on religious holidays (including Sundays and saints' feast days); while the woman was menstruating, pregnant, or nursing; and for reasons other than procreation. Multiple marriages, **divorce**, and **remarriage**, which were practiced among the Germanic peoples of northern Europe, were another frequent target of the penitentials. As large areas of Europe converted from Paganism to Christianity, the Christian clergy attempted to change the sexual practices of the new converts. Given that this was as much an attempt to change traditions as it was to change laws, the Christian model of human sexuality spread slowly and with some difficulty, although by the eleventh century it was the dominant model throughout most of Europe.

Another area of concern in early medieval canon law was the sexual behavior of the clergy. Like all other Christians, priests were expected not to engage in sexual activity outside of marriage. Although there was a long-standing tradition of clerical celibacy, as well as rulings by several fourth- and fifth-century church councils and popes that priests should not marry, by the tenth century it was not uncommon for priests to marry and even father children. In the mid-eleventh century, as part of the wider reform movement known as the Gregorian Reform, the papacy attempted to enforce the older decrees against clerical marriage. Although there was a considerable amount of resistance, celibacy for priests eventually became the norm in the Latin west. (Priests in the Greek churches were, and still are, allowed to be married.)

The twelfth century saw major changes in the way the canon law was created and transmitted. More reliable, systematic collections of canon law began to appear. The most comprehensive of these collections was the *Decretum*, compiled around 1140 by an Italian monk named Gratian. This became the main textbook for the teaching of canon law in the new universities that sprang up in the twelfth century. Legal scholars known as the decretists began producing commentaries on the *Decretum* within a decade or so of its publication. As the study of canon law was becoming more systematic and professionalized, control of the creation of canon law became more and more the responsibility of the papacy. In 1234, Pope Gregory IX issued his *Decretales*, the first official canon law collection. From the thirteenth century on, the creation and collection of canon law for the Western church was left in papal hands.

Despite these changes, the basic content of the canon law of sexuality remained essentially the same. All nonmarital sexual activity was considered sinful, and even marital sex was closely restricted. One area that did see considerable development, however, was marriage law. The jurists of the twelfth and thirteenth centuries were very concerned to properly define and regulate the institution of marriage. The major topics of discussion were **consanguinity**; when a marriage became valid; and divorce. In the early Middle Ages, marriage between persons related by seven degrees was forbidden, that is, if they could be connected on a family tree by seven or fewer links (for example, second cousins once removed). This was reduced to four degrees in the late twelfth century. The question when a marriage became valid, and thus theoretically unbreakable, was a matter of contention throughout the later Middle Ages. The two main positions were that a marriage became valid when the two parties agreed to be married (consent), or that it was completed when the two parties engaged in sexual intercourse (consummation). The eventual consensus was that consent made the marriage, but consummation was an essential part of a marriage that made the bond stronger. While divorce was never fully accepted by the medieval church, the canon lawyers did make some attempts to define when a marriage could legitimately be ended and how that was to be done.

Canon law was, and is, the law of an independent legal system, enforced by ecclesiastical tribunals and courts. While separate from the laws of nations and other secular governmental bodies during the Middle Ages, canon law did influence the development and content of civil law, especially as far as marriage was concerned. *See also* Catholic Europe; Catholicism.

Further Reading: Boswell, John. *Christianity, Social Tolerance, and Homosexuality.* Chicago: University of Chicago Press, 1980; Brundage, James. *Law, Sex, and Christian Society in Medieval Europe.* Chicago: University of Chicago Press, 1987; Bullough, Vern L., and James A. Brundage. *Handbook of Medieval Sexuality.* New York: Garland, 1996; Payer, Pierre J. *Sex and the Penitentials.* Toronto, ON: University of Toronto Press, 1984.

Stephen A. Allen

CANTIGAS DE SANTA MARIA. *Cantigas de Santa Maria* is a thirteenth-century collection of poems to the Virgin Mary. It was written during the reign of Alfonso X, king of Castile, who is himself believed to have written some of the poems. Out of the 420 poems in the book, 356 are narrative poems that tell stories of miracles performed by the Virgin to save her adherents from sin. Though many types of sins are mentioned throughout the text, a significant proportion, thirty-two in all, deals specifically with sexual sins. A partial listing includes **rape, incest, adultery,** and promiscuity in addition to several tales of runaway nuns and priests involved in sexual relationships.

A wide range of sins of the flesh are exhibited throughout the collection, and the Virgin's attitude toward them varies. She might either accept or condemn acts of **lust**, forgive repentant or nonrepentant sinners, dissuade the sinner by suggestion or action, or in some cases even help her devotees to commit a sin.

Very typically, a *cantiga* will teach by example the importance of refraining from committing a sin of the flesh. A case in point is *cantiga* 15, about an empress who, throughout her life, is the object of sexual advances by a variety of men including her brother-in-law. Remaining chaste, she never falls into temptation, and as a reward for her virtue the Virgin grants her the power of healing leprosy.

The Virgin uses a variety of methods to prevent her followers from falling into sin. In *cantiga* 58, a nun is tempted by the devil to fall in love and leave the convent to be with the lover. The night before her flight, Mary appears in her dreams showing her the horrors of hell, whereupon the nun decides not to leave. Other *cantigas* demonstrate how an image of the Virgin or even something connected to her can halt a devotee's slide into sin. *Cantiga* 42 is a fascinating case in which the Virgin lies down between two lovers in order to prevent a carnal act because the man had earlier pledged his chastity to her.

Sometimes the Virgin prevents the committal of a sin, but sometimes she intervenes afterward. She might either forgive or help repentant sinners like Pope Leon who cut his hand after being kissed by a woman, but she also helps nonrepentant sinners like the priest she resuscitated after he drowned on his way to meet his lover.

In some poems the Virgin fails to condemn wrongdoing and actually helps her followers to cover up sins of the flesh. *Cantigas* 55 and 94 portray two cases of runaway nuns who had eloped from the convent to be with their lovers. Deciding to come back to the convent, they discovered that Mary had taken their places so that nobody noticed their absence or their sinful acts. Perhaps most provocative of all is the portrayal, in *cantiga* 135, of Mary as facilitator for two young lovers coming together and consummating their relationship despite being unwed, her favor being earned by virtue of their having sworn their love in front of her. *See also* Marianism.

Further Reading: Alfonso X. *Cantigas de Santa Maria*. Madrid: Castalia, 1986; Burke, James. "Virtue and Sin, Reward and Punishment in the Cantigas de Santa Maria." In *Studies on the Cantigas de Santa Maria: Art, Music, and Poetry*, edited by Israel Kats and John E. Keller, 247–52. Madison, WI: Hispanic Seminar on Medieval Studies, 1987; Sturm, Sara. "The Presentation of the Virgin in the Cantigas de Santa Maria." *Philological Quarterly* 49 (January 1970): 1–7.

Claudia M. Mejía

CASTRATION. Origen, a third-century church father, castrated himself in order to live a strictly ascetical life. His act was condemned by almost all of his contemporaries who emphasized the importance of the necessary sacrifices that men had to make to live a celibate and ascetic life. Castration, however, continued to be performed by the state on criminals, slaves, and others, and this action was never condemned by the religious authorities. Castrated men, or **eunuchs**, also served important roles in the Byzantine army and the state. They, however, could not hold the position of emperor. Most of those castrated simply lost their testicles, but in **China** and elsewhere total castration was performed, in which the penis was also removed. This operation had a higher mortality. Eunuchs served in the imperial court in China as they did in the Byzantine empire and Islamic states. In **India**, asceticism and renunciation of sexual desire led some to practice total castration.

In late medieval and early modern Europe, castration was practiced on boys in order to preserve their soprano voices since women were forbidden to sing in the choir. Technically, the Christian church in the West had banned castration in the fourth century, but there was no ban on using the services of the *castrati*. The *castrati* thus continued to be important in churches mainly in Italy and southern Europe until 1878, when Pope Leo prohibited their use in choirs. Some *castrati* singers survived into the twentieth century and some of them were recorded.

Further Reading: Bullough, Vern L. "Eunuchs in History and Society." In *Eunuchs in Antiquity and Beyond*, edited by Shaun Tougher. Swansea, Wales: Classical Press, 2002.

Vern L. Bullough

CATHARS. See Manicheans and Cathars

CATHOLIC EUROPE. In the beginning of the Middle Ages, the European continent—with the exception of the classical world—was occupied by an amorphous group of tribes and peoples. Yet by the end of the period, a unified Catholic Europe had emerged, and the organization of many present-day European states had been put into place.

THE FOUNDATION OF CATHOLIC EUROPE. The year 410, in which Alaric (king of the Visigoths) sacked Rome, officially marks the fall of the Roman empire. No longer sheltered by the *Pax Romana* (Roman Peace), western Europe was plagued with the invasion of barbarian hordes. By the end of the fifth century and beginning of the sixth, Clovis, king of the Franks, subdued many of the tribes surrounding his territories. After his own conversion to Christianity, Clovis facilitated the spread of the new faith in the lands that belonged to him, thereby laying the foundations of the Franco-Christian empire.

The spread of Christianity in Europe was achieved through intense monastic activity. As early as the fourth century, St. Martin (c. 316–397) traveled from Panonnia (present-day Hungary) to France to study under Hilary of Poitiers, and established a monastery at Tours. The *Life of St. Martin* composed by Sulpicius Severus documents Martin's fearless efforts to convert the inhabitants of the region to Christianity, breaking pagan altars with his own hands, and standing up to local druids and cults.

The successful conversion of the Irish is credited to St. Patrick (c. 387–493). Briton by birth, Patrick was kidnapped at a young age and taken as a slave to Ireland. (Some legends claim that Patrick was the nephew of St. Martin of Tour.s) In the *Confession*, Patrick records how he prayed day after day, until the love of God grew in him so strong that he heard the voice of an angel commanding him to flee from his master. Patrick escaped from Ireland by sea and, after sailing to the Continent, returned home to Britain. Soon, he was called by God to go once again to Ireland and minister to the people there. A later section of the *Confession* presents Patrick's admonition to his compatriots to become fishers of men and cast out their nets over all nations in Europe, so that those people may be converted to Christianity. Furthermore, Patrick ordered his abbots to answer directly to the pope in Rome, and not to local secular or religious powers. In so doing, Patrick prepared the way for the creation of a truly Catholic and European religious identity, answering to the papacy and extending beyond national borders.

Two of Patrick's most notable followers were St. Columba (The Dove of the Church), who founded the renowned monastery on the Scottish island of Iona in 563, and St. Columbanus (The Little Dove, c. 543–615). Jonas of Bobbio's *Life of St. Columbanus* (c. 643) recalls how the holy man was tempted by **lust** in his youth and sought out the advice of a religious woman. Reminding him that Samson, David, and Solomon were all led astray by women, she urged Columbanus to flee the earthly world and its corruption. Columbanus resolved to become a monk, choosing the love of God and of heavenly things over the love of the earthly world. After sailing to the Continent, he founded during his lifetime religious houses in Burgundy (Annegray, Luxeuil, and Fontaines), Switzerland (St. Gall), and Italy (Bobbio). Together, Columbanus and his disciples established between forty and one hundred religious houses, thereby laying down the infrastructure for a pan-European network of monasteries. It comes as no surprise that the twentieth-century French minister of foreign affairs, Robert Schuman, credited St. Columbanus as being the patron saint of those seeking to construct a unified Europe.

The spread of the Order of St. Benedict of Nursia (c. 480–543), encouraged by Pope Gregory the Great (c. 540–604), also played an important role in the establishment of Catholic Europe. Augustine, one of the most influential and famous Benedictine missionaries, was sent by Rome to England, where he established the Sees of Canterbury, York, and London. St. Boniface dedicated his life to spreading the faith amongst the Germanic peoples, thereby earning the title Apostle to the Germans. Those mentioned above are but a few amongst many women and men of tremendous religious conviction and vocation who spread Christianity throughout Europe.

THE CHRISTIAN EMPIRE AND THE THREAT OF ISLAM. Wars, invasions, and disputes over succession continuously jeopardized the solidity and predominance of the Franco-Christian kingdom. In 732, Charles Martel (Charles the Hammer) defeated Islamic invaders at the battle of Poitiers and was hailed as the defender of Christendom. In turn, Charles's son, Pepin the Short, solidified the relationship between political and religious spheres by proclaiming the union of church and state. Pepin's rule marked the beginning of the Frankish monarchs' close support of the papacy. This alliance was further solidified by Pepin's son, Charlemagne (Charles the Great), who was crowned Holy Roman Emperor by the pope on Christmas Day in the year 800. In the name of God, Charlemagne conquered an immense empire, extending from the Ebro and the Apennines to the Eider River, and from the Atlantic to the Elbe and the Raab. As God's chosen ruler on earth, Charlemagne was charged with leading all nations and races according to God's will. During his rule, many new dioceses and monasteries were founded throughout Europe. Although political unity in the West was never fully restored after the end of the Carolingian empire, the religious unity of Europe, fostered by Charlemagne, remained in place until the Reformation. Charlemagne also encouraged a revival of classical learning, thereby laying the foundations for the later Renaissance of the twelfth century. New scripts were developed to facilitate the efficient copying of damaged manuscripts and disintegrating papyri. Carolingian minuscule, which would be used by European scribes for centuries, survives even today in the modern font Times New Roman.

By the end of the first millennium, the Greek church was also gaining considerable influence in eastern Europe. In 955, the first Christian princess of Russia, Olga, was baptized at Constantinople. During the rule of her grandson, Vladimir (baptized in 989), Christianity became the official religion of Russia. Hence, by the year 1000, the majority of the European continent was Christian. Parts of Spain, however, were ruled by the Arabs, who had been occupying the peninsula since 711. Likewise, Sicily had been under Saracen rule since 878.

As a response to the increasing Islamic threat, both in Europe and in the Holy Land, a series of concerted and collaborative expeditions were organized by the papacy. These Crusades lasted nearly 200 years (1061–1244). Political leaders, monks, and bishops from all of Europe—such as Richard the Lionheart of England and St. **Bernard of Clairvaux**—actively supported the venture. Although the crusaders' goal of freeing Palestine from the hands of non-Christians was not met, **Islam** was gradually driven out of Catholic Europe. Sicily was freed by a lengthy Norman expedition led in 1061–1091. Then, in 1212, the Spanish Arabs were pushed back to Granada. That city was not reclaimed by the Christians, however, until 1492. For hundreds of years, Arabic thought and art forms profoundly influenced the Spanish intellectual tradition; from Spain they spread to the rest of Europe.

CATHOLIC EUROPE AND LOVE (CARITAS). The emergence of a deeply personal faith, centered upon God's love for the world, as presented in the Gospel of John (or Gospel of Love), dominated religious inquiry from the year 1000 onward. Much of this shift in religious sensibility has been associated with the writings of St. Anselm of Canterbury, who in the *Cur Deus Homo* (*Why God Became Man*) reflected upon the necessary sacrifice of God's son, Jesus Christ, given through love to the world so that humankind could be reconciled with their creator. In turn, the writings of St. Bernard of Clairvaux emphasized the importance of achieving a mystical union with God through love. Anselm and Bernard were succeeded by a long and flourishing tradition of medieval mystics, including, for example, Catherine of Siena (1347–1380), Julian of Norwich (1342–c. 1416), Meister Johannes Eckhart (1260–1327), and Thomas á Kempis (c. 1380–1421).

Beginning in the eleventh century, religious art evolved to reflect the newly placed emphasis on the humanity of Christ. This is especially evident in the evolution of depictions of the Crucifixion, which take on increasingly human expressions of pain and suffering. In contrast to the unemotional crucifixion scenes of the sixth through tenth centuries, depicting an upright and serene God-like figure nailed to the cross, greater emphasis was now placed upon the affliction of the crucified Christ, whose body bleeds, and whose head hangs agonizingly to the side. The colors of the passion, white and red—which recall Christ's pallid body and crimson blood, and which are closely associated with the bread and wine of the Eucharist—came to symbolize, throughout the Middle Ages, both the love of God for humankind and also the love between a man and a woman. The colors have been adapted by writers of religious and secular works, as well as artists and designers of stained glass. One of the most famous uses of the color scheme in vernacular literature survives in the Arthurian *Quest for the Grail* or *Perceval* (c. 1190) by Chrétien de Troyes. As Perceval rides toward Arthur's camp, he leaves the path to follow a wounded goose. When he arrives at the place where the bird fell, it had already departed, leaving three drops of (red) blood on the (white) snow. This vision leads Perceval to become lost in deep contemplation, during which the blood drops and the snow merges to create, in his mind, the image of his beloved's face.

The rise of **Marianism**, directly linked to the new-found emphasis on Christ's humanity, also profoundly influenced European religious and vernacular poetry as well as other art forms. Throughout Europe, countless churches and cathedrals constructed first in the Romanesque style, and then in the elevated Gothic style, were dedicated to the glory of Our Lady. These earthly palaces of the Blessed Virgin solidified the privileged place occupied by the female sex in the process of salvation. Depictions of the Lady as saint or savior are overwhelmingly present in Latin religious poetry, the songs of the **troubadours**, and the immense corpus of courtly literature. The excesses of **courtly love** were, however, soon critiqued and parodied in such works as the anonymous thirteenth-century *Aucassin and Nicolette*. *See also* Catholicism.

Further Reading: Jordan, William Chester. *Europe in the High Middle Ages*. New York: Penguin, 2004; Keen, Maurice. *The Penguin History of Medieval Europe*. New York: Penguin, 1991; Southern, Richard W. *The Making of the Middle Ages*. New Haven, CT: Yale University Press, 1961; Southern, Richard W. *Western Society and the Church in the Middle Ages*. New York: Penguin, 1990.

K. Sarah-Jane Murray

CATHOLICISM. The sexual doctrine of the medieval Catholic Church originated in patristic reflection, elaborating concepts from **Judaism** and stoic philosophy, transforming them, and bringing them to a conclusion. Christian writers, beginning in the second century CE, insisted on the obedience to God's wishes, expressed not only in the words but also in the actions of Jesus. The Christian should imitate Christ. The right sexual attitude is the same as that Jesus practiced: absolute chastity. Tertullian in the third century wrote that Christians are God's temple consecrated by Holy Spirit, and chastity is the priestess and victim of it. Tertullian also claims that **virginity** is a wedding with Christ, an imitation of the church as the bride of Christ. **Marriage** is the only alternative to total virginity. However, being the figure of the union of Christ with church, and of Mary with the Holy Spirit, even in marriage, virginity should be the rule.

In the third century, Cyprian wrote that with Christ's arrival, marriage had exhausted its function, and he recommended virginity to everybody. The doctrine of chastity handed down by Basil of Caesarea, Gregory Nazianzen, Gregory of Nissa and **John Chrysostom**, Ambrose and **Jerome** reached the apex with **Augustine**, who reassumed and rehandled it, emphasizing **lust** and the doctrine of marriage as a remedy to it. The doctrine of the perpetual virginity of Mary, proclaimed by the Council of Ephesus in 431, furnished in Mary and later, beginning only from the ninth century in Europe, also in her chaste bridegroom Joseph, other perfect models of virginity close to that of Christ. Other models of chastity were offered by the **virgin martyrs**, who were faithful to their union with Christ, and sacrificed their lives.

On the other hand, sexuality in marriage became not a pleasure but a duty to the consort who demanded the "conjugal debt" or rather the rightful share to sexual action from the legitimate partner. From here, a whole satirical literature exalted poor husbands exhausted from the insatiable desires of their wives. The presence of prostitutes was tolerated as an excuse to avoid greater sin.

Monasticism, especially the Benedictine, institutionalized the union, with Christ and the church, of women and men who spent their hard-working life within the monasteries. Beginning in the thirteenth century, the idea of offering their virginity was carried on to the mendicant orders, especially the Franciscan and Dominican, the orders that gave **scholastic philosophy** its greater representatives. The greatest exponent of scholasticism, **Thomas Aquinas**, considered for the first time in the Middle Ages the pleasure of the sexual action in marriage as a positive fact, retaining nevertheless rigid positions on sexual actions outside the matrimonial tie, particularly **sodomy** and **masturbation**. In the medieval society they could not find a place for other categories beyond the legitimate ones of continent spouses and virgins, even if sexual habits were changed with the demographic growth of the cities.

Franciscans in particular preached a sexual ethic. Fasts and bodily penitences were recommended to preserve chastity and to mortify the desires of the body. Hagiography exalted the virtue of chastity in all the models proposed to the veneration of the believers, handing down episodes such as that of Francis of Assisi throwing himself among the thorns of roses in a moment of carnal temptation, or Mary Egiziaca rejected by an invisible hand from the doors of a church because she was a prostitute, or Thomas Aquinas sending away a woman sent him by his brothers to corrupt him using a brand of fire, or Anthony the Abbott fighting against the sensual visions the devil showed him in the desert. The saint is seen like an angel in human body, who succeeds in maintaining his separation from carnal pleasures thanks to a severe penitence. The fear of pestilences and cataclysms, which medieval preachers associated with the presence of sinners, made possible the legislation included in imperial laws and town statutes that punished sexual dissidents, sodomites, and prostitutes as corrupt. Lay penitential movements publicly practiced scourging and bodily mortifications to implore divine punishments. The sin against chastity was particularly diffused in ecclesiastical institutions, where persons forced into vocations, a bachelorhood and seclusion by their families, often engaged in secret relationships, sometimes homosexual. **Peter Damian**, Catherine of Siena, and **Bernardino of Siena** wrote and preached against these relationships. Families also often publicly promised their children marriage when they were infants. These marriages were generally founded on economic agreements and provoked more clandestine adulterous relationships. In these marriages, often between consorts of very different ages, sincere love was rare.

Connected to sexual sins were those of **contraception**. Frequent **confession**s, approved and recommended, not only failed to limit sexual sins but rather encouraged them due to the facility with which committed sins could be canceled through penitence. Confession and spiritual direction were powerful methods of social control by the church. Theologians like John Gerson wrote works on how a confessor should question penitents so as not to put curiosities that they would not have had otherwise into their heads. The conflict between religion and sex led to the marginalization and sometimes the physical elimination of people who practiced sex not in the way conforming to the norm. Medieval institutions, pretending to act in the name of Christ, often seemed to forget the love and compassion of Jesus for sinners. Serious sexual scandals committed in ecclesiastical institutions also influenced literature, for example, in Italy the *Divina Commedia* of **Dante Alighieri** and the *Decameron* of **Giovanni Boccaccio**, which exposed in different ways sexual sins and clerical corruption. Reading the sources gives the idea of a society with severe laws inspired by the epoch's Catholic doctrine of a sex-phobic ethic, rules that were generally not observed. *See also* Catholic Europe; Marianism; Monasticism, Female; Monasticism, Male; Scholastic Philosophy.

Further Reading: Baldwin, John W. *The Language of Sex: Five Voices from Northern France around 1200*. Chicago: University of Chicago Press, 1997; Flandrin, Jean Louis. *Il sesso e l'Occidente*. Milano: Mondadori, 1983.

Elvio Ciferri

CELIBACY. Celibacy refers to either complete abstinence from sexual activity or the state of being unmarried. In this article, the former definition will be used. Celibacy should not be confused with chastity, which refers to limiting sexual activity but not necessarily completely avoiding it.

Medieval Christianity inherited from the Patristic period the idea that celibacy was the preferred sexual state. Those who were unwilling to remain celibate were to limit their sexual activities to **marriage**. Within marriage, sexual activity was limited, and some Christian writers even proposed the idea of a celibate marriage for those forced into marriage for social or dynastic reasons but felt the call to a celibate life, or for those who had already had children and thus fulfilled the purpose of marriage, which in medieval Christian thought was procreation. The ideal held by many medieval theologians and writers on sexual matters was that of monastic life, where individuals not only avoided sexual contact but also swore not to marry. Monasticism was very popular throughout medieval Europe and also in the Christian East. From the tenth century onward, the monastic ideal was applied increasingly to other persons in the religious circle, such as parish priests. Although there was a considerable amount of resistance to making clerical celibacy the norm, by the end of the twelfth century all priests in western Europe were expected to be unmarried and celibate. Priests in the Greek churches could marry before entering the priesthood, but if they did not, they were expected to remain celibate after ordination.

Comparatively little is known about the sexual practices of the Germanic tribes of northern Europe before their conversion to Christianity, but celibacy does not appear to have been a major, or even significant, part of their sexual practices. The prevalence of **concubinage** and other socially recognized nonmarital unions suggests that celibacy was not considered normal or desirable. In fact, the continued existence of concubinage was one of the major obstacles facing Christian reformers in the struggle for clerical celibacy: priests would agree in principle not to marry, but would maintain concubines and even families.

Celibacy did not hold as important a place in medieval **Judaism** as it did in medieval Christianity. The sexually abstentious teachings of late antique Jewish groups such as the Essenes had more of an effect on the development of Christian sexual teachings than of Jewish ones. Though sexual activity was closely regulated, there was no requirement of celibacy for religious leaders, and abstinence was not held up as the highest sexual ideal for most **Jews**. Premarital sex was forbidden, and the virginity of women was carefully guarded, but the sexual ideal for medieval Judaism was marriage and reproduction, not celibacy. Sexual activity was thus not broadly condemned, but it was regulated to maximize procreation.

Like Judaism, medieval **Islam** regulated sexual activity and promoted the ideals of marriage and the production of children, but with few exceptions it denigrated celibacy. The only major group within Islam that promoted celibacy was the Sufi tradition, and Sufis were generally regarded with suspicion and even outright hostility by other Muslims in the Middle Ages. Although Muslim sexuality gradually became more closely regulated after the twelfth century CE, and there was a substantial misogynist strain in much medieval Islamic thought, this did not lead to the promotion of celibacy.

It is difficult to define precisely the role of celibacy in medieval **Hinduism**, as that religious tradition is complex and has many different subdivisions, each with its own teachings. In general, it can be said that ascetic self-denial, including the rejection of sexual activity, was viewed with respect but considered the purview of an enlightened few, while for most individuals sexual activity was considered enjoyable and laudable. During the medieval period, the Indian subcontinent produced several classics of sexual literature, including the *Kama Sutra*, which suggests that celibacy was not a major concern of medieval Hinduism.

With the exception of a few schools, such as the Mi-tsung tradition in **China** and Tantrism in **Tibet** and Nepal, medieval **Buddhism** emphasized celibacy as a way of avoiding earthly entanglements. Large monastic settlements were common, and both men and women were encouraged to enter the religious life, albeit in separate communities. Medieval Buddhism was closer to medieval Christianity than it was to Judaism, Islam, or Hinduism in the high value it placed on celibacy, and together they were the only two major medieval religious traditions to place celibacy above marriage as the preferred sexual state for the majority of practitioners. *See also* Monasticism, Female; Monasticism, Male.

Further Reading: Abbot, Elizabeth. *A History of Celibacy*. New York: Scribner, 2000; Bullough, Vern L. *Sexual Variance in Society and History*. New York: John Wiley and Sons, 1976; Elliott, Dyan. *Spiritual Marriage: Sexual Abstinence in Medieval Wedlock*. Princeton, NJ: Princeton University Press, 1993.

Stephen A. Allen

CENTRAL ASIA. A profusion of faiths has flourished in central Asia. Most of the main creedal religions, as well as various indigenous religions such as shamanism and animalistic cults, have been represented here. The spread of creedal religions gradually submerged—often eradicating by force—the indigenous religions of the steppe peoples and their customs relating to love and sexuality. Yet, in many cases, the ancient traditions survived, usually in semi-disguised form, sometimes renamed and reinterpreted to conform to the new religious norms. In addition to the ensemble of diverse faiths, physical geography has influenced central Asian culture. The mountain ring and the absence of any significant body of water lead to sparse precipitation, resulting in very low humidity and a wide variation in annual temperature. Two main rivers, the Amu Darya (Oxus River) and Syr Darya (Jaxartes River) provide water for the region.

Most of the population lived either along the fertile banks of rivers and streams or in the foothills of the mountains. Very few people lived in the vast arid interior. Medieval central Asia's population could be divided into the agrarians and nomads. Since antiquity, the relationship between the two groups has been marked by conflict. The nomadic lifestyle was well suited to warfare, and the steppe nomads, such as the Mongols, were among the most militarily potent people in history. However, territorial gains were short lived as the nomads lacked internal unity. They were also typically fewer in numbers and would quickly be assimilated into the culture of those they had conquered.

Military campaigns and east-west trade through the oases led to a flux of people, products, and ideas in and out of central Asia. By the fourth century CE, central Asians were a heterogeneous mixture of cultures and religions. Shamanism was everywhere, and where it was not practiced as a religion, its rituals profoundly influenced local customs and traditions. **Buddhism** was concentrated in the east. Around Persia, Zoroastrianism was prominent. Christianity and Manichaeism were also practiced. In the eighth century, Muslim conquest brought **Islam** to central Asia, where it began to replace Zoroastrianism, Christianity, and Manichaeism.

Shamanistic and geographic factors are all-important in religion, myth, ritual, and epic. Elsewhere in the world, fertility rites for the promotion of agriculture were dominant, but in central Asia rituals to ensure success in hunting and breeding livestock were primary. Whereas elsewhere the male-female opposition is prominent, as symbolizing the union of the forces of nature in producing crops, in central Asia there was an emphasis on the opposition between summer and winter.

Islamic law makes generous provisions for male sexual needs, and Islamic religious institutions strongly condemned illicit love—but the realities of daily living were different. Attitudes toward sex ranged from viewing its public discussion as taboo to celebrating it as a life-giving force. Central Asian literary works display an ongoing tension between sacred (*haqiqi*) and profane (*majdzi*) love. Sufi influences that emphasize feeling make use of profane imagery when describing the sacred. This makes classification more difficult, and in some instances meaningless. Alongside the boastful and insensitive prowler, one finds the submissive adorer for afar professing a more ethereal passion—a compromise between sensual love and mystical experience.

Central Asian love poetry, whether profane or sacred, employs common images of the beloved's body such as hot lips; broad chests; breasts (voluptuous and small); strong arms; long, black locks; golden faces; white bodies; as well as the nature imagery of flowers, gardens, and nectar. Love poetry covers themes ranging from the erotic ("I grant you entrance into the scented, moist garden of my body") to the theoretical. Theoretical discourses on love draw from Platonic ideas regarding its ethical dimensions, which places good over pleasure and profit as the ultimate goal of true love. These works distinguish between love, sex, and **marriage**, although there can be considerable overlap in these categories.

Much of central Asian literature was written by men and reflected the particular milieu in which they functioned. Many central Asian societies were ostensibly Islamic, but often infused with distinctive local traditions that added new dimensions to the classical literary heritage, most notably, works on love between individuals who are incompatible in some way, by belonging to a different tribal, social, or religious group. Later works—especially those of Sufi persuasion—transfer the relationship of lover and beloved to express multiple sets of power relationships: slave and master, poet and patron, or man and God. There are also works that switch the role of lover and beloved while exploring power relationships.

In some of this literature, the male author desires (and sometimes makes love to) a married woman. One such genre is the *misra*. *Misras* are supposed to be sung in one breath, the singer winding up, when his breath gives out, in a piercing sound, half yell and half gasp, much higher than the song itself. Many *misras* are difficult to translate, and even the mildest ones are very explicit. Mothers would sing lullabies (*landay*) to their sons, where they would describe the youth's prowess in battle (another popular theme in central Asian literature), followed by an illicit affair with a maiden from the vanquished tribe (typically the chief's daughter). The descriptions are highly detailed. For instance, the maiden is described as having a "smooth face, all hair shaved off her body, small pointed breasts, each large enough to fill a hand." The maiden tells the youth that she will secretly meet him and "lie down beside you, my lips to yours, my thighs to yours." Central Asian love literature ranged from the sacred to profane, practical to theoretical, and is written for audiences in the princely courts to the countryside, for adults and children.

Further Reading: Abdullah, Achmed. *Lute and Scimitar*. New York: Payson & Clarke, 1928; Baldick, Julian. *Animal and Shaman: Ancient Religions of Central Asia*. New York: New York University Press, 2000; Chaliand, Gerard. *Nomadic Empires: From Mongolia to the Danube*. Translated by A. M. Berret. New Brunswick, NJ: Transaction Publishers, 2003; Devereau, R. "XIth Century Muslim Views on Women, Marriage, Love, and Sex." *Central Asiatic Journal* 11 (1966): 134–40; Gross, Jo-Ann. *Muslims in Central Asia: Expressions of Identity and Change*. Durham, NC: Duke University Press, 1992; Lazar, M., and N. Lacy, eds. *Poetics of Love in the Middle Ages: Texts and Contexts*. Fairfax, VA: George Mason University Press, 1989; Manz,

CHASTITY IN MARRIAGE. The fathers of the church, like St. Ambrose, clearly stated that the virgin state is superior to the matrimonial one. The Christian marriage, nevertheless, is to be considered chaste, if its principal objective is reproduction and not sexual pleasure. **Marriage** is chaste if it fights **lust** with an honest use of sex, according to **Augustine**. Abstaining from sex during festivals such as **Lent** is also important. Obviously, a chaste marriage implies total loyalty between the consorts and allegiance to the goals that God has chosen for the matrimonial institution.

Medieval ecclesiastical authors also described another type of matrimonial chastity—the virgin marriage—which lacked carnal union between the two consorts. The example of Mary and Joseph's marriage brought the matter to the attention of moralists and jurists who discussed whether a marriage without sex is a true marriage or not. According St. Ambrose it is a true marriage, because the wedding consists in not the deprivation of **virginity** but swearing a communion of life. The marriage of Mary and Joseph had all the perfections and signs of a true marriage: the issue, fidelity, and sacrament. **Thomas Aquinas** also saw in the union of the souls and in the cohabitation of Joseph and Mary a perfect union without sexual union. The long and complex debate on the virgin marriage of Mary and Joseph inevitably brought with it the question whether this type of matrimonial union was imitable and more perfect than that which involved physical action.

There were two answers to this question. The first, the heretical one, practiced by Cathars and other heterodox groups, considered marital sex a sinful and negative act, as opposed by the Roman church. The second, the ascetic-mystical one, was the marital couple who with mutual consent, expressed either before or after the matrimonial union, chose to live in complete virgin chastity throughout the marriage. Couples who have followed this type of marriage have attracted the veneration of believers, as in the case of St. Elzearius of Sabràn (1284–1323), Count of Ariano Irpino and his wife, the blessed Delfina of Signe (1282–1360), both members of the secular third Franciscan order. Another famous couple, who after years of marriage chose to live in virgin chastity, was the blessed John Colombini from Siena (1304–1367) and his wife Biagia: the two however separated before Colombini founded the religious mendicant order of the Jesuats or Poor Brothers. Analogous were the seven holy founders of the order of the Servants of the Holy Virgin Mary in the thirteenth century. See also Celibacy.

Further Reading: da Crispiero, Massimo. *Il matrimonio cristiano*. Torino: Edizioni Marietti, 1976; da Crispiero, Massimo. *Teologia della sessualità, approfondimenti sui temi del matrimonio e della verginità*. Bologna: Edizioni Studio Domenicano, 1994; Moioli, Giovanni. *Per una rinnovata riflessione sui rapporti tra matrimonio e verginità* La Scuola Cattolica 95 (1967): 201–55.

Elvio Ciferri

CHAUCER, GEOFFREY (c. 1343–1400). Geoffrey Chaucer had a perceptive and comprehensive eye for love and sex in fourteenth-century England, as he did for society at large. A man of the world whose experiences cut across all classes from commoners to monarchs, he was ideally suited to observe human relations and relate them in his poetry.

Chaucer celebrates married love in his first major poem, "The Book of the Duchess" (1369–1370), a dream vision that functions as an elegy for the deceased wife of Prince John of Gaunt. At about the same time, Chaucer may have been translating the *Roman de la rose*, which by then had come to be seen as an assault on women and the God of Love. Hence, Chaucer claims that his *Romaunt of the Rose* is one of the transgressions for which he is ordered by cupid to compose *The Legend of Good Women*, stories about women who remained faithful to the religion of love.

Another of Chaucer's transgressions was his *Troilus and Criseyde*, which tells the story of Criseyde's betrayal of Troilus in favor of the Greek Diomede during the Trojan War. Troilus is strong, brave, and generous, the ideal courtly lover, and considerably more faithful than Criseyde. *The Parliament of Fowls* is a dream vision in which several species of birds meet on Saint Valentine's Day to choose their mates. The ensuring dialogue parallels the ways in which human classes view and talk about love.

Chaucer's treatment of love and sex culminates in *The Canterbury Tales*. In "The Knight's Tale," the Knight, befitting his role, tells of two young Thebans who both desire the same woman, and of the ultimate triumph of courtly honor when Arcite, on his deathbed, commends Emily to his erstwhile adversary. Yet many of the tales depict less nobility in matters of the heart and bed. In "The Wife of Bath's Tale," the heroine survives five husbands, and to win a sixth concocts a tale about an old hag who appears beautiful. Despite her deceit, she can be seen as something of a feminine heroine. "The Miller's Tale" tells a ribald story about a young wife cuckolding her older husband. In "The Reeve's Tale," two young Cambridge clerks trick their miller host by sleeping with his wife and daughter. In "The Sompnour's Tale" Sompnour proves adept at seducing young girls and his traveling companion, the Pardoner, with a voice as small as a goat's and no beard, may be, Chaucer suggests, a gelding or a mare.

Other characters, although not evil-minded, care altogether too much about earthly love for their vocations. The Prioress wears a broach containing the slogan "Amor vincit omnia" (Love conquers all). The Monk fastens his hood with a pin containing a love knot. As he does with other aspects of fourteenth-century England, Chaucer offers as thorough a view of the relations between the sexes as one is likely to find anywhere.

Further Reading: Bowden, Muriel. *A Reader's Guide to Geoffrey Chaucer*. New York: Farrar, Straus, 1964; Ellis, Steve. *Chaucer: An Oxford Guide*. New York: Oxford University Press, 2005.

Edward J. Rielly

CHILDBIRTH. The history of medieval childbirth is difficult to recover. Generally speaking, as historian Peter Biller has noted, in Europe obstetrics has followed the pattern of written **medicine**. Initial advances were made in the Greco-Roman world (especially during the Greek period). Medical knowledge survived in **Byzantium**, where Muslim doctors built on it. But in western Europe obstetrical knowledge declined after the fall of the western Roman empire, despite its limited presence in the Benedictine monasteries that spread across the continent. Western Europeans did not make significant contact with Greek medicine again until the twelfth century, a time when childbirth in Europe may have undergone important changes. For example, as Greek medicine filtered into Western Europe, universities were established where physicians and surgeons were trained. At the same time, hospitals were founded to serve the destitute; some of the poor these hospitals served were pregnant women needing obstetrical support.

The Roman church also had significant impact on childbirth during the later Middle Ages. **Marriage** and family became focuses of the church and marriage became a sacrament. Baptism also became a church concern as it struggled to convince Christians of the necessity of baptism for salvation. Throughout the thirteenth century, the church emphasized the need for **midwives** and others who assisted in births to know how to baptize newborns in danger of dying. This tendency of the church to raise the dignity of marriage and its generally positive view of children might have had significant benefits for many medieval women; unlike the Cathars, whose antisex and antiprocreation stance might have disturbed some women, the Roman church sent relatively positive signals to married women who wanted to conceive and bear children.

Poor women often gave birth in their homes, although by the later Middle Ages they had the option of visiting the growing number of hospitals established to support pregnant women. Since childbirth entailed real risks to the mother's and baby's well being, women often prepared themselves physically and spiritually. Christian women, for example, were encouraged to make **confession** and receive communion in advance of their labors. Among Christians of noble rank the preparation for birth appears to have had something of a ritualistic character. A pregnant noblewoman would remove herself from the outside world approximately one month before her baby was due, entering the chamber where she decided to give birth. This process would be preceded by a mass (and possibly more than one) celebrated in a nearby chapel. During the liturgy the woman would receive communion (which emphasized the importance of the occasion since laypeople did not routinely receive communion at this time). Once the mass ended, she would enter the room where the birth would take place. From this time on, she would be in the company of the women who would assist her when the labor began.

Once the child was born, a medieval woman entered a "lying in" period, which could last up to six weeks. This gave the new mother time to recover and acclimate to her new responsibilities while enjoying the support of a network of female friends and relatives.

AID FOR MOTHERS IN PREGNANCY AND LABOR. Midwives and mothers employed several strategies to help women prepare for and cope with a difficult time. Muslim and Christian sources recommended baths and eating easily digestible foods, though they differed on the use of frequent sexual intercourse to ensure easy delivery. While 'Arib ibn Sa'id's *Book on the Generation of the Fetus and the Treatment of Pregnant Women and Newborns (Kitab Khalq al-Janin wa-Tadbir al-H'abala wa'l-Mawludin)*, a tenth-century work of Muslim provenance that was commissioned by Caliph al-Hakam II of Cordoba, agreed with this advice, it was difficult for Christians to follow since a complicated calendar regulated when husbands and wives could be intimate with one another. Several sources suggest that Christian spouses were prohibited from sexual relations when they were expecting a child.

During the labor itself, Jewish, Christian, and Muslim women prayed. For Christian women there are records of many other aids as well. They touched relics hoping that the saint's (or saints') intercession might help the woman deliver safely. Charms were also used. Amulets and scrolls—some with crosses on them—could be held and girdles and belts worn. Among **Jews** women could wear their husbands' belts, which were sometimes embroidered with protective formulas; Christian belts appear to have been associated with saints—such as St. Anselm's belt at Canterbury, and the belts of the Virgin at Westminster Abbey and Bruton Abbey. Even food could be used creatively; the pregnant woman could eat foods that had inscriptions on them. At times mineral stones like malachite, jasper, iris, and eaglestone could be placed near the woman in labor. And saints could be invoked directly; the most popular were the Virgin Mary, St. **Mary Magdalene**, St. Anne, and, perhaps most famously, St. Margaret of Antioch. Though these were Christian intercessors, the sources reveal cross-cultural influence, as when a Jewish woman in labor was chastised by the women attending her for calling on the Virgin Mary for help.

THE ROLES OF MEN. With some exceptions, men were not present at deliveries. They were, however, involved indirectly. Educated men wrote many of the medical treatises that provided information on fertility and birth. Priests, physicians, and surgeons could supervise births, especially by the later Middle Ages. Male relatives, particularly fathers, were clearly interested in the births of their children. In wealthy families fathers chose the wet nurses who would feed their children. This was an important job because many medieval people believed that the nurse could transfer personal qualities to the child via her milk. Of course, male friends and relatives also played supportive roles by visiting newly delivered mothers. Thus, in the Middle Ages, just as in today's world, childbirth was an occasion in which men and women were deeply invested.

Further Reading: Baumgarten, Elisheva. *Mothers and Children: Jewish Family Life in Medieval Europe*. Princeton, NJ: Princeton University Press, 2004; Biller, Peter. "Cathars and Material Women." In *Medieval Theology and the Natural Body*, edited by Peter Biller and A. J. Minnis, 61–107. Rochester, NY: York Medieval Press, 1997; Biller, Peter. "Childbirth in the Middle Ages." *History Today* 36 (1986): 42–49; Deegan, Marilyn. "Pregnancy and Childbirth in the Anglo-Saxon Medical Texts." In *Medicine in Early Medieval England: Four Papers*, edited by Marilyn Deegan and D. G. Scragg, 17–26. Manchester: Manchester Centre for Anglo-Saxon Studies, 1989; Lee, B. R. "A Company of Women and Men: Men's Recollections of Childbirth in Medieval England." *Journal of Family History* 27 (2002): 92–100; Musacchio, Jacqueline Marie. *The Art and Ritual of Childbirth in Renaissance Italy*. New Haven, CT: Yale University Press, 1999; Orme, Nicholas. *Medieval Children*. London: Yale University Press, 2001; Rawcliffe, Carole. "Women, Childbirth, and Religion in Later Medieval England." In *Women and Religion in Medieval England*, edited by Diana Wood, 91–117. Oxford: Oxbow, 2003.

Dawn Marie Hayes

CHINA. China has a long tradition of celebrating love between consenting adults. One of the oldest collections of Chinese literature, the *Shijing*, contains a significant amount of erotic poetry. Prior to the dissemination of **Buddhism** to China, none of the Chinese systems of thought condemned sexuality. For the Confucian tradition, sexuality within the context of **marriage** was a responsibility that one should not abjure, while the Daoist tradition developed sexual yogic practices that were thought to aid one in the pursuit of immortality. Later, however, under the influence of both Buddhism and Neo-Confucianism, the Chinese developed more conservative attitudes toward sexuality.

LOVE AND MARRIAGE. Love and sexuality was viewed as a positive force in traditional China. According to the Confucian tradition, marriage and sexuality were essential for the fulfillment of an obligation that children had to their parents: the production of grandchildren. Most Chinese marriages were arranged, yet love between married couples was highly valued; it was discussed with approval by the Confucian philosopher Mencius (c. fourth century BCE). Chinese literature, particularly poetry, has, from ancient to modern times, celebrated love in all of its forms, including love between married people as well as forbidden or furtive love between the unmarried.

Although some non-Chinese peoples on the fringes of the Chinese cultural world practiced polyandry and **polygamy**, the Han Chinese officially practiced monogamy.

However, among the wealthy, de facto polygamy was common. Wealthy men often married several times, although subsequent wives were legally considered to be concubines. Marriage was seen as an alliance between families, and engagements were often conducted when the couple was in their infancy or early childhood. Marriage would be conducted following puberty. In most parts of China, marriage was virilocal, with the couple living in the groom's household. Marriage by choice or by love was extremely rare among the upper classes, but more common among the lower classes.

Female chastity was extolled in Confucian literature, and unmarried women were guarded by their family members. Female infidelity was often punished harshly; however, male infidelity was highly tolerated. **Prostitution** was common in medieval China, and also legal. During the Song (960–1278), Yuan (1206–1368), and Ming (1368–1644) dynasties, the imperial government owned and operated brothels, which competed with privately operated brothels. Chinese histories reveal the presence of influential courtesans, particularly during the Tang (618–907) and Song dynasties. Unlike common prostitutes, courtesans were often highly educated. A number of courtesans became involved with extremely powerful men, including emperors, and several had serious impact on Chinese history. These include Xue Dao (768–831), a lover of the great general Wei Gao, as well as Li Shishi, a paramour of the Huizong emperor (r. 1101–1125) Marco Polo estimated that there were 20,000 prostitutes in Beijing during his visit there in the thirteenth century.

The Neo-Confucian philosopher Zhu Xi (1130–1200) advocated a more conservative social ethic, calling for the **seclusion of women** so as to preserve their chastity. His ideas gained acceptance under the Yuan dynasty, partly because the occupation of China by a foreign power, the Mongols, led to greater conservatism in Chinese society. As a result, the Chinese began to sporadically censor erotic literature, particularly during the Yuan and Ming dynasties.

This change was accompanied by the rise of the practice of footbinding during the Song and Yuan dynasties. Footbinding was begun in childhood around age eight. Young girls' feet were repeatedly bound in increasingly tighter bindings that pressed the toes downward toward the heel, in order to break and deform the bones of the feet. This violent breaking process would typically last about two to three years, and was excruciatingly painful. The process created a sharp upward curve in the foot, and forced the smaller toes downward and against the heel. The big toe would project forward, creating the triangular effect that was maintained by wearing rigid, shaped shoes.

The deformed feet were euphemistically called "golden lotuses." This practice greatly reduced a woman's mobility, and also rendered her unable to work. This made women completely dependent upon male relatives, and enforced their seclusion. This practice was uncommon among the lower classes that depended upon women's labor. Women with bound feet were highly eroticized, in part due to the belief that they were both more lustful and more sexually pleasing.

MEDICAL AND RELIGIOUS VIEWS OF HETEROSEXUALITY. The union of men and women was considered natural in China. Male and female were seen as manifestations of complementary but inseparable cosmic forces, *yang* and *yin*, respectively. Sex between men and women was also deemed positive, provided that it was performed properly and moderately, as well as at the appropriate times. The Chinese were not prudish about sex, but wrote numerous works describing it. These works include popular erotic novels, such as Li Yu's *The Carnal Prayer Mat*, and also manuals on the topic of sex, instructing men and women on the proper techniques for enjoying sexual union without negative consequences.

The Chinese developed a very sophisticated system for understanding human sexuality, and also concomitant practices to safeguard and augment sexual function. In the Chinese worldview, sexuality involved the exchange of vital essence, known as *jing*. Manifesting in men as semen, *jing* would leave the man's body and enter the woman's, where, if conditions are right, it would combine with her *jing* to produce an embryo. Ordinary sexuality was viewed as draining for men, as it necessarily involved the loss of vital essence. Sex, however, was not seen as draining for women.

Men were viewed as the more vulnerable sex, for they tended to be afflicted by strong sexual desire, leading them often to engage in excessive sexual activity. The Chinese were very concerned with the loss of vital essence experienced by men, and developed various methods to counteract it, such as regimens of diet and exercise to replace lost *jing,* and the consumption of tonics, usually concocted from herbs and/or animal parts. Since male vital essence was identified as being *yang* in nature, these tonics contained substances rich in *yang* energy. These were often phallic in nature, either literally (such as tiger and bear penises) or phallic representations (such as rhinocerous horns, antlers, etc.). The Chinese also developed sexual techniques to aid men in prolonging erections, or avoiding ejaculation, in order to minimize the loss of *jing*. This literature was largely, but not entirely, written from the male perspective. The Chinese also composed several **sex manuals** specifically for women. However, there was a tendency to demonize women as sexual vampires who drained men's *jing*. A good deal of the Chinese literature on sex is agonistic, depicting sex as a battle. As men were naturally disadvantaged in this arena, much of this literature described techniques that men could use to turn the table on women, and absorb the female partner's *jing*, rather than losing his own.

This perspective is common in Daoist literature. By the early medieval period, that is, during the period ranging roughly from 420 CE through the Tang dynasty, Daoists had composed a number of texts that describe sexual techniques for achieving immortality. They are included under the rubric of "inner alchemy," which required that *jing* be stored and purified. Some texts call for the theft of *jing* from female sex partners, and encourage the adept to engage in sex with multiple sex partners, who should be, ideally, virgins.

Buddhists however taught that sexuality, or, more precisely, attachment to sex and other sensual pleasures, was a major obstacle to spiritual development. Buddhists thus advocated monastic renunciation, which required the practice of **celibacy**. Under Buddhist influence, some schools of **Daoism**, such as the Complete Perfection (*quanzhen*) school, also adopted the practice of monasticism, and developed systems of "inner alchemical" meditation that did not require the violation of the vow of celibacy. However, **Tantric Buddhism**, in much the same manner as Daoism, advocated the use of sexual yogic practices for the purpose of achieving enlightenment. In fact, there appears to have been significant mutual influence among Tantric Buddhist and Daoist groups in this area.

Tantric forms of Buddhism arrived in China during the eighth century, but the initial transmission does not seem to have involved the texts and traditions that advocated sexual yogic practices. These texts and traditions arrived in China during the late tenth and early eleventh centuries. However, given the increasing conservatism of Chinese society during this time, the texts themselves were translated in a bowdlerized fashion that minimized their erotic impact, and there is no proof that the sexual yogic practices that some of them describe were transmitted to China. However, Chinese records indicate that during the Yuan dynasty, under the reign of the Shundi emperor (1333–1367), Tantric rituals involving nudity and (possibly) sexuality may have been performed at the court under the tutelage of a Tibetan Buddhist lama. But it is not clear if these accounts are reliable.

ALTERNATE SEXUALITIES. Although the Chinese tended to strongly advocate heterosexual relationships and sexuality, there is significant evidence indicating that homosexuality was widely tolerated, particularly during the early medieval period. Chinese historical and literary writings record numerous instances of male homosexual love, such as the relationships between the scholars Xin Deyuan and Pei Rangzi during the Northern Wei dynasty (386–535), the poet Yu Xin (513–581) and the politician Xiao Shao, as well as that which occurred between Wendi, the second Chen emperor (r. 559–566) and his general Chen Zigao. The Tang poet Bai Xingjian (776–846) wrote explicitly about homosexual love in his work *Poetical Essays on Supreme Joy*. During the late medieval and early modern periods, as Chinese society became more conservative, homosexuality came to be viewed as socially unacceptable.

Given the greater surveillance of women in Chinese society, female homosexuality was less accepted than male homosexuality, and descriptions of lesbianism are less common in Chinese literature. However, men and women with homosexual inclinations apparently often found refuge in the monastic orders. Monks and nuns were widely believed to frequently develop homosexual relationships. *See also* Bo Xingjian; Chinese Paintings of Elite Women; *New Songs from a Jade Terrace*; Sun Simiao; Wu Zetian; Yang Guifei; Zhang Boduan; Zhang Zhuo.

Further Reading: Gernet, Jacques. *Daily Life in China on the Eve of the Mongol Invasion, 1250–1276*. Stanford, CA: Stanford University Press, 1970; Hanan, Patrick, trans. *The Carnal Prayer Mat, Li Yu*. Honolulu: University of Hawaii Press, 1996; Ruan, Fang Fu. *Sex in China: Studies in Sexology in Chinese Culture*. New York: Plenum Press, 1991; Van Gulik, R. H. *Sexual Life in Ancient China*. Leiden: Brill, 1961; Wang Ping. *Aching for Beauty: Footbinding in China*. Minneapolis: University of Minnesota Press, 2000; Wile, Douglas. *Art of the Bedchamber: The Chinese Sexual Yoga Classics, Including Women's Solo Meditation Texts*. Albany: State University of New York Press, 1992.

David B. Gray

CHINESE PAINTINGS OF ELITE WOMEN (*Shinü hua*). The genre of Chinese painting known as "paintings of elite women" (*shinü hua*) emphasizes the depiction of court ladies, courtesans, and educated women as figures experiencing erotic longing or desire.

An early use of the term *shinü hua* appears in Zhu Jingxuan's (fl. c. 806–840) *Record of Famous Painters of the Tang Dynasty (Tangchao minghua lu)*. In later periods, the genre would be recast as "paintings of beautiful women" (*meiren hua*).

Members of the imperial courts of the Tang (618–907), southern Tang (937–975), and Song (960–1279) dynasties frequently commissioned paintings of elite women. The high regard given these paintings may reflect the long-standing popularity of palace-style poetry (*gongti shi*), first compiled at the courts of the southern dynasties (420–589). This poetry focused on the lovelorn female persona. During the Song dynasty, literati painters and poets also became interested in this theme, resulting in the rise of a new form of poetry, song lyrics (*ci*), written by scholars and courtesans and detailing their encounters.

Renowned painters of the genre include Zhou Fang (fl. 713–742), Zhang Xuan (c. 730–c. 800), Zhou Wenju (fl. 961–975), and Su Hanchen (fl. c. 1101–1163). A fourteenth-century connoisseur of painting, Tang Hou, writes in *Painting Critique (Hua jian*) that these court painters were particularly skilled at representing women's emotions. Chinese art critics typically use the style of one of these masters, especially Zhou Fang or Zhang Xuan, as the basis for assessing the quality of later *shinü hua* paintings, and sometimes attribute an early painting of unknown authorship to one of them.

Paintings of elite women tend to represent them in particular settings enjoying one of a circumscribed range of activities, most of which can be traced back to palace-style poetry. One typical setting is a secluded garden, where an erotic relationship could be encoded in the interaction or juxtaposition of natural elements with metaphorical meanings; for example, the interaction of butterflies (which represent wandering men) and flowers (which represent waiting women), or the juxtaposition of garden rocks (a metaphor for scholars) and blossoming plum trees (a sometime metaphor for beautiful women). Another possible setting is the inner quarters of palaces or elite households, where women were imagined to pass their leisure hours pining for men.

The activities female figures take part in include seductive dancing or musical performance (presumably of love songs), dressing or applying makeup (seemingly in preparation for a tryst), gazing upon their faces in mirrors (as if imagining how lovers might view them, or mourning lost beauty), and making clothes for absent men (understood as the sublimation of erotic desire). Because all of these situations derive from poetry, an educated viewer would immediately recognize the connotations of each.

Although such paintings are sometimes misunderstood as paintings of daily life, they are very much idealized visions of women and of erotic relationships. Moreover, because the majority of painters working in this genre were men and often court painters, the paintings tend to give a one-sided, exaggerated view of such relationships and reveal more about the taste of the paintings' patrons than about the realities of women's lives in the Tang through Song periods.

Further Reading: Birrell, Anne M., trans. *New Songs from a Jade Terrace: An Anthology of Early Chinese Love Poetry.* London: George Allen & Unwin, 1982; Laing, Ellen Johnston. "Chinese Palace-Style Poetry and the Depiction of *A Palace Beauty*." *Art Bulletin* 72, no. 1 (March 1990): 284–95; Liu Fangru, ed. *Glimpses into the Hidden Quarters: Paintings of Women from the Middle Kingdom (Shinü hua zhi mei).* Taipei: National Palace Museum, 1988.

Lara C. W. Blanchard

CHRISTINE DE PISAN (1363–1430). Born in Venice in 1363, Christine was the daughter of a Bolognese physician and astrologer, Thommaso de Pisan, and his wife, the daughter of a Venetian councilor. Christine moved to the court of Charles V of France in 1368, where her father was the king's advisor and doctor. In 1378, Christine married Etienne du Castel, a royal notary, with whom she had two surviving children and enjoyed an extremely happy **marriage**. Her life shifted dramatically with the accession of Charles VI in 1380, who dismissed her father, and the death of her husband in 1389. To attract patrons to aid her in securing her husband's arrears in pay, Christine began writing ballades and rondeaux, which won her the admiration of powerful nobles like Louis of Orleans and his wife, Valentine Visconti.

After a reading program in her patrons' libraries, meant to make up for a haphazard education, Christine produced *L'Epistre au Dieu d'Amours* (1399), a critique of the **Romance of the Rose**, stressing the loyalty and honesty of women rather than the chivalric *belle dame sans merci*. Her *Cite des Dames* took these ideas further, citing historical examples of women who profited from equal educations to rule wisely, perfect their virtues and act in Christian piety. All of her writing stands apart from the medieval tradition of placing women on a pedestal while attacking them for fickleness and deception. Referring to admirable women like Penelope and Zenobia, she argued the equality of the human soul regardless of gender and the place of women as responsible partners of their spouses and families.

Her writing shows a familiarity with Aristotle and **Dante Alighieri**, and an experience with contemporary manners and court politics. Other works include a prose history of Charles V's reign; advice to the royal children on wise rule; a guide to military practice and chivalry; and a popular guide to wifely behavior, stressing honesty, financial responsibility, and attraction to and respect for one's spouse. Several of these remained in print until the mid-sixteenth century, showing constant demand in English and French.

Christine was admired widely in elite French circles, as well as by Henry IV of England and the Visconti Dukes of Milan. Her poems on the religious Great Schism and pleas for peace amongst French noble factions were widely circulated. Distressed by France's political turmoil and the invasion of Henry V of England in 1415, Christine withdrew to the convent at Poissy, joining her daughter. She emerged from seclusion in 1429 to compose a celebratory poem on the coronation of Charles VII as king of France and the role played by **Joan of Arc**, a woman who seemed to represent the virtues cited in her works. Christine died at Poissy.

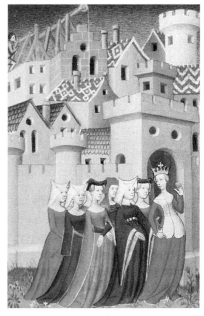

Christine de Pisan and a group of women outside the city walls, 15th century. From *The Works of Christine de Pisan*. © HIP/Art Resource, NY.

Further Reading: Brown-Grant, Rosalind. *Christine de Pisan and the Moral Defense of Women*. Cambridge: Cambridge University Press, 1999; McLeod, Enid. *The Order of the Rose: The Life and Ideas of Christine de Pizan*. Totowa, NJ: Rowman and Littlefield, 1976; Willard, Charity. *Christine de Pizan: Her Life and Works*. New York: Persea Books, 1984.

Margaret Sankey

CHRYSOSTOM, JOHN (349–407). Born in Antioch, Syria, in 349, John Chrysostom rose to prominence during the tumultuous fourth century, becoming the bishop of Constantinople and one of the most influential figures of the Eastern church.

As a child, Chrysostom enjoyed an elite education in Antioch under the prominent scholar Libanius, thus leaving him well prepared to enter public service like his father, a military commander. However, at the age of eighteen, John decided to embark on a spiritual life instead. Attracted to asceticism, he spent time in the Syrian deserts before returning to Antioch, where he was made a deacon in the church. He advanced quickly to the rank of presbyter or preacher, and his moving sermons earned him the adoration of his congregation and growing fame. In 397, he was made bishop of Constantinople, a see that ranked second to Rome in importance.

As bishop, John was drawn into secular affairs and intrigues of the empire, eventually earning Empress Eudoxia's animosity and losing the imperial protection he once enjoyed. In addition, John's efforts to elevate the See of Constantinople earned him the enmity of the powerful bishop of Alexandria, Theophilus. In 403, this tension escalated following John's return to Constantinople after an extended visit to a troubled church in Asia Minor. At the Synod of the Oak in 403, John failed to answer the summons to appear and was subsequently deposed and exiled from Constantinople. He challenged the ruling, arguing that the synod was comprised of his enemies, but to no avail. In 404 he was exiled to Armenia. His enemies forced him to move from city to city, and in 407, en route to the city of Pithyus, he became ill and died.

In his sermons, John was noted for eloquence, earning him the name *Chrysostom* or "golden-mouthed." Unlike earlier theologians such as Origen of Alexandria, who used allegory extensively in their exegesis, John emphasized literal interpretations. John also left several biblical commentaries, numerous letters written largely during his exile, and *opuscula*, works devoted to defining terminology and practice. He emphasized moral issues, though he is also known for virulent attacks on **Jews** and **Judaism**.

John's works reflect his views on his society and culture. Often shocked by the lack of discipline and the opulent lifestyle of church officials, John encouraged the clergy to limit opportunities for overindulgence. He recommended that his congregation adopt similar standards, warning against the dangers of wealth and urging women to avoid ostentatious dress. The latter position earned him the hostility of the empress and the female members of her court.

John's views on **marriage** and sex stem partly from his views on extravagance. Holding **virginity** and **celibacy** as the ideal, John counseled widows against **remarriage**. He taught that fornication defiled the body, resulting in divine punishment. Marriage was good insofar as it prevented fornication, though people should strive to remain chaste. Because he did not advocate **divorce**, John advised people to be careful in selecting their spouses, paying special attention to temperament. *See also* Orthodox Christianity.

Further Reading: Kelly, J.N.D. *Golden Mouth: The Story of John Chrysostom—Ascetic, Preacher, Bishop.* Ithaca, NY: Cornell University Press, 1998; Mayer, Wendy, and Pauline Allen. *John Chrysostom.* London: Routledge Press, 1999; Wilken, Robert. *John Chrysostom and the Jews: Rhetoric and Reality in the Late 4th Century Church.* Berkeley: University of California Press, 1983.

Lisa R. Holliday

CIRCUMCISION. Circumcision of males involves removing all or part of the prepuce, or foreskin, from the penis. The procedure has been in existence for longer than recorded history and has been linked to several religious traditions. Although the origins of this practice are ancient and in question, by the Middle Ages male circumcision was widespread in Jewish and Islamic cultures. It was also practiced in parts of Australia, as well as in the Aztec and Mayan societies in the Americas. With few exceptions, Christians eschewed the practice; so most of western Europe was uncircumcised in the medieval period.

Some scholars believe that the practice started as a cleanliness issue, but circumcision was so widespread, even among cultures where cleanliness was not as important, that the theory is questionable. **Judaism** cites the covenant between God and Abraham for the origin of their tradition. God commanded Abraham to circumcise himself and all the males of his household as a physical sign of the promise that Abraham would be the father of a great nation. Originally, the circumcision ceremony among the **Jews** was *brit milah*, which involved the excision of only the tip of the foreskin on the eighth day after birth. After the second century, the *brit periah*, the excision of the entire foreskin, was the usual method, and this has survived into modern times. One reason for the change seems to be that Hellenistic Jewish men, in an effort to look more like Gentiles, developed weighted devices to stretch their foreskins. Rabbis retaliated by making it impossible for them to do this. In the twelfth century, **Moses Maimonides** (1135–1204), a rabbi and a physician, gave a moral reason for circumcision beyond the traditional covenant, arguing that the procedure reduced sexual gratification and weakened the male penis, making it easier for man to resist **lust** and violence.

Although circumcision has long been associated with Judaism, Arab nations also practiced it. Islamic lore even asserts that the prophet Mohammed (570–632) was born circumcised. Although it has become a tradition in Islam to circumcise infant boys on the seventh day after birth, pre-Islamic societies regularly performed the rite on boys entering puberty. Although the traditions surrounding the practice changed with the advent of **Islam**, circumcision itself is more of a cultural practice than a religious one in Arabic societies. Most other societies circumcised pubescent, or older, males instead of infants. In several aboriginal societies in Australia, males were not allowed full membership in their tribes or to marry before they were circumcised.

Further Reading: Boyle, Gregory J., Ronald Goldman, Steven J. Svoboda, and Ephrem Fernandez. "Male Circumcision." *Journal of Health Psychology—Men's Health.* www.moondragon. org/articles/malecircumcisionpain.html; Kimmel, Michael. "The Weights of Tradition." Circumcision Information and Resource Pages: http://www.cirp.org/pages/cultural/kimmel1/.

Jennifer Della'Zanna

CLITORIDECTOMY. In one of the most common forms of female genital mutilation (often incorrectly referred to as female **circumcision**), all or part of the clitoris, the female organ viewed as the primary source of sexual pleasure, is removed. Clitoridectomy originated in **Africa**, specifically Egypt, and is known to have been practiced in parts of Asia and throughout most of Africa. Greek physicians and historians recorded the specifics of the practice after traveling to Egypt throughout the Middle Ages. It was not generally associated with religious rites, but it spread within Islamic culture following the Arab conquest of Egypt in 642. (Mohammed's own daughter, Fatima, was not mutilated.) During the eighth century, clitoridectomy reached Indonesia, and it was practiced in various parts of Europe for centuries to cure diseases. Because the reason behind the practice of clitoridectomy is largely social, beliefs on why it is a necessary rite of passage for girls to womanhood vary from culture to culture.

Many who practice this form of female genital mutilation believe that it will keep a girl chaste and ensure her future husband and family of her **virginity**. It is believed that women who have not been mutilated are, by nature, prostitutes, with no power over their sexual desires and no regard for their family name. The risk of being ostracized by the community for not undergoing a clitoridectomy is too much for most girls to bear, especially considering that no man will marry them if they go uncut. It is believed that only men should experience sexual pleasure, and by removing the clitoris from the female, any chance of sexual pleasure for her is impossible.

Clitoridectomy is still widely practiced today, and the procedure has not changed much from that during the Middle Ages. The manner in which clitoridectomy was performed varied from region to region. Sharp objects such as seashells, stones, and knives were used to perform the operation. Some communities held ceremonies for the girl being mutilated, in which only women were allowed to attend. The age for clitoridectomy also widely varied; infant girls to women well into their first pregnancy have all been cut. The common age ranged from four to eight years, and the tradition was typically performed by an elder of the community to an entire group of girls at the same time. The only medicinal treatment a girl might receive after the mutilation was a paste made of animal dung and raw eggs to stop the bleeding.

Further Reading: Boyle, Elizabeth Heger. *Female Genital Cutting*. Baltimore: Johns Hopkins University Press, 2002; Kelly, James Martin. *Female Genital Mutilation: A Search for Its Origins*. Ann Arbor: UMI, 1993; Lightfoot-Klein, Hanny. *Prisoners of Ritual: An Odyssey into Female Genital Circumcision in Africa*. Binghamton, NY: Haworth Press, 1989.

Vanessa Yosten

COLLATIO LEGUM MOSAICARUM ET ROMANARUM (392/395). The *Collatio Legum Mosaicarum et Romanarum* (or "Collation of the Laws of Moses and the Romans"), which is also known in the manuscript tradition as the *Lex Dei* (or "Law of God"), is an important collection of **Roman law**s that was used in the Middle Ages. The work of an anonymous collator writing around 392–395, the *Collatio* is divided into sixteen titles or sections. Each title starts with an injunction from the Hebrew Bible, followed by excerpts from Roman law codes or statements by Roman jurists regarding aspects of Roman laws similar to the biblical laws.

Several titles deal with sexual issues. Title IV (*De Adulteris*) treats **adultery**, Title V (*De Stupratoribus*) concerns those who engage in illicit intercourse (especially male homosexuality), and Title VI (*De Incestis Nuptis*) deals with incestuous **marriage**s. Of these, Title V is of special interest because it preserves a fuller text of a Roman law against homosexuality from the late empire than that which survives in the *Theodosian Code* (*CTh* 9.7.6). While there was probably an earlier Roman law against homosexual **rape** (the so-called *Lex Scantina*, dating from sometime during the Roman republic), the law preserved in Title V and *CTh* 9.7.6, emanating from Emperor Theodosius I in 390, condemns homosexuality itself, and especially concentrates on capital punishment involving burning of homosexual prostitutes.

The *Collatio* was apparently adopted by the library of the church in the early Middle Ages. Recent scholarship has shown that it was used in Merovingian church councils as early as the sixth century. Early in the manuscript tradition, it was bound together with the *Epitome Iuliani* (an early Byzantine law book written c. 554). Bishop Hinkmar of Rheims cited Titles V and VI of the *Collatio* in the famous **divorce** trial of Lothar II and Theutberga in the ninth century. The *Collatio*, then, was an important source for Roman laws of marriage and sexual behavior in the Middle Ages.

Further Reading: Frakes, Robert M. "*Item Theodosianus?* (Observations on Coll. V. 3. 1)." *Quaderni Urbinati di Cultura Classica* n. s. 71 (2002): 163–68; Hyamson, Moses. *Legum Mosaicarum et Romanarum Collatio*. Oxford: Oxford University Press, 1913; Kaiser, Wolfgang. *Die Epitome Iuliani*. Frankfurt am Main: Vittorio Klostermann, 2004.

Robert M. Frakes

CONCUBINAGE. Concubinage is a socially accepted relationship between a man and a woman that is conjugal, but inferior to legal **marriage**. Concubinage was permitted in innumerable medieval societies either as a substitute for or as a supplement to regular marriage. Usually, the male partner could terminate the relationship at will and, unlike the concubine, he was not obliged to remain faithful. The position of concubines in relation to wives and the status of their children varied considerably, but normally concubines were secondary to formally married spouses. In some societies concubines were slaves or war-captives; in others they could be free—even highborn. Despite possible disadvantages concerning status, in some societies, families were eager to place their daughters as princely concubines because it was an honor, and royal favor could incur benefits to the whole family.

In Europe, during late antiquity, concubinage was a licit but secondary legal institution for those who could or would not contract matrimony. Concubinage was basically a monogamous union of some duration, but distinguished from marriage by its lack of marital affection (marital intent) and the difference in status. Concubines were usually slaves or freed women; if freeborn, they were usually of lower status than their partners. If a cohabiting couple was socially unequal, the assumption was concubinage rather than matrimony. Taking a concubine entailed no special ceremonies. She had no protected legal status; nor did her possible children have any inheritance rights. Byzantine clerics criticized concubinage, yet long-term monogamous unions between two single persons were an accepted legal institution. This notion was later rejected by the Orthodox Slavs.

In Germanic lands concubinage had no special legal status. Concubines were assimilated to slave girls, and free women entering concubinage relationships without family consent risked losing their inheritance rights. Later, in the High Middle Ages, the difference between wife and concubine became blurred as Catholic doctrine enabled marriage without formalities. Canonists ambivalently used this term when speaking of temporary and illicit sexual liaisons. They also regarded concubinage as a permanent monogamous relationship with marital affection a secondary type of marriage, but, inconsistently, children of concubines were considered illegitimate. Later in the Middle Ages, ecclesiastical and lay authorities started to increasingly discourage and punish concubinage.

When the Catholic Church forbade priests' marriages, it created the class of clerical concubines. While all nonmarital sexual activities were explicitly prohibited in ecclesiastical law, judging by later medieval evidence, clerical concubinage was more or less overtly practiced in many European regions.

Concubinage was licit according to Jewish law. Among **Jews** living in Christian areas, the trend was toward compulsory monogamy, while traditional **polygamy** and concubinage persisted in Jewish communities under Islamic rulers. In Islamic culture a man was allowed to keep an indefinite number of his own slave girls as concubines in addition to four wives. As slavery contained no lasting social stigma, men could marry their manumitted slave-concubines. In the Qur'an and *hadîths*, a dower, a wedding banquet, and veiling differentiated between wives and concubines. Slave-concubines, mothers of their masters' recognized children, were automatically freed at their masters' death.

Concubines (*qie*) were commonplace in wealthy Chinese households. Although their children were on par with the offspring of legal wives, the concubine was something between maidservant and wife. Often bought from a dealer or hired, she entered the household unceremoniously as a servant or concubine, depending on her attractiveness and skills. She addressed her mate as "master," not "husband." She was subject to the wife's, her mistress's, authority in the women's quarters and was promptly to obey both her and the master. The inferior legal position of concubines was visible in the only limitedly applicable ancestral mourning obligations and the denial of protection awarded to widows after the death of their spouse. Widowers were also forbidden to marry their concubines.

In addition to their formally married principal or official wife, Aztec rulers and aristocracy also had concubines. The wife's offspring were preferred as successors, but all children were considered legitimate and potential heirs. Rulers cemented alliances through marriages, but kept up to dozens or hundreds of attractive female slave-concubines. King Nezahualpilli of Teczoxo had reputedly over two thousand concubines.

Emperor Moctezuma II, another owner of an impressive **harem**, fathered 150 children. The Incas and Mayas also kept slaves legally as concubines, and Inca rulers had harems of two to three hundred women.

Further Reading: Arjava, Antti. *Women and Law in Late Antiquity*. Oxford: Oxford University Press, 1996; Brundage, James A. *Law, Sex, and Christian Society in Medieval Europe*. Chicago: University of Chicago Press, 1987; Ebrey, Patricia Buckley. *Women and the Family in Chinese History*. London: Routledge, 2003; Falk, Ze'ev W. *Jewish Matrimonial Law in the Middle Ages*. Scripta Judaica 6. London: Oxford University Press, 1966; Soustelle, Jacques. *Daily Life of the Aztecs*. Mineola, NY: Dover Publications, 2002.

Mia Korpiola

CONFESSION. Confession is the sacrament of penitence, revealing one's own sins to a priest to be absolved by him. Sexual sins find their own place in the discipline of this sacrament. In the ancient church, an extremely rigorous penitential system gradually emerged, known as public penitence: whoever embraced it became a penitent and was in turn submitted to a public trial under the authority of the bishop who privately listened to their sins. The penitence was hardly repeatable.

By the beginning of the sixth century, this original penitential regime had fallen into disuse, replaced by a repeatable private penitential routine. It is believed that this routine was conceived in the monasteries of the British Isles, from where the name insular penitence is derived. Thanks to the missionaries, private penitence passed on to the Continent. The two fundamental characteristics of the new system of administering penitence were its secretiveness and repeatability; the sinner confessed his or her sins privately to the priest, not to a bishop. Another aspect of this new approach was the system of precise penalties for the guilty; every type of sin corresponded to a set of obligations that the sinner had to carry out, recorded in manuals called **penitentials**.

Sex finds a particular position in the discipline of confession. Sexual sins, generally considered as very serious, needed to be confessed in detail to understand the quality and the quantity of the guilt and therefore to inflict the exact penitence for repentant sinners once they had received sacramental absolution. If a penitent was not clear in confessing his or her sins, the priest could question him or her to know all the circumstances in which the guilt had been committed. The penitent must find the correct words to confess exactly this type of sin without offending the holiness of the sacrament with scurrilous language and without revealing the sin of others, therefore maintaining secret the exact identity of accomplices in sexual sin. It was also important that the penitent intend to break completely with the past, to totally repent and not repeat the committed sins. Many penances also performed the function of "mortification" of the senses, or the sensual nature of man, such as fasting or undertaking long pilgrimages to weaken the wish to engage in sexual relations.

To prevent the moral decadence of the clergy, priests were strictly forbidden to acquit their accomplices in sexual sins, otherwise they could have promised sexual partners absolution. The sacramental seal affixed to the secrecy of the confession, the punishment for violating which was excommunication, guaranteed a great trust in the process of confession, at least up to the Protestant reform, with the only exception being heretical groups. The legend of John of Nepomuk in the fourteenth century, confessor of the Queen of Bohemia, who was killed by King Venceslaus for not revealing the secret of the confession, is symbolic of the importance attributed to the secrecy of sexual sins within the confession box.

Further Reading: Tanquerey, Adolfo. *Brevior synopsis theologiae moralis.* Torino: Marietti, 1934.

Elvio Ciferri

CONSANGUINITY. Consanguinity, or relationship by blood, is a means of identifying relationships between individuals descended from a common ancestor. It differs from other categories such as affinity (relationship by **marriage** or sexual intercourse) and compaternity (spiritual relationship, as between godparents and godchildren). Restrictions on marriages or sexual relationships between consanguineous partners are a form of **incest** prevention in many societies. In Jewish and Christian traditions, the explicit ban on sexual activity between close family members, laid out in chapters eighteen and twenty of Leviticus, established rules for relations between consanguineous partners. Similarly, explicit bans in the fourth *sura* (section) of the Qur'an underpinned Islamic views. Consanguineous marriages are described as endogamous (marriage to someone within a defined kin group) as opposed to exogamous (marriage to someone outside the group).

From approximately the tenth to the twelfth centuries, consanguinity became a central issue in the negotiation of royal and noble marriages in Christian Europe because the church imposed a restriction on marriages between partners related within seven degrees. Historians have debated the reasons for this excessive restriction, but it undoubtedly created tensions between a church trying to impose its will more thoroughly on marital practices and the fathers and families who were the traditional arbiters of marital negotiations. Contradictions also abounded within church policy, given the desire to overturn marriages between consanguineous partners while still upholding the idea of the indissolubility of the sacred marriage bond. In practical terms, church authorities tended to be more lenient on consanguineous marriages contracted in the remoter degrees of relationship, while acting against those between closer relatives.

Part of the problem arose from the variety of methods of calculating the relationship between the marital couple. Under the Germanic system, each generation from the common ancestor was counted as one degree of consanguinity. Siblings were therefore related in the first degree and first cousins in the second degree. In the earlier Roman system, each act of procreation counted as one degree. Under this method, siblings were related in the second degree, and first cousins in the fourth. This calculation was done by counting the generations from the first party back to the common ancestor, and then continuing down to the second party. At times Roman civil law banned only those marriages contracted within the fourth degree of relationship, meaning those to first cousins (or closer). This was the equivalent of marriages within the second degree under the Germanic system, and was therefore far less restrictive than the situation prevailing in the tenth to twelfth centuries, by which time Germanic counting had become the standard model in **canon law**.

The severe restrictions on marriages within seven degrees of consanguinity were respected at first, but later led to much abuse of the spirit of the rules. In a famous example, King Louis VII of France arranged an annulment of his marriage to Eleanor of Aquitaine (in effect, a **divorce**) in 1152 on the grounds of a previously ignored relationship. They were related in the fourth and fifth degrees: there were four generations from Louis and five from Eleanor back to their common ancestor, King Robert II. Similar annulments of convenience were rife during the period. In reality, this was merely an excuse to extract Louis from a marriage that had failed to produce a male heir. The cynicism of the episode is demonstrated by Eleanor's marriage two months later to Henry Plantagenet, to whom she was equally closely related. Such issues were recognized in 1215, when the Fourth Lateran Council under Pope Innocent III reduced the ban to marriages within four rather than seven degrees. Although this eased the problem of misuse of consanguinity rules, it did not disappear completely and disputes over consanguineous marriages occurred throughout the later Middle Ages at all levels of society.

In other cultures, consanguineous marriages were viewed more positively. Jewish communities encouraged marriage to kin (beyond the immediate family group) as a way of maintaining Jewish identity in the midst of the larger and often hostile Christian or Islamic populations. In **Islam**, marriage of cousins (who fell outside the restrictions imposed on marriage between closer relatives) enabled family assets and religious values to remain under the control of the wider kin group. Byzantine law banned the marriage between first cousins in the late seventh century and the marriage of second cousins (those related in the sixth degree according to the Roman calculation) in the eighth century, but these restrictions were far less onerous than those that later came into force in the Christian West. *See also* Catholicism.

Further Reading: Archibald, Elizabeth. *Incest and the Medieval Imagination*. Oxford: Oxford University Press, 2001; Bouchard, Constance B. "Consanguinity and Noble Marriages in the Tenth and Eleventh Centuries." *Speculum* 56 (1981): 268–87.

Lindsay Diggelmann

CONTRACEPTION. Jewish and Christian teachings of the medieval period agreed that contraception and **abortion** were not only wrong but also sinful. The Jewish position was based upon the belief that it was a crime to waste "seed" or semen. This concurred with the position of both the Eastern and the Western Christian church that to prevent conception or prevent a birth was homicide. Christian scholars taught that procreation was the sole purpose of sexual intercourse and then only within **marriage**. In the Eastern Orthodox church, even miscarrying required a woman to perform penance. What was more, contraception was perceived as a greater sin than even abortion or infanticide because with contraception it was impossible to know how many lives had been lost as a result.

Islam differed in that it did not consider contraception to be sinful. One of the primary causes for this divergence was that Islam viewed pleasure as a legitimate reason for sexual intercourse. Muslim jurisprudence also recognized several practical reasons for not wanting to produce an infant, economic and health concerns being the most important. Muslim medical practitioners had adopted a Galenic view that both a male and a female seed were necessary to produce a child. Thus, the loss of one or the other was not serious because separately neither amounted to much. Conversely, the Christian church of the later medieval period adopted an Aristotelian position that the male semen activated the female matter and thus played the primary role in procreation. Abortion was similarly contentious for medical thinkers, an issue that may be traced to classical antiquity. According to some scholars, the Hippocratic oath forbade abortion. However, other scholars argue that the proper translation of the oath is that a doctor will not provide an abortive pessary (e.g., a vaginal suppository that induces miscarriage). Indeed, in antiquity, doctors themselves were uncertain as to the intention of the oath. They were also unclear about the difference between contraception and abortion as they did not understand when, exactly, conception took place.

This is mirrored in the question of ensoulment. There was debate within both Islam and Christianity during the Middle Ages as to whether an abortion performed in the early part of a pregnancy was an illegal, sinful act or not. The controversy revolved around the issue of when the fetus was believed to receive a soul (that is, become human). The Koran was quite explicit about when this occurred—after 120 days or four months. Many Western Christians felt that "quickening" (first movement indicating life and ensoulment) occurred at around the same time, too. Nonetheless, there was still much debate on whether it was sinful (and, if so, to what degree) to prevent ensoulment from occurring. The Orthodox church believed that it was sinful because ensoulment occurred at the moment of conception.

Despite religious proscription, contraception was practiced and abortions did occur throughout the medieval world. Modern scholars continue to debate premodern knowledge of natural birth control. There is little evidence that earlier societies practiced an effective form of the rhythm method as there was inaccurate knowledge regarding the menstrual cycle. One of the primary forms of contraception was *coitus interruptus*, or withdrawal before ejaculation. This method was not highly effective. Nonvaginal forms of intercourse were also employed, whether oral, anal, manual, or interfemoral (between the legs). There is evidence that prostitutes used these methods to avoid pregnancy and venereal disease. There is also evidence that some new mothers used lactation-induced amenorrhea. This, however, is not a reliable form of contraception—the introduction of any solid foods to the child and the use of wet nurses at some levels of society will have decreased its effectiveness.

One of the chief sources for contraceptive methods was the work of Soranus (c. 120), a doctor in the Roman empire. His most significant surviving work is *Gynecology*, which discusses such topics as pregnancy and its prevention, **childbirth**, and selecting a wet nurse. Although not all of his theories were accurate by modern standards (Soranus's recommendation on the time for "fruitful intercourse" is in opposition to modern science's view of the menstrual cycle and the time of ovulation), his work remained the standard treatise on women's health and midwifery in the Western world well into the sixteenth century. Soranus is exceptional in the ancient world and beyond for his distinction between abortifacients and contraceptives. The difference between the two caused puzzlement before and after Soranus—in the fourth century and beyond, there was still uncertainty about the difference among many. The church father **John Chrysostom** commented on this confusion. In Christian Europe, the connection between contraception and paganism was strong and likely played a role in establishing the church's position against the use of contraceptives.

While the type of female contraception mentioned most frequently in Muslim writings is the intravaginal suppository, Christian texts focus primarily on oral medications. Despite many surviving recipes for plant-based contraceptives, modern scholars continue to debate the ability of premodern cultures to accurately use these herbal agents. The work of John Riddle demonstrates the use of efficacious herbal forms of contraceptives and abortifacients. Plants could be administered orally in a drink or placed in the vagina as a contraceptive or abortive suppository; some were also spread on both the male and female genitalia and could have acted as spermicides. It is recognized now that many flora and fauna act as emmenagogues (meaning that they induce a woman's menstrual cycle). Many of these plants also contain female sex hormones, which prevent implantation if taken within the first few days after intercourse—much like the modern emergency contraception pill. Modern laboratory studies on animals argue for the efficacy of the ingredients in these ancient recipes though exact dosage by premodern cultures is undetermined.

Despite the church's position, it is clear that women continued to use contraception and abortion, the reasons and means varying from woman to woman. We will likely never know with certainty how widespread this knowledge was or how effectively it was practiced. What is clear from the surviving works by ancient and medieval physicians, the **penitentials** and other religious writings of the Christian theologians and canonists, as well as the works of Muslim jurists, is that knowledge of contraceptives and abortifacients did exist in the medieval era and was widespread enough to provoke comment in a number of areas.

Further Reading: McLaren, Angus. *A History of Contraception from Antiquity to the Present Day*. Cambridge: Basil Blackwell, 1990; Musallam, B. F. *Sex and Society in Islam: Birth Control before the Nineteenth Century*. Cambridge: Cambridge University Press, 1983; Noonan, John T., Jr. *Contraception: A History of Its Treatment by the Catholic Theologians and Canonists*. Cambridge, MA: Harvard University Press, 1965; Riddle, John M. *Eve's Herbs: A History of Contraception and Abortion in the West*. Cambridge, MA: Harvard University Press, 1997; Soranus. *Soranus' Gynecology*. Translated by Owsei Temkin. Baltimore: Johns Hopkins University Press, 1956. Reprint 1991.

Alison Jeppesen

COURTLY LOVE.   Courtly love is a code of love that developed in the eleventh century in southern France, spread throughout France in the twelfth century, and appeared in other European countries, including England, during the remainder of the Middle Ages. Although not completely absent from actual life, courtly love primarily existed within the confines of literature.

Courtly love originated in Provence among the **troubadours**, lyric court poets who borrowed heavily from Ovid's *Art of Love*. One of the most prominent of the troubadours, Bernart de Ventadorn, enjoyed a romantic relationship with Eleanor of Aquitaine, who married Louis VII, king of France, in 1137. As queen of France, Eleanor's influence expanded, and both she and her daughter, Marie of Champagne, encouraged the courtly love conventions, which positioned love exclusively within adulterous relationships.

The two most important writers of courtly love were closely associated with Eleanor and her daughter: Chrétien de Troyes, Marie's court poet; and **Andreas Capellanus** (the name means Andreas the chaplain), often assumed to have been a chaplain in the court of Champagne.

Courtly love literature features specific character types. There is the beautiful, aristocratic, and married woman with blond or golden hair, white, unblemished skin, rosy lips, and a slender and graceful body. Her lover is usually a knight, enraptured by her beauty, who pledges absolute fidelity and submission with the hope of winning her love and physical intimacy. It is obviously necessary to keep the adulterous relationship secret, especially from her husband. Despite the illicit nature of the relationship, the love, far from being sordid, is depicted as ennobling and the source of all that is good and true. The knight proves his honor through absolute faithfulness to the lady, demonstrates his courage through any martial contests she desires of him, and, except for **adultery**, manifests impeccable Christian values.

Gaining the lady's love, though, is not easy. The lady is cold and aloof. He grows pale in her presence and stumbles in his speech. He pleads for her mercy, kneels in her presence, and prays that she will grant him her favor. The knight thus adopts a manner similar to two important contemporary relationships, those of a feudal vassal and his lord and of a Christian and God.

In fact, courtly love is presented as a type of love, paralleling or even parodying Christianity. Courtly love also has its deities, saints (the great lovers of the past), and commandments. The afterlife includes rewards and punishments for those who have loved well or badly, and these future rewards and punishments may be made visible in a love vision paralleling religious visions.

One of the great works on courtly love is Chrétien's **romance** *Lancelot*, which he composed somewhere around the late 1170s at the request of the Countess of Champagne. His contributions to courtly love include elaborating in richer detail ideas treated briefly by the troubadours, such as the way in which the lady's beauty affects the knight (entering through his eyes and striking his heart, leaving a wound that only the lady can heal) and the inability of the knight to leave his beloved (the knight's heart staying with her as he journeys elsewhere). In *Lancelot*, Chrétien also wedded courtly love to the **Arthurian legend**, making the court at Camelot the ultimate embodiment of courtly love. Lancelot, for example, seeks Guinevere in the land of Gorre, where she is held captive. When Lancelot finally reaches the queen, she will not speak to him, and when she finally deigns to address him, orders Lancelot deliberately to lose in the lists, a command that, despite the humiliation it entails, he unquestioningly obeys. The religion of love is also clearly present. When Lancelot approaches the queen's bed, he kneels to adore her, and when he leaves her chamber, he genuflects.

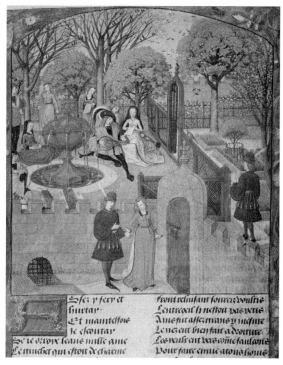

Courtly garden scene. From *The Roman de la Rose*, ca. 1440. © Snark/Art Resource, NY.

As Chrétien became the great poet of courtly love, so was Andreas Capellanus its theoretician. His *De Arte Honeste Amandi*, written in Latin in the late twelfth century, includes eight dialogues between different types of lovers explaining how a man may win over the woman he loves. The title of his work has been translated in many ways, but it means the art of loving honestly or truly; that is, it describes how to manifest true love. Andreas codifies the art with a set of thirty-one rules describing many of the characteristics described above. Widely translated and studied, it combined with Chrétien's Arthurian romances to establish courtly love as a major dimension of medieval literature.Courtly Love

Further Reading: Hopkins, Andrea. *The Book of Courtly Love: The Passionate Code of the Troubadours*. New York: HarperCollins, 1994; Lewis, C. S. *The Allegory of Love*. 1936. Reprint, New York: Oxford University Press, 1985; Swabey, Ffiona. *Eleanor of Aquitaine, Courtly Love, and the Troubadours*. Westport, CT: Greenwood Press, 2004.

Edward J. Rielly

CROSS-DRESSING. *See* Transgenderism and Cross-Dressing

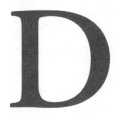

DANTE ALIGHIERI (1265–1321). Dante Alighieri focused much of his creative efforts, including *The Divine Comedy* and *The New Life* (*La Vita Nuova*) on the great love of his life, Beatrice Portinari. Differing sharply from the adulterous and physical nature of **courtly love**, Dante expressed his love for Beatrice in ideal, spiritual terms, culminating not in physical union but in an imaginative entry into the heavenly paradise. Dante first met Beatrice, whose name means "a bestower of happiness or blessings," in 1274 when they were both nine years old. When, nine years later, Dante saw her dressed in pure white, he experienced a sense of blessedness. The time, Dante noted, was nine o'clock, the number nine conveying spiritual meanings he consistently associated with Beatrice, including symbolic meanings of three (the root of nine), such as the Trinity.

Dante's brief encounter with Beatrice was followed by a dream vision in which he saw the figure of a lord (Love) holding Beatrice in his arms. Love awakens the lady and feeds her Dante's heart. Dante is thus embarking upon both a lifelong spiritual love for Beatrice and the new spiritual life that he writes about in *The New Life*. That Beatrice married a banker named Simone dei Bardi seems not to have affected Dante's perception of her. Beatrice died at the age of twenty-four in 1290.

By 1295, Dante had written *The New Life*, in which he records the occasions when he saw Beatrice, as well as visions of her future death. Beatrice becomes a Christ figure in the work, in one scene preceded by another woman whom Dante likens to John the Baptist preparing the way for Christ. When Dante is attracted by a woman gazing at him from a window, he is reclaimed by a vision of Beatrice in glory clothed in red and looking as young as in their first meeting. The final section of *The New Life* sets the stage for Beatrice's reappearance in *The Divine Comedy* as Dante commits himself to studying in preparation for writing of Beatrice in a manner no man had ever attempted writing of a woman.

Dante apparently began writing *The Divine Comedy*, a poem describing his journey through the realms of the afterlife, as early as 1307. He completed the first part, *Inferno*, by 1314 and continued with *Purgatory* and *Paradise*, the latter concluding shortly before his death in 1321. In Dante's masterpiece, Beatrice represents divine revelation and wisdom while also functioning as a Christ figure. Dante encounters Beatrice once he has reached the earthly paradise near the conclusion of *Purgatory*. Beatrice descends from heaven, coming to Dante as Christ does to individual sinners, to bring salvation. She judges Dante, rebukes him for his failings, and following his repentance leads him forward. As they move through the heavenly spheres of the Ptolemaic system, Beatrice instructs and strengthens him.

Reaching the Empyrean, the heavenly paradise, Dante finds that Beatrice has left him, and looking around sees her on her throne in the third circle from the highest. Beatrice smiles at Dante, having granted her favor, not sexually as in the **courtly love** tradition, but spiritually. Dante is now in a position to see the Virgin Mary and through her gain the privilege of observing the Divine Majesty and glimpsing the Holy Trinity and the union of God with human nature in Christ. *See also* Catholicism.

Further Reading: Hollander, Robert. *Dante: A Life in Works*. New Haven, CT: Yale University Press, 2001; Williams, Charles. *The Figure of Beatrice: A Study in Dante*. New York: Farrar, Straus and Cudahy, 1961.

Edward J. Rielly

DAOISM. Daoism has had a complex attitude toward sexuality. During the medieval period, some Daoists advocated sexual practices as essential for attaining longevity or immortality, while others rejected these practices, advocating asceticism and/or celibate monasticism.

DAOIST SEXUAL CULTIVATION. Daoist attitudes toward sexuality are rooted in Chinese preconceptions. Ancient Chinese texts indicate that sexuality was viewed as a basic human need, one that contributed to the good, both by producing happiness and by maintaining the social order. Sexual practices have been integrated into Daoism in two ways.

The first is a practice of ceremonial sexual union that was conducted by members of the Celestial Masters tradition in the early medieval period. This practice involved groups of up to twenty people, who would engage in prayer and visualization. Then, in couples, the participants would recite formulas, and practice dance and massage followed by ritualized sexual union. This practice had political implications, as it was thought to usher in a new era of great peace. This is described in the *Ritual for Passing, from the Yellow Book of the Shangqing*, which may date to the third century CE. Rites of this sort were apparently observed during the early medieval period. A Buddhist convert from Daoism, Chen Lun, describes rituals of this type in his polemical work *Ridiculing the Daoists*, composed in 570 CE.

Sexual practices were more commonly included into the programs of spiritual cultivation advocated by Daoist alchemists. Many Daoists believed that sexual cultivation was essential for achieving mental and physical balance. The Daoist tradition sees both the universe and the human body as consisting of complementary forces, *yin* and *yang*, which are correlated to the feminine and masculine, respectively. These forces ultimately derive from the *dao*, a singular ultimate reality that is the source of all that exists. By bringing them into harmony, the Daoist

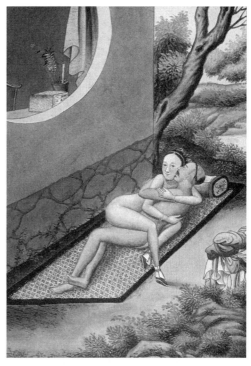

Detail from *Sou Nu King*, Chinese Taoist treatise on sexual initiation. © The Granger Collection, New York.

adept comes closer to the desired goal of achieving union with the *dao*. This balance could be achieved either within one's own body, or through sexual union.

Many Daoists held a positive attitude toward sexuality. Deprivation and excessive indulgence were both thought to lead to negative physical and mental health consequences. Sexual cultivation, if practiced properly, could enable one to live far longer than normal. Daoist alchemists such as Ge Hong (283–363) believed that the time it would take to produce the elixir of immortality was considerably longer than the average lifespan. Sexual cultivation would buy the alchemist the extra time needed to perfect the art. This cultivation entailed the retention of the vital essence (*jing*), which is identified with sexual fluids. In some practices, it would also involve absorbing one's partner's vital essence, which could then be transformed into vital energy (*qi*), promoting health, vigor, and youthfulness.

Daoist texts on sexual practices, such as the *Secrets of the Jade Chamber*, composed during the Sui dynasty (581–618), advocated that one engage in these practices in a calm state of mind, free of passions that disturb the energies of the body and mind. This text called for multiple sexual partners, who should ideally be young. These practices became a fad during the Tang dynasty (618–907). Reports say that during this period there were courtesans who specialized in Daoist sexual cultivation exercises.

DAOIST ASCETICISM AND MONASTICISM. Not all traditions of Daoism advocated sexual practices. Many early Daoists believed that asceticism and an eremitic lifestyle were essential for the achievement of immortality. Living in isolation and maintaining an extremely austere dietary regimen, these Daoists saw sex as an entanglement to be avoided. This lifestyle is supported by classical Daoist texts such as the *Dao De Jing* (c. fourth century BCE), which problematized desire, and advocated rejection of the goal-oriented, egocentric behavior typical of ordinary people.

The ascetic tendency of Daoism was strengthened by its encounter with **Buddhism**. Buddhists ridiculed Daoist sexual practices, and under Buddhist influence some Daoist traditions eventually established monastic orders. This trend came to its fruition with the rise of the Complete Perfection school of Daoism, which was founded by Wang Chongyang (1112–1170). This tradition borrowed from Buddhists the practice of celibate monasticism, and advocated contemplative techniques. They were particularly known for their advocacy of inner alchemical practices that jettisoned the need for sexual practices. *See also* China; Zhang Boduan.

Further Reading: Eskildsen, Stephen. *Asceticism in Early Taoist Religion*. Albany: State University of New York Press, 1998; Schipper, Kristofer. *The Taoist Body*. Berkeley: University of California Press, 1993; Wile, Douglas. *Art of the Bedchamber: The Chinese Sexual Yoga Classics, Including Women's Solo Meditation Texts*. Albany: State University of New York Press, 1992.

David B. Gray

DEVADASIS. The term *devadasis* may be translated as "the maidservants of God." Devadasis form part of the religious practices of southern **India**, especially Andhra Pradesh. As part of the convention, parents marry their daughter to either a deity or a particular temple. Usually, the **marriage** is solemnized before the girl attains puberty. The ceremony makes the girl fit to become a prostitute for the upper-caste community members. The devadasis are supposedly dedicated to Gods. The priests can henceforth lay claim on them, and later others too have a right on them. They can be better understood as courtesans in God's court, even though this sounds like an anomaly. A devadasi cannot marry a human being or lead a normal family life since she is already common property. Therefore, she has foregone all rights to any personal form of expression. Such girls are also called *joginis*. It is a voluntary system of offering oneself to the service of the gods in Brahmanical temples, seemingly a very noble vow.

In *Castes and Tribes of Southern India* (1987), Edgar Thurston recognizes seven kinds of devadasis: *datta* (who gives herself to the temple), *vikrita* (who sells herself to the temple), *bhritya* (who offers herself for the sake of the prosperity of her family), *brita* (who is enticed away and presented to the temple involuntarily), *bhakta* (who enters the tradition out of devotion for the deities), *alankara* (who is presented to the temple by kings and noblemen after being trained and perfected in her "profession"), and the *rudraganika* or *gopikas* (who are employed to sing and dance).

It was believed that devadasis were earthly incarnations of the mythical Urvashi, the celestial nymph. According to legend, Urvashi, while dancing in Indra's court, noticed his son Jayanta and faltered for a brief moment. This error aroused the anger of the sage Agastya, who had observed their infatuated exchange of looks. Agastya cursed the pair, and Indra and Jayanta had to accept, the result of which was banishment to earth for purposes of performance pleasures. So, for a small mistake of a celestial dancer, generations of devadasis were exploited.

The origin and spread of this system has been variously explained: religious beliefs, caste orthodoxy, male domination, and economic conditions have all been held responsible for the growth of this practice. In many areas, the emergence of this system has been identified with the downfall of **Buddhism**. There is evidence suggesting that devadasis were originally Buddhist nuns. Works of ancient writers like Jaatakas, Kautillya, or Vatsayana do not mention them, but later puranas do list some instances. In this light, the myth of Urvashi can be seen as a legitimizing tool for the evil inherent in the very system.

According to a report in the *Times of India* (November 10, 1987), the devadasi system originated as a result of a conspiracy between the feudal class and the priests (Brahmins). Brahmins influenced peasants and craftsmen to give **prostitution** a religious sanction by devising the devadasi tradition. Young girls from poor families were sold at private auctions, then dedicated to the temples, and eventually initiated into prostitution.

Over the centuries, the system has continued in some form or other due to the persistent sociopolitical conditions that led to its birth in the first place. In fact, it is still alive in certain parts of Maharashtra and Karnataka. The devadasi system was declared illegal in India as late as 1988.

Further Reading: Chakraborthy, Kakolee. *Women as Devadasis: Origin and Growth of the Devadasi Profession.* Delhi: Deep & Deep, 2000; Sadasivan, K. *Devadasi System in Medieval Tamil Nadu.* Nagercoil, South India: CBH Publications, 1993; Thurston, Edgar, and K. Rangachari. *Castes and Tribes of Southern India.* Vol. 4. New Delhi: Asian Educational Services, 1987.

Jitendra Uttam

DIVORCE. Although uncommon, medieval Christianity did permit divorce in very special circumstances. The church authorized two forms of divorce: *Divorce a vinculo matrimonii* (divorce from the **marriage** bond), essentially an annulment, could be granted in situations where a preexisting impediment to the marriage could be proven. *Divorce a mensa et thoro* (divorce from table and bed), in effect a court-sanctioned separation, might also be awarded in certain extreme circumstances.

MEDIEVAL "DIVORCE." In theory, marriages contracted in a valid fashion according to the church were indissoluble. A marriage created a union of flesh, and, as Matthew 19:6 proclaimed, "What therefore God hath joined together, let no man put asunder."

Nevertheless, even in the Middle Ages, provisions for divorce existed and were carried out under the aegis of the medieval church. This essentially differed from modern divorce: a couple could not simply divorce because their personalities were incompatible. Rather, divorce was rigidly regulated, and only available in a limited number of circumstances; thus, a church-approved divorce was not a common occurrence.

ANNULMENTS. A *divorce a vinculo matrimonii* is what we would call today an annulment. Basic to this form of divorce is the idea that the marriage should never have taken place. Plaintiffs in litigation of this nature sought to prove the existence of a canonically sanctioned impediment to marriage. The following six impediments tended to dominate litigation for annulments:

1. *Incest*. At the Fourth Lateran Council in 1215, the church resolved all questions about **incest**. It declared that anyone related within four degrees (generations to the common ancestor) by blood (**consanguinity**), by sexual relationship (affinity), or by sponsorship (being a godparent at a baptism or confirmation) was prohibited from marrying. In order to avoid the possibility of contracting marriages where an impediment existed without a couple knowing, the church introduced the concept of the reading of the banns at church on three consecutive Sundays before the ceremony was to take place. Since the nineteenth century, it has been argued that medieval couples frequently exploited the rules of incest in order to dissolve an unhappy marriage. More recent studies, however, suggest that this may not have been the case.
2. **Impotence**. Since the time of **Augustine**, the church understood marital sex as fulfilling two important roles: first, as the only licit outlet for the relief of **lust**; second, procreation, as without procreation as a goal even marital sex was sinful. Thus, sex was central to marriage, and a spouse's inability to perform was a serious impediment. Because sexual intercourse created a union of flesh, however, the condition had to exist prior to the marriage. If it developed after the marriage was consummated, it was unfortunate, but not an impediment.
3. *Force and Fear*. The church's insistence that only the consent of the bride and groom were necessary to create a valid marriage conflicted with the more traditional notions of arranged marriages. Because marriage involved the exchange of substantial portions of family land, it is not surprising that families, especially parents or guardians, believed they, too, should have a voice in spousal selection. With such a long tradition of family involvement in the formation of marriages, most couples married at the advice and supervision of their families. Consequently, it is rare to find cases of force and fear, where individuals alleged that they had been compelled into marriage against their will. Cases of marriage litigation on these grounds tend to represent a clashing of strong wills, or a woman forced into marriage by a suitor.
4. *The Impediment of Crime*. The impediment of crime was the most complicated of all impediments. Because the church upheld the indissolubility of marriage, it was necessary to recognize the possibility that some individuals might end a marriage through unlawful means. Thus, if, for example, a married woman had a lover, and then was somehow involved in her husband's death and wished to marry that lover, she was prohibited from the subsequent marriage by the impediment of crime. In the same way, if she had sworn to marry her lover after her husband's death, then also she was prohibited (since there was no way to prove definitively that she was innocent of her husband's death). The rarity of cases of this nature suggests that the church did not regularly enforce this impediment.
5. *Infra annos nubiles* (under-aged marriage). According to **canon law**, a couple could be betrothed as early as the age of seven, although upon reaching the age of marriageability (twelve for a woman, fourteen for a man), the individual had the choice

of reclaiming or rejecting the contract. Any child "married" before the canonically sanctioned age could take his case to court and request an annulment, although this, too, was exceptional.

6. *Precontract.* By far the most common grounds for an annulment were allegations of precontract, or **bigamy**. Cases on these grounds attest to a lingering custom of self-divorce, in which unhappy couples simply "divorced themselves" and then went on to remarry other people. If the church became aware of a previous marriage (often at the suit of the former spouse who had since changed his or her mind), it was required to test the validity of that first marriage and, if necessary, dissolve the subsequent marriage in favor of the first.

Further impediments (among others, error of condition, solemn religious vows, holy orders) also existed, but rarely produced litigation.

JUDICIAL SEPARATIONS. The other recognized form of divorce, *divorce a mensa et thoro*, included a judicial separation. The church awarded a couple the right to live separately, and released them from the demands of the conjugal debt, but neither was permitted to remarry. In theory, there were only three acceptable grounds on which the court might award a judicial separation: flagrant **adultery**, heresy or apostasy, and cruelty (*saevitia*). In practice, the church was determined to uphold the bonds of marriage at all costs, and was hesitant to award separations except in the most extreme situations, usually where the life of one of the spouses was in danger.

Further Reading: Helmholz, R. H. *Marriage Litigation in Medieval England.* London: Cambridge University Press, 1974; Phillips, Roderick. *Putting Asunder: A History of Divorce in Western Society.* London: Cambridge University Press, 1988.

Sara M. Butler

DOMESTIC VIOLENCE. Despite the rigid social and familial hierarchy of medieval society, domestic violence in the form of spousal abuse was recognized as a problem and addressed by the medieval church courts. Judicial separations on the grounds of cruelty were sometimes awarded. Involvement of family and friends played an important role in reducing the levels of violence within **marriage**. Moreover, literature in this period representing the need for patriarchal control of the home probably led to a toleration of some level of violence. Jewish attitudes toward domestic violence share many of the same characteristics, although they were much subject to regionalism.

SOCIAL HIERARCHY. Medieval Europe was a remarkably hierarchical society. The feudal system reinforced the notion that every individual is subject to the will of his lord. Although women and children existed outside this system, the patriarch was expected to fill this role in the home. Accordingly, **canon law** and secular law permitted husbands and fathers to use a reasonable degree of force to discipline and instruct members of their households. The difficulty lay in determining the boundaries of what was considered "reasonable."

VIOLENCE AGAINST CHILDREN. Child abuse does not seem to have been considered a problem in the medieval context. R. H. Helmholz's study of intrafamily violence highlights the absence of cases of child abuse in the English courts (apart from the occasional case of infanticide); in fact, the only cases of violence between parents and their children treated parents as the victims, and urged children to repent and reform. Misericords depicting students having their bottoms birched by schoolmasters would tend to strengthen the notion that the beating of children was considered a necessary part of a good education.

Domestic Violence in the Church Courts. If not officially, the jurisdiction of the Christian church courts was thought to include all acts of violence within the family. The church courts assumed the role of marriage counselors, routinely addressing cases of marital violence and requiring husbands to treat their wives decently, and to provide guarantors for their future good behavior. Moreover, the church permitted separations on the grounds of cruelty (*saevitia*). In the English context, the courts were reluctant to grant separations on these grounds except in those cases where a spouse's life was in danger. A more lenient attitude can be found on the continent; separations were more frequently awarded in France, Germany, and Italy. The *Corpus juris civilis*, which formed the base of continental law, also permits separation for violence between spouses with the intent to kill; thus, it is likely that continental courts were marginally more receptive to the notion of separation for violence.

Marriage as a Public Institution. Today, domestic violence often goes unpunished because it is considered a private problem. This was not the case in the medieval world. Although marital violence did not frequently appear in medieval courts of law, men and women would not generally have found legal resolution necessary or even appropriate. Not only were families, neighbors, and friends instrumental in contracting marriages, they also played a continuing role as arbitrators throughout the marriage, in order to prevent violence from spiraling out of control.

Domestic Violence in the Arts. Although artwork from the period is more likely to depict a "world turned upside down," in which tyrannical wives mercilessly beat their downtrodden husbands, the literature of the period advocates the opposite. Sermons, ballads, conduct books, and fabliaux urge husbands to keep their homes in order by controlling their wives with physical force. The disobedience of wives, a legacy of Eve's fall from paradise, is highlighted as a recurring problem that can best be resolved through the use of force. The proliferation of this ideology may have normalized violence in marriage.

Jewish Attitudes toward Domestic Violence. Medieval Jewish communities exhibited a wider range of attitudes about the beating of wives. This disparity is most likely a result of regionalism and the immersion of Jewish communities within gentile environments. For example, Jewish sages living in Muslim countries tended to condone occasional incidents of cruelty and only punish husbands guilty of habitual violence. Abusive husbands were subject to fines payable directly to their wives. This lax treatment fits in well with Muslim teachings about marital violence. The Qur'an urges husbands to beat their wives for any suspicion of immodest or disrespectful behavior. Jewish communities in France and Germany seem to have been the most intolerant of domestic violence. Jewish sages supported a beaten wife's right to demand a **divorce**, even against her husband's will. Some sages also advocated corporal punishment for abusive husbands (from beating to amputation), although it is not known how frequently this was enforced.

Further Reading: Grossman, Avraham. "Medieval Rabbinic Views on Wife-Beating, 800–1300." *Jewish History* 5, no. 1 (1991): 53–62; Helmholz, R. H. "And Were There Children's Rights in Early Modern England? The Canon Law and 'Intra-Family Violence' in England, 1400–1640." *International Journal of Children's Rights* 1 (1993): 23–32.

Sara M. Butler

DROIT DU SEIGNEUR. According to popular belief, the *droit du seigneur* (Fr. "right of the lord") or *jus primae noctis* (Lat. "right of the first night") was a feudal lord's right to claim the **virginity** of his vassal's wife on the night of her wedding.

No compelling historical evidence attests to the actual existence of *droit du seigneur* in medieval Europe, yet the theme is reflected in many writings of the period.

Perhaps the belief in such a practice evolved from the custom that all vassals were required to obtain the permission of their lord in order to marry. In Germany, the bridegroom paid a fee to the bride or her family in exchange for the right to have intercourse with her. Unfree men obtained the fee from their lord as a loan. The latter symbolically acquired the right to the maiden's virginity and performed a ritual known as the *Beilager*. (Intercourse between the lord and the bride was not, however, a part of the legal **marriage** ceremony.) Other marriage fees and taxes were levied throughout Europe, such as the *cullage* in France.

If the custom of *droit du seigneur* is probably legendary, it nevertheless reflects a harsh reality of medieval life and attests to the precarious place women occupied in medieval society. The eighth-century *Annals of Clonmacnoise* records how Viking conquerors claimed the right to have sex with Christian brides in Ireland. And, according to the early sixteenth-century chronicler Boece, King Ewen III established such a custom in Scotland during the late ninth century. (Modern historians doubt that Ewen ever existed.) Literary works also present the *droit du seigneur* as commonplace. In the fourteenth-century French epic *Baudoin de Sebourc*, a tyrannical lord will excuse a bride from her sexual obligations to him only in exchange for a large portion of her dowry. Other texts suggest that, in the medieval world, powerful men did not hesitate to **rape** their female serfs. For example, Odo of Cluny's *Life of Count Gerald of Aurillac* recalls how Gerald informed a maiden belonging to him of his intent to deflower her. Through divine intervention, when the count arrives in the virgin's room, she appears to him so ugly that he abandons his plan.

Further Reading: Boureau, Alain. *The Lord's First Night: The Myth of the Droit de Cuissage*. Translated by Lydia G. Cochrane. Chicago: University of Chicago Press, 1998.

K. Sarah-Jane Murray

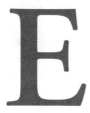

EDWARD II, KING OF ENGLAND (1284–1327). Edward II of England (r. 1307–1327) was the most famous example of the trouble that close emotional relationships with men of considerably lesser rank could cause a medieval king. The love between the king and the nobleman Piers Gaveston, possibly sealed in some kind of ceremony or vow, may or may not have been sexual but was described by contemporary chroniclers as immoderate and excessive. The political problems Edward faced were caused by the impression that Gaveston, the son of a mere knight, had too much influence over the king's decisions. Gaveston was regent of the kingdom when the king was absent from France, and played a very prominent role in the coronation ceremony in 1308. Later that year, a coaliton of English barons forced Gaveston into exile. The struggle between the nobility and Gaveston culminated in 1312, when he was kidnapped and killed.

Edward II's second controversial male favorite was Hugh Despenser the Younger, the son of a knight who had served his father. Despenser was appointed chamberlain of the king's household in 1318 and they became inseparable companions, although Edward's relationship with Despenser does not seem to have been as passionate as his relationship with Gaveston. Like Gaveston, the greedy and ambitious Despenser was the focus of opposition from English nobles, joined in his case by Edward's queen Isabella of the royal family of France. Isabella charged that Despenser was driving her and her husband apart. Late in 1325, Isabella became the lover of a nobleman named Roger Mortimer, enraging her husband. Edward and Despenser were captured by French-backed rebels allied with Isabella and the king's own son late in 1326. Despenser was executed, and Edward deposed the following year. He died shortly afterward while in captivity. The exact means are unknown, but the story appears in one chronicle that a red-hot poker was inserted into his body through his anus. Although anti-Edward writers in his own time focused more on Gaveston's and Despenser's inappropriate political influence on the king, Edward was also charged with having them as lovers. The portrayal of Edward as a lover of men culminated in the sixteenth-century play *Edward II* by dramatist Christopher Marlowe. *See also* Homosexuality, Male.

Further Reading: Haines, Roy Martin. *King Edward II: Edward of Caernarfon, His Life, His Reign, and Its Aftermath, 1284–1330.* Montreal, Canada: McGill Queens University Press, 2003.

William E. Burns

EJACULATION. *See* Orgasm, Male

ERMENGAUD, MATFRE. The southern French Franciscan Friar Matfre Ermengaud, of whom little is known, was the author of a long encyclopedic poem, *Breviary of Love*, begun in 1288 and finished in the following decade. Beginning with the Trinity, Ermengaud covered various topics in theology and natural philosophy using love, including the love of God for humanity, as an organizing principle. The last 8,000 lines, a little under a fourth of the poem's total length, consist of advice to women on the subject of love in dialog form. Ermengaud drew heavily on the **courtly love** tradition and **troubadour** literature, with over 250 direct quotations from troubadour poets. He recommended that women should show friendliness and receptiveness to declarations of love while avoiding any stain of dishonor. He claimed that praise from troubadours brought glory to women. The *Breviary* was widely circulated and translated into Catalan and Castilian.

Further Reading: Bornstein, Diane. *The Lady in the Tower: Medieval Courtesy Literature for Women*. Hamden, CT: Archon, 1983.

William E. Burns

EUNUCHS. Castrated males, or eunuchs, played many roles in medieval societies. In both **Islamic society** and **China**, eunuchs were often members of peripheral or foreign ethnic groups. Europe and Japan did not have large foreign immigration in the medieval period, which may explain the minor (in the case of Japan, nonexistent) role of eunuchs in these culture.

Eunuchs exercised political influence through their connections to courts in many polities, particularly the late Roman and Byzantine empires, Islamic states, and China under the Tang and later the Ming dynasty. Court eunuchs played a particularly prominent role in the late Roman empire as the court assimilated to Hellenistic and Persian models, despite the occasional efforts of reforming emperors such as Julian to expel them. The widely hated eunuch Eusebius during the reign of Constantine II was believed to be the effective ruler of the empire. Attitudes toward eunuchs became more positive under the Byzantine empire. Eunuchs were everywhere in the Byzantine power structure. The only office forbidden to them was the post of emperor, but eunuchs could and did become patriarchs of the Orthodox church. Byzantine eunuchs also served outside the court as generals and administrators. The best-known Byzantine eunuch soldier was General Narses, leader of the reconquest of Italy in the reign of Justinian. Writers on eunuch generals in **Byzantium** generally credited their successes to intelligence, organization, and loyalty to the emperor rather than martial valor.

Eunuch power waxed and waned in China according to different dynastic settings. It was its early height during the Tang dynasty. Eunuch power was always opposed by the Confucian literati, who saw eunuchs as aspiring dictators or unprincipled imperial tools. Eunuchs, particularly in the Tang, responded by often participating in anti- or non-Confucian movements, such as **Buddhism**. It was customary for old eunuchs to retire to Buddhist monasteries.

Eunuchs did not play a significant political role in the Song and Yuan dynasties, but this changed again in the Ming, despite the loudly proclaimed antipathy of the founder of the dynasty, Hongzi, to eunuchs who engaged in politics. Beginning with Hongzi himself, the Ming made extraordinarily heavy use of eunuch royal servants as generals, admirals, arms manufacturers, trade supervisors, mining superintendents, engineers, and

EUNUCHS

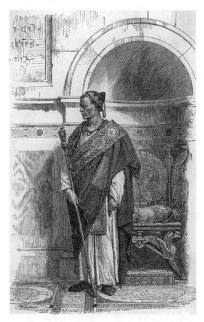

Undated engraving of Narses, Byzantine general and eunuch. © Mary Evans Picture Library.

judges, the most notable being the admiral Zheng He, the leader of the massive Ming expeditions in the Indian Ocean in the early fifteenth century.

Castration had been prohibited by early Arab and Islamic cultures, and eunuchs played little role in Islamic society in the age of the early caliphs and the Umayyad dynasty. However, with the ascension of the Abbasid caliphs and the move from Damascus to the new eastern capital of Baghdad, the caliphate adopted a more elaborate court culture influenced by Persian and Byzantine traditions and the eunuchs that went with it.

Some societies accorded eunuchs a sacred status. A leading example was the *hijra* community of **India**, males (not all of whom were castrated) who adopted female garments and were associated with a particular goddess. In **Islam**, the Eunuchs of the Prophet were a sacred community charged with guarding Mohammed's tomb at Medina. They date from the twelfth century and were initially part of an effort by the Sunni rulers of Egypt, who were also suzerains of Mecca and Medina, to establish Sunni presence in Shia-dominated Medina. (The idea of eunuch guardians of sacred tombs was also present among the Shia, however. The tomb of Ali, the Shia hero, was guarded by eunuchs.) Some Medina eunuchs received admiring biographies from Sunni scholars and were treated as particularly close to God. In the Byzantine empire, the originally hostile attitude toward eunuchs expressed by early Christian writers became more positive, as eunuchs became prominent leaders of the church from the eighth century on. The role of eunuchs as imperial servants promoted the idea that they alone were able to serve perfectly, helping people to accept the idea that they could be perfect servants of God. By the tenth century, Byzantine writers identified the revered Old Testament prophet Daniel as a court eunuch. Eunuchs were often associated with the angels, who, it was believed, played the same role in the court of heaven that eunuchs played in the emperor's court on earth. Latin **Catholicism** had a schizophrenic attitude toward eunuchs, admiring their chastity and freely using the biblical metaphor of those "who made themselves eunuchs for the kingdom of God," but was very suspicious of actual eunuchs. Castration of humans was forbidden by the Council of Nicea in 325.

Some viewed eunuchs as desirable sexual partners. One Abbasid prince was allegedly so enamored of young eunuchs that his worried mother dressed slender, boyish girls in male clothing and paraded them in front of her son in hopes of changing his tastes. Several Chinese emperors had eunuch lovers in addition to their wives and concubines.

Further Reading: Ayalon, David. *Eunuchs, Caliphs and Sultans: A Study in Power Relationships*. Jerusalem: Magnes Press, Hebrew University, 1999; Marmon, Shaun. *Eunuchs and Sacred Boundaries in Islamic Society*. New York: Oxford University Press, 1999; Ringrose, Kathryn M. *The Perfect Servant: Eunuchs and the Social Construction of Gender in Byzantium*. Chicago: University of Chicago Press, 2003; Tsai, Shih-Shan Henry. *The Eunuchs in the Ming Dynasty*. New York: State University of New York Press, 1996.

William E. Burns

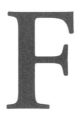

FERRER, VICENTE (1350–1419). Vicente Ferrer was a Spanish preacher of the Dominican order, famous for his work in promoting moral values, and instilling them within the ethos of the society of his day. He was born in Valencia (Spain) in 1350, the son of Guillermo Ferrer and Costancia Miguel. In 1363 he became a Dominican and studied in Barcelona. He taught philosophy and theology in the universities of Barcelona and Paris. He was one of the greatest preachers of his time, and was also greatly appreciated for his ascetic writing. He travelled in Italy, France, Switzerland, and elsewhere in Europe. Vicente's spiritual works, such as the severely ascetic *Treatise on Spiritual Life*, centered on despising and renouncing "earthly joys and pleasures." He died in 1419 in Vannes (France). He was renowned for his holiness and miracles, and was canonized by Pope Callistus III in 1455.

Vicente's position on sexuality is described in contemporary biographies and accounts of his legendary life, where the saint appears as the victim of terrible temptations by women, or devils disguised as women. There are similarities with the temptations of St. Anthony, "Abbot in the desert." Vicente was also the author and instigator of extraordinary conversions of sinners and prostitutes. Women are often considered in his preachings as instruments of perdition. With women he had a double face in the sexual context; they were often condemned, but were also portrayed as "sweet" when they renounced their sexual nature. One of the most famous episodes of his legend tells of the miracle of a woman who, after her spiritual conversion, became physically beautiful thanks to the prayers of Vicente. He was particularly adverse to the prostitutes who lost clients after his preaching, and women, who, inquisitive about his private life and sexuality, invaded his closed convent to spy on him. Women's loquacity often causes fights with their husbands: Vicente frequently reproached women for this vice. He often helped those who were unjustly accused of unfaithfulness, and as a miracle worker he was famous for freeing parturient women from the pains and dangers of **childbirth**. *See also* Catholicism; Misogyny in Latin Christendom.

Further Reading: Tomarelli, Ubaldo. *San Vincenzo Ferreri apostolo e taumaturgo*. Bologna: Edizioni Studio Domenicano, 1990.

Elvio Ciferri

FIFTEEN JOYS OF MARRIAGE. *Fifteen Joys of Marriage* is an anonymous French book written in the first half of the fifteenth century and primarily devoted to the relationship of a married man with his wife. It is attributed to Gilles Bellemère, bishop of Avignon from 1380 to 1408, an expert in law and matrimonial problems. The work introduces itself as a satirical treatment of **marriage**, valid in every epoch. The clerical author looks on marriage with a rational eye and describes it ironically. A married couple's relationship is described as one of conflict, often as a struggle for power over the family, initiated by the wife and inevitably concluding with the defeat of the husband. *Fifteen Joys of Marriage* is a book for men who want to defend themselves from the malice of their wives, but also for wives who want to know their husbands better. The text describes not only the malice and shrewdness of wives, but also the psychological vulnerability of their husbands. It is misogynistic, but without going far from raw realism. The husband's role in marriage as a loser is viewed with pity, and marriage is ironically compared with penitence.

Five scenes are represented, each signifying different phases within a marriage. Repeated references to sexuality demonstrate how ephemeral pleasure precedes the great punishment that marriage inevitably carries. Some chapters discuss the wife's motives, as she avoids sexual contact with her husband, excusing herself because she does not feel well, in order to reserve all of her energies for meeting her lover the following day. The lover will fill her with those delights she desires and those her husband would never be able to give her. This betrayal is consummated in the early morning, while her husband still sleeps, with the wife's excuse of having to do domestic chores. The unlucky husband remains alone, since the maid is the wife's accomplice and their daughter follows in the footsteps of her mother. All of female humanity is indicted.

The author's knowledge of female psychology is amazing: the wife is not only antagonistic but also the protagonist with her whims, her inventions, her arrogance, her disguised unfaithfulness, her interested seductions, her sensuality, and her egoism. The married couple's relationship is also described during their most intimate and secret moments, revealing their conversations in their bedroom and the pretence and strategies used by the wife to hide her betrayal. The author does not want to find a remedy to the unhappiness that he sees as inherent within marriage, but rather describes the sad reality as inevitable. *See also* Misogyny in Latin Christendom.

Further Reading: Crow, Joan, ed. *Les quinze joyes de mariage*. Oxford: Blackwell, 1969.

Elvio Ciferri

FOOTBINDING.   *See* China

FREYA/FRIGG.   Freya and Frigg are the two main goddesses in the northern European pantheon. In the Icelander Snorri Sturluson's compendium of mythological lore, the *Prose Edda* (1179–1241), Frigg is held to be the wife of Odin, the all-father of the gods, and from these two descend the Aesir, the race of gods who reside in Asgerd. Frigg is typically associated with **marriage** and **childbirth**. Although represented as a mother goddess by Snorri, she has a more obscure existence in northern European lore than the goddess Freya. Freya, daughter of the sea god Njord, and sister of Frey, numbers among the Vanir, a race of gods who are primarily associated with fertility. Snorri describes Freya as renowned, and indeed she appears to have been more popular than Frigg. Snorri identifies her with poetry, notes that women are called "fru" (madam) because of her, and recommends her as a divine ally in matters of love. Freya's husband is the otherwise obscure Od, who, according to Snorri, undertakes long journeys during which Freya seeks after him and weeps tears of red gold because of his absence. Her cult in Scandinavia appears to have been especially popular and long-lived.

Both goddesses are subject to accusations of sexual promiscuity in the surviving literature. The mythological poem *Loki's Quarrel* depicts the trickster-god Loki accusing Frigg of having improperly received Odin's brothers Ve and Vili into her embraces. In his *Saga of the Ynglings*—the Ynglings are a legendary Swedish dynasty and the eventual progenitors of the line of Norwegian kings—Snorri elaborates on Frigg's alleged infidelity. He relates that during one of Odin's particularly long absences from Asgerd, Ve and Vili assume their brother has died and subsequently divide his possessions among them except for Frigg, whom they share equally. Accusations of divine **adultery** are similarly leveled against Freya by Loki, when Freya speaks on behalf of Frigg in *Loki's Quarrel*. Loki quickly turns his attentions to Freya, whom he accuses of having been the lover of elves, of all of the Aesir, and even of her own brother, Frey. It is also worth noting that Freya's promiscuous behavior is defended by her father Njord, whom Loki in turn accuses of having begotten his children upon his own sister. *See also* Pagan Europe.

Further Reading: Jochens, Jenny. *Old Norse Images of Women*. Philadelphia: University of Pennsylvania Press, 1996; Orchard, Andy. *Cassell's Dictionary of Norse Myth and Legend*. London: Cassell, 2002.

John T. Sebastian

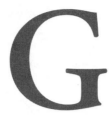

GENITAL CONTACT IN ISLAMIC LAW. Medieval Islamic law stipulates certain forms of ritual purification for sexual contact and for contact with genitals. Before performing obligatory rituals (e.g., prayer, fasting, offering, pilgrimage), Muslims must be ritually pure. There are two main purification rituals, one or both of which must be performed depending upon the types of impurity and the state of the person to be purified.

The first ritual is called the *Wudu*, usually translated as "ablution." It is mentioned in Qur'an 5:6, which specifies the washing of the face, and hands to the elbows, wiping the head, and the feet to the ankles. Traditional practice also includes using a toothpick, rinsing the mouth, snuffing, wiping the ears, and combing the beard with the fingers. This ablution is required following urination, defecation, nonmenstrual bleeding, and other substances that might exit from the body (pus, vomit, etc.). It is also mandatory after sleep, madness, and other forms of unconsciousness.

Most medieval Muslim jurists agreed that ablution was also necessary for contact with genitals, although there was much discussion of the details. According to some jurists, **masturbation** and genital contact done for pleasure required ablution. Other jurists maintained that any genital contact, even nonintentional, necessitated ablution. Intentional genital contact, whether for pleasure or not, is usually defined as touching one's own genitals with the palm of the hand, but can also include contact between the genitals and the back of the hand or other body parts that makes one conscious of the contact. Muslim jurists define genitals as the penis, vagina, anus, and attached areas. Although most jurists limit the requirement of ablution to those cases where contact is between the hand and genitals of a single person, some jurist hold that ablution is necessary for touching the genitals of another person, animals, or corpses, severed genitals, and pieces of genitals.

The second major type of ritual purification is the *Ghusl*, often translated as "washing." This ritual washing is supposed to remove actual physical impurities from the surface of the entire body. It is required after ejaculation, contact between genitalia without ejaculation, **menstruation**, and **childbirth**.

It is important to note that these purification rites are symbolic in character and emphasize different aspects of the natural human condition. The ablution focuses on the human need to sleep and eat. The washing focuses on sexual reproduction. Muslim jurists use certain test cases to illustrate the differences between ablution and washing: a nose-bleed requires ablution but menstruation requires washing because it is related to sexual reproduction, ejaculation requires washing but the emission of prostatic fluid requires ablution because it is not related to sexual reproduction. Both ablution and washing must be temporary since it would not be possible for people to discontinue eating and sleeping (ablution) or for human society to continue without sexual reproduction (washing).

These purification rites are closely related to the mythology of Adam and Eve in the Garden of Eden. According to the Qur'an and Muslim exegesis, Adam and Eve were not aware of their genitals before their fall from Eden since they did not use them to urinate, defecate, or have sex. It was only after Adam and Eve fell and met in Mecca that they began to practice sexual reproduction and eat food that caused the elimination of bodily wastes. *See also* Islam; Sharia.

Further Reading: Katz, Marion Holmes. *Body of Text: The Emergence of the Sunni Law of Ritual Purity*. Albany: State University of New York Press, 2002; Wheeler, Brannon. "Touching the Penis in Islamic Law." *History of Religions* 44 (2004): 89–119; Zannad, Traki. *Le lieux du corps en Islam*. Paris: Publisud, 1994.

Brannon Wheeler

GERSHOM BEN JUDAH (c. 960–c. 1040).   Gershom ben Judah founded rabbinical studies in northern Europe among Ashkenazi **Jews**. His edict against **polygamy** has been permanently influential. Gershom was born around 960 at Metz, Lorraine (now in France). He studied with Judah ben Meir ha-Kohen (Sir Leontin), one of the great Jewish scholars of the age. Among Gershom's numerous students from many countries were Eleasar ben Isaac (ha-Gadol), nephew of Simeon ha-Gadol and Jacob ben Yakar who became the teacher of Rashi. After his first wife died Gershom married a widow named Bonna and settled in Mayence (Mainz), where he headed the Yeshivah (rabbinical school). Gershom was able to bring the Talmudic learning of the academies in Babylon and Palestine to western Europe. He wrote a critical work on the Talmud and the Masora. He also gave extensive oral commentary on the Talmud to his students. So dominating was Gershom's influence that all subsequent Ashkenazi Jewish scholars are considered his students.

As a rabbinical scholar, Gershom was presented with numerous legal issues. His legal decisions (*taqqanot* or *takkanot*) molded northern medieval Jewish life and practices. The impact of his decisions led others to honor him with the titles "Me'or ha-Golah" ("Light of the Exile") and "Rabbeun" ("Our Teacher").

Around the year 1000, Gershom called leading Jewish scholars to a rabbinical synod that was to decide a number of issues, including a prohibition against reading another person's mail. The major issues related to family life that the synod settled were polygamy and **divorce**. Polygamy was debated with biblical and Talmudic references. In Gershom's time Ashkenazic Jews did not practice polygamy. However, it was common in the books of the Law, the Prophets, and the Writings and was not prohibited by the Babylonian *Halakah*. The Babylonian *Mishnah* and the *Talmud* permitted a man to have up to four wives as long as he could provide food, shelter, clothing, and other necessities, and keep all four sexually satisfied.

Gershom gained the day with a *taqqanot* that prohibited polygamy despite the precedents of earlier times. The *taqqanot* became a *herem* (ban) against **bigamy**. This ruling was to produce a major split between the Ashkenazian and Sephardic Jews. Gershom was also able to eliminate the right of a husband to divorce his wife without her consent. He was able to extend the rights of wives so that a woman had to agree to a divorce before a man could obtain a *get* (writ of divorce). Gershom died at Mainz in either 1028 or 1040.

Further Reading: Eidelberg, Shlomo. *The Responsa of Rabbenu Gershom Meor Hagolah.* New York: Yeshiva University, 1955; Weis, J. Max. *Great Men in Israel: Sketches from Rabbinic and Medieval Jewry.* New York: Bloch Publishing, 1922.

Andrew J. Waskey

GHAZAL. Ghazals are lyric poems about different aspects of love. The term is originally Arabic and literally means "talking with women." Sometime in the eleventh century in Iran the term became applied to a strict verse form in Persian. The Persian ghazal is composed of *Sher* (couplets), numbering from seven to thirteen, sharing *qafiya* (rhyme) and *radif* (refrain). Although the couplets are in the first person, the last one, known as *makhta*, often gives the name or some other identification of the poet. Some of the most brilliant expositions of the Persian ghazal are found in the writings of medieval Persian poets such as **Nizami, Rumi,** and **Hafiz.**

The ghazal spread to South Asia in the twelfth century. The tradition of ghazal writing began there with Amir Khusrau (1253–1325), who is credited with bringing about a cultural rapprochement between Persia and the Indian subcontinent. The *Tuhfa-tus-Sighr* (*Offering of a Minor*), *Wastul-Hayat* (*The Middle of Life*), *Khamsa-e-Khusro* (*Five Classical Romances*), and *Nihayatul-Kamaal* (*The Height of Wonders*) were some of his notable works.

Further Reading: Mirza, Wahid. *Life and Works of Amir Khusrau.* Calcutta, India: Baptist Mission Press, 1935; Yarshater, Ehsan, ed. *Persian Literature.* Albany, NY: Bibliotheca Press, 1988.

Patit Paban Mishra

GILES OF ROME (c. 1243/7–1316). Giles of Rome, an Italian and a member of the Augustinian order, was an influential and sometimes controversial professor in the faculty of theology at the University of Paris. He became archbishop of Bourges in 1295. A former student of **Thomas Aquinas,** Giles was an independent and original thinker not content to follow others blindly. As a theologian, Giles's understanding of sexuality is strongly influenced by **Augustine** and Aquinas. Giles maintains that sexual intercourse is natural and therefore good. In his reflections on the creation account in Genesis, he observes that Eve was created to serve as a helpmate to Adam, and this primarily for the purposes of procreation. The pleasures of intercourse were greater for human beings in the state of innocence than after the Fall, since their bodies were superior and their sense powers more acute. With the arrival of original sin, a fundamental disorder was introduced into human nature; no longer was sensuality under the control of reason.

Giles's interest in the scientific aspects of human reproduction is evident in his *De formatione corporis humani in utero* (*On the Formation of the Human Body in the Uterus*). Much of this work examines Galen's theory that females produce a seed, correlative to the sperm of males, which then plays an active role in human reproduction. The existence of a female seed was thought to be suggested by the presence of testes (ovaries) in females, by the white seed-like color of vaginal secretions, and by the fact that children bear a physical resemblance to both parents. Giles argues that females produce no seed; vaginal secretions have as their true purpose the facilitation of the process of conception by creating a friendly environment in the womb for the sperm, and increasing the pleasures of intercourse. It is the male alone who provides the active principle in generation; the female is passive, contributing by means of her menstrual fluid the matter for the fetus. By their sperm exerting dominion over the menstrual fluid, males transmit their characteristics to the fetus; the resemblance of a child to its mother is explained by the weakness of the sperm and the degree of resistance offered by the menstrual fluid. *See also* Scholastic Philosophy; Theories of Sexual Difference.

Further Reading: Hewson, M. Anthony. *Giles of Rome and the Medieval Theory of Conception: A Study of the De formatione Corporis Humani in Utero.* London: Athlone Press, 1975.

Mark D. Gossiaux

GOLIARD POETS. The Goliard poets were wandering scholars who composed and recited their poetry for money during the twelfth to fourteenth centuries. Being former university students, the Goliards composed in Latin. Among their favorite topics was love, usually treated in a physical, sexual sense.

Also known as vagantes or vagi (vagabonds) because of their wandering, often in the university towns and religious centers, the Goliards plied their trade in taverns and abbeys, wherever they could find someone willing to buy their entertainment. Sometimes a vagus might find a powerful patron, like the poet referred to as the Archpoet in the twelfth century, who benefited from the financial support of Archbishop Reginald of Cologne.

The Goliards, the names of almost all of them unknown, rose simultaneously with the European universities. They were from various European nations, including England, France, Italy, and Germany. Whatever their national origin, they were inevitably clerics, that is, members of the church, for the university curriculum was directed exclusively toward preparing men for service in the church. Most of the poets, though, either were in low orders or had not entered orders, and had no position in a church or religious community.

Along with poems celebrating wine and gambling, and poems written in imitation of religious hymns and satirizing the church, the Goliards celebrated physical love in their poems. Typically set in springtime in the woods or fields, the poems portray the beauty and allure of a Phyllis, Floris, or Caecilia, her cheeks like roses or lilies, her hair tawny or black. The pursuer is unnamed, but seeks, often in frankly sexual terms, to win the woman, almost always lower class rather than of noble birth.

The Council of Rouen in 1231 sought to curtail the Goliards by issuing a decree of degradation, an official lowering of their status from cleric. The position of the Goliard in society steadily declined so that by the fourteenth century the term "Goliard" came to mean a procurer for prostitutes. Although the Goliards largely disappeared in that century, many of their poems remain. An especially important collection that includes many love poems is the *Carmina burana*, a thirteenth-century manuscript that was preserved in the abbey of Benedictbeuern in Germany.

Further Reading: Symonds, John Addington. *Wine, Women and Song.* New York: Cooper Square Publishers, 1966; Waddell, Helen. *The Wandering Scholars.* 7th ed. London: Constable, 1947.

Edward J. Rielly

GONORRHEA. *See* Sexually Transmitted Diseases

GOWER, JOHN (d. 1408). The English poet John Gower wrote several significant works dealing with romantic and sexual issues, most notably, the massive English poem *Confessio Amantis* (*The Lover's Confession*), of over 30,000 lines. Gower's French-language *Fifty Ballads* draws on the courtly tradition to paint a picture of a love affair between the poet and a lady. Like other of Gower's works, it exalts steadfast and constant love. Another set of French and English verses from late in his career exalt married love founded in reason rather than passion (Gower married late in life) in similar terms.

Confessio Amantis, probably completed in 1390, tells the story of a lover wounded by the arrow of Cupid. Cupid's mother, the goddess Venus, instructs the lover to confess to her priest, Genius, who tells many tales of lovers arranged under the headings of the seven deadly sins, each of which is related to particular aspects of love. The stories are meant to give moral lessons again emphasizing the importance of constant and mature love, what Gower refers to as "honest love." (Gower's friend **Geoffrey Chaucer** referred to him as "moral Gower" in *Troilus and Criseyde*.) Like many medieval European poets writing of love and sensuality, Gower draws heavily from the ancient Roman poet Ovid as well as other classical writers, the Bible, and medieval sources for his anecdotes. At the conclusion of the poem, Cupid removes the arrow from the lover, now too old for love. *Confessio Amantis* was one of the most popular long poems in English during the later Middle Ages, surviving in forty-nine manuscripts and even being translated into Portuguese and Spanish. *See also* Ovidianism.

Further Reading: Bakalian, Ellen Shaw. *Aspects of Love in John Gower's "Confessio Amantis."* New York: Routledge, 2003.

William E. Burns

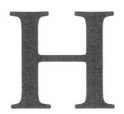

HAFIZ (1327–1391). Khwaja Shams ud-Din Mohammad Shirazi, better known as Hafiz, was the preeminent writer of love poetry in Persian. He was born in the Iranian town of Shiraz, where his father Baha-ud-Din was a coal merchant. Hafiz studied Arabic and theology in Shiraz, an important center of learning. As he learned the Qur'an by heart, he received the status of a *Hafiz*. He had a passionate love affair with a woman of extraordinary beauty, Shakh-e Nabat, and dedicated some of his **ghazal**s to her. He called her "branch of sugar-cane." The romantic poet even prayed for forty days in the tomb of a Sufi saint, Baba Kuhi, to become successful in his love.

Hafiz became famous under the patronage of Shaikh Abu Ishak Inju and wrote romantic poetry. But under the new puritan ruler Muzaffarid Mubariz al-Din Muhammed, his fortune began to languish from the year 1353. Writing dissenting odes, he gave the title *muhtasib* (one who restricts, or censor of public morals) to the ruler, who had imposed restrictions on the wine-loving Hafiz. After falling out from favor, he went to a self-imposed exile to Isfahan and Yazd. His poems reflected his longing for his beloved Shakh-e Nabat and his hometown. He returned five years later to Shiraz and got back his earlier position under King Shah Shoja, and wrote spiritual poetry. In 1387, he was imprisoned by Timur, but freed. Toward the end of his life, he was more concerned with communion with God and held a forty-day vigil inside a circle he drew. A beautiful mausoleum was erected after his death inside the Musalla Gardens on the banks of Ruknabad River. The Hafiziyya became a tourist center.

Hafiz wrote only when he was inspired and authored ten ghazals per year. Embellished with Sufi symbolism and imagery composed for a long period of time, his *Divan-e-Hafiz* consisted of 500 ghazals and 42 rubaiyees. His ghazals are characterized by ambiguity and different interpretations of the identity of the subjects of his poems, who could be God, a spiritual master or a beloved. He was given the title of *Tarjuman al-asrar* ("analyzer of mysticism") and *Lisan al-ghayh* ("tongue of the invisible zone"). *See also* Sufism.

Further Reading: Arberry, A. J., ed. *Persian Poems: An Anthology of Verse Translations*. New York: Dutton, 1964; Browne, E. G. *A Literary History of Persia*. Vol. 3. London: Cambridge University Press, 1920; Gray, E. T. *The Green Sea of Heaven*. Ashland, OR: White Cloud Press, 1995; Yarshater, Ehsan, ed. *Persian Literature*. Albany, NY: Bibliotheca Press, 1988.

Patit Paban Mishra

HAFSA BINT AL-HADJDJ (c. 1135–1190). Hafsa Bint al-Hadjdj, along with **Wallada bint al-Mustakfi**, was the most esteemed woman poet of Islamic Spain, particularly noteworthy for her passionate love odes and her long relationship with the poet Abu Ja'afar Ibn Said. She lived at a time when freedom for women in Islamic Spain were being curtailed due to the rise of puritanical North African Berber dynasties, the Almoravids and the Almohads. Hafsa managed to have a public role for some time, openly visiting Ibn Said's house and even winning the favor of the Almohads. One Almohad caliph, Abu Said Uthman, even fell in love with her, provoking Ibn Said's jealousy. In 1163, Ibn Said was imprisoned and executed for plotting against the Almohads. Hafsa wrote verses mourning his death and dressed in black to express sorrow, an action for which she was widely condemned. Shortly afterward, she abandoned poetry and became a tutor of Almohad princesses at the court of Marrakesh in North **Africa**.

Further Reading: Walther, Wiebke. *Women in Islam from Medieval to Modern Times.* Princeton, NJ: Markus Wiener Publishers, 1995.

William E. Burns

HALEVI, JUDAH (c. 1075–1141). Judah Halevi, a Spanish Jew, was a physician, merchant, poet, and philosopher. His love poems and **marriage** songs were so beautiful that they were, and still are, often included in wedding services. He lived in the Iberian peninsula and received a solid education in both Hebrew and Arabic at a time when **Jews** there lived under precarious conditions, constantly attacked by both Muslims and Christians. He married and had one daughter. Devastated by the death of his wife, he set off for the Holy Land (which was under crusader rule at the time) to fulfill his life's highest and last aspiration, *aliyah*, or "the return from the diaspora." Legend varies as to whether he actually made it to Israel or died on the way.

His most renowned work, *The Kuzari* (*The Book of Argument and Proof in Defense of the Despised Faith*), is a polemic against the use of Aristotelianism as a refutation of **Judaism**. It is a theological defense of Judaism in the face of Greek philosophy. Halevi also wrote over eight hundred poems, roughly eighty of which are considered love poems. His themes are common to Arabic-Hebrew love poetry of the time and include praise of female beauty, yearnings for love, the angst of separated lovers, and songs in honor of bride and bridegroom. Much of his poetry is replete with biblical citations and allusions, but his descriptions of female beauty more often come from nature. Occasionally, he includes a graphic comparison such as that of breasts to sweet apples or pomegranates, but the poems remain sensual or gently erotic, never lascivious or crass. Often the love poems address a deer or a gazelle. Like the *Song of Songs*, several of his love poems can be read as describing the love between God and Israel rather than the relationship between two people. Halevi's love poems accentuate female beauty and sensuous relations between man and woman; sin and guilt are absent in these verses, as is an overtly Jewish philosophy. Halevi's love poems are universally romantic.

Further Reading: Brody, Heinrich. *Selected Poems of Jehudah Halevi.* Translated by Nina Salaman. Philadelphia: Jewish Publication Society of America, 1924; Kayser, Rudolf. *The Life and Time of Judah Halevi.* New York: Philosophical Library, 1949.

Deborah Thalheimer Long

HAREM. In the Middle Ages, the harem as an institution developed in royal palaces, particularly in the Islamic world. The harem was a place of residence for wives, female slaves, war captives and servants, concubines, female relatives, and **eunuchs**. (In **India**, *hijras* were sometimes employed in harems as porters and bodyguards.)

Similar special quarters were also marked for *zennana* (females) in many aristocratic households. A classic work of Arabic literature, **the Thousand and One Nights**, depicts a female slave, Shahrazad, telling stories to the sultan in the harem, depicted as a place of intrigue, infidelity, amorous affairs, and sexual pleasure. Harems existed in the pre-Islamic world in parts of Asia, and although strongly associated with the Muslim world in popular imagination, were never limited to it. Similar institutions existed in **China**, Mesoamerica, and Hindu India. Harems were not pleasure houses—many of the women there were expected to work at household maintenance or to engage in textile production or other such activities. *See also* Islamic Society; Shajarat ad-Durr.

Further Reading: Hambly, Gavin. *Women in the Medieval Islamic World: Power, Patronage, and Piety.* New York: St. Martin's Press, 1998; Kausar, Zinat. *Muslim Women in Medieval India.* Patna, India: Janaki Prakashan, 1992.

Patit Paban Mishra

HELOISE. *See* Abelard, Peter, and Heloise

HERMAPHRODITES. The term "hermaphrodite" comes from the Latin *hermaphroditus*. This in turn derives from the Greek Hermaphroditos, originating from the ancient Greek figure, Hermaphroditos, son of Hermes and Aphrodite. Hermaphroditos was a beautiful young man who was raised by the Phrygian nymphs. Salmacis, a lake nymph, fell in love with him. He refused her advances but dove into the lake to swim. Salmacis desired never to be separated from him and prayed to the gods for help. Their response was to fuse them into one body. Realizing what had happened, Hermaphroditos asked the gods that any man who bathed in this lake should lose his virility.

The figure of Hermaphroditos would be seen today as a simultaneous hermaphrodite, one person possessing both male and female sexual organs. The other form, a sequential hermaphrodite, is one who begins life as one sex and transforms (naturally) into the other over time. This does occur in nature, and although there has never been a case of a human sequential hermaphrodite, the ancient Greek legend of Tiresias, who changed from a man to a woman and back again over the course of his life, fulfills this definition. These images are represented in the Middle Ages mainly through Ovid, who tells the story of Hermaphroditus (*Metamorphoses* 4.285–388) and whose work was frequently invoked by medieval poets and theologians alike.

Using the myth of Hermaphroditos as a starting point, the earliest definition of a hermaphrodite evokes a union of masculine and feminine identities as well as a loss of virility and masculine potency. Technically, a hermaphrodite is one who is born with the condition of gonadal dysgenesis, the appearance of both masculine and feminine sexual organs at birth. This condition occurs naturally in plants, fish, and birds, although rarely in mammals. It is common (and benign) among plants and fish but

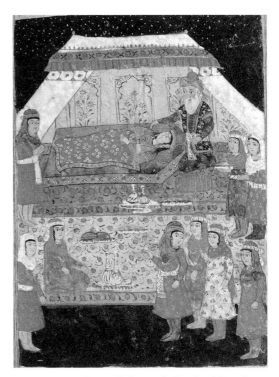

Harem scene. From *Shah-nameh* (Book of Kings), an epic poem by the Persian poet Firdausi. © The Art Archive/Dagli Orti.

when it occurs in mammals it usually results in neither set of organs being functional. The word *hermaphrodite* first appeared in English in 1398 in John Trevisa's *Bartholomeus de proprietatibus rerum*: "In harmofroditus is founde bothe sexus male and female: but alway vnperfyte." In modern times, hermaphroditism (now called *intersexuality* or *sexual bipotentiality*) is often "corrected" cosmetically through gender reassignment surgery and therapy. The irony in the medieval perceptions of hermaphroditism is that often the condition was seen as metaphorically balanced, confused with the androgyny or gender harmony of the divine. Often, too, the hermaphrodite is included among figures who, by modern definitions, should be seen as homosexuals or transvestites. This failure of medieval philosophers to fully understand the hermaphrodite, combined with their obvious desire to do so, further represents a central paradox of medieval thought: simultaneous engagement with potential spiritual interpretations while often rejecting genuine physiological reality.

Critics and medieval scholars of the last century have represented both extremes in their treatment of the medieval hermaphrodite. Some, showing the characteristic anxiety of variant sexuality of early-twentieth-century scholarship saw the hermaphrodite as a thinly veiled male homosexual. They followed the Ovidian story that Hermaphroditus retained some degree of masculine consciousness. Others, inspired by the growing critical attention to medieval mysticism and the work of Julian of Norwich, saw the hermaphrodite as an allegory of the incarnation; he has, like Julian's "Jesus as Mother," a metaphor for Christ whose sexuality is evenly distributed between the male and female nature of humanity, simultaneously embodying and fulfilling both masculine and feminine desire. *See also* Ovidianism; Theories of Sexual Difference.

Further Reading: Long, Thomas L. "Julian of Norwich's 'Christ as Mother' and Medieval Constructions of Gender." March 2005. http://members.visi.net/~longt/julian.htm; Nederman, Cary, and Jacqui True. "The Third Sex: The Idea of the Hermaphrodite in Twelfth-Century Europe." *Journal of the History of Sexuality* 6 (1996): 497–517; Silberman, Lauren. "Mythographic Transformations of Ovid's Hermaphrodite." *Sixteenth Century Journal* 19 (Winter 1988): 643–52.

Susannah Mary Chewning

HIJRAS. Hijras or **eunuchs** are castrated or cross-dressing males who maintain a third-gender role in Indian society. Neither man nor woman, hijras have performed varied functions in Indian society through different periods.

In Urdu, hijra means an impotent person. In ancient Indian texts and religious beliefs, there are examples of the third sex and even Gods taking on female attributes. Shiva has assumed the form of a woman, and the androgynous Shiva is worshipped by hijras. Arjuna in the epic *Mahabharata* led the life of a hijra in his exile. Vatsyayana's ***Kama Sutra*** (approximately third century CE) has described about the third-natured persons putting on dresses of women and performing oral sex with other men. In this homoerotic act, the hijra becomes a passive partner. The hijras worked as bodyguards and porters in the courts and **harem**s of medieval kings. They were taken into confidence because of their fierce loyalty.

The hijras sing and dance in female apparel when a new baby is born. They have become indispensable in the christening ceremony and also in marriages. They are held in contempt by some because they are aggressive in nature, and often demand money and curse a miser host. There have been cases where the hijras exposed their private parts, if ridiculed. But generally they are tolerated and their presence is seen as a good omen in family functions. The negative view toward the hijras stem from the fact that some indulge in **prostitution**, a legacy from earlier times. Many nonhijra men become their husbands. Working as pimps in brothels is another profession. Some hijras lead the life of a recluse by becoming ascetics, whose blessings are sought for begetting a child. **Transgenderism** thus leads to the power of generativity.

Living in separate communes, the hijras refer to themselves with female pronouns. There is a strong sense of kinship with each household having a master. Apart from worshipping gods and goddesses like Saraswati, Besraji, Arjuna, **Krishna**, Shiva, Amba, Shikhandin, and others, the hijras' main deity is mother goddess Bahuchara Mata. With the coming of **Islam**, hijra culture blended Muslim and Hindu elements. Both Muslim and Hindu hijras are devotees of Bahuchara Mata and bury the dead according to Islamic rites rather than the Hindu system of cremation.

Further Reading: Jaffrey, Zia. *The Invisibles: A Tale of the Eunuchs of India*. New York: Pantheon, 1996; Nanda, Serena. *Neither Man nor Woman: The Hijras of India*. Belmont, CA: Wadsworth Publishing, 1990; Sharma, Satish Kumar. *Hijras, the Labelled Deviants*. New Delhi: Gian Publishing House, 1989.

Patit Paban Mishra

HILDEGARD OF BINGEN (c. 1098–1179). Born probably near Bermersheim, Rhineland, Hildegard was the tenth child of wealthy commoners, and was given as an oblate to the church at birth. At age eight, she was sent to Jutta von Sponheim, an anchoress at Disibodenberg, who educated her in spoken Latin, psaltery, and scripture. Hildegard took the **veil** in 1112, and became abbess of Disibodenberg on Jutta's death in 1136. Although Hildegard had had visions since the age of three, her life was transformed in 1141 by an experience in which she was granted special understanding of biblical writings and prophetic visions. For the rest of her life, Hildegard dictated these revelations, primarily to her secretary, the monk Volmar. She quickly drew the attention of Pope Eugenius III, **Bernard of Clairvaux**, and numerous local nobles. She wrote three books based on her visions, *Know the Way of the Lord*, *The Book of Life's Visions*, and *Book of Divine Works*, all of which are mystical and apocalyptic, and illustrated with vivid scenes of the end time.

Although Hildegard became famous in the twentieth century for a revival of her unusual musical compositions for the convent choir, she was also widely regarded as an expert in cosmology, **medicine**, and botany. Her books *Physica* and *Causae and Curae* are works of natural history and practical medicine, based on the medieval belief in the four humors. Her interest in cataloging native plants and animals was to classify their "qualities" as hot/cold or moist/dry and thus their medical use. Hildegard dispensed frank sexual advice, promoting the role of pleasure in conceiving children, and emphasizing the contributions of the mother to the potential child's strength and character. Children conceived by passionate parents were more likely to be male and strong and healthy. Her writings may contain the first Western description of a female orgasm, described in terms of heat descending into the female genitals.

In 1148 she moved to her own convent at Rupertsburg (Bingen on Nahe), where she attracted crowds of admirers and advice seekers and dispatched letters of criticism and admonition to secular rulers like England's Henry II. Her autocratic temper sometimes irritated male church officials, who resented her influence and her performance of healings and exorcisms. She attacked heretical groups like the Cathars and met with pilgrims, although increasingly weak and suffering from lifelong migraines (which modern experts feel contributed to her visions). Volmar, her longtime friend, died in 1174, and Hildegard followed in 1179. Despite several attempts, she was never canonized, although her bones and relics are venerated and her feast day (September 17) is celebrated in Germany. *See also* Catholicism; Manicheans and Cathars; Monasticism, Female; Orgasm, Female.

Further Reading: Flanagan, Sabina. *Hildegard of Bingen*. London: Routledge, 1989; Maddocks, Fiona. *Hildegard of Bingen*. New York: Doubleday, 2001.

Margaret Sankey

HINDU LITERATURE. The medieval period was especially significant for the development of the manifold concepts of love (*kama*) in **India**. It was during this period that *kama* was recognised as one of the four objects of human life (De 1959, 91), and love surpassed the boundaries of the profane to enter the sacred sphere, engulfing both spheres equally.

In early medieval literature in Sanskrit, Prakrit, and Tamil, love was described in its purest form without any encumbrances of the society. Love and sex were discussed openly and formed part of philosophical debates. It was essential to understand and experience love even for a mendicant to obtain superior knowledge and liberation. Knowledge is incomplete unless *kama* is known and understood, as seen in the legend of Sankara (eighth century CE), one of the greatest teachers of **Hinduism**. He was asked questions on *kamasastra* by Bharati, wife of Mandana, whom he had previously defeated in philosophical debate. Since Sankara had no knowledge of love and sex, he sought a month to prepare to answer her questions. Sankara then preserved his body in the hole of a tree and his soul entered the body of a dead king, Amaru, about to be cremated. As Amaru, he experienced the many facets of love with his numerous wives and finally answered the questions of Bharati, thus displaying the superiority of his knowledge. As Amaru, he is said to have composed his Sanskrit work, the *Amaru Sataka* (700 CE), edifying his experiences and understanding of love. This is one of the earliest Sanskrit texts to discuss love in its varied forms. Amaru describes the emotion of love and the relation of lovers in isolation, without connecting it to the other aspects of life. This exemplifies one of the conventions of love, that lovers become oblivious to the other factors of life.

Another early text on love, Hala's *Gathasaptasati* (100 CE), was composed in Prakrit and contains a number of tales of romance describing the various forms of love. The depth and variety of love stories in this text captured the imagination of later poets, and a number of similar works were composed in Sanskrit. The *Brihatkathamananjari* (1100 CE) of Ksemendra, the *Kathasaritsagara* or "Ocean of Story" (1100) of Somadeva, the *Vetala Pancavimsati* (1600) of Shivadasa, and the *Sukasaptati* (1400) are some narratives of this nature.

South India has its own tradition of love poetry. The poetry of love was termed *Aham* poetry (*aham* meaning home or heart). The subject of this poetry is human love set in natural circumstances. A majority of poems in the *Ettuthokai* or "eight anthologies" of early Tamil verse (100–500 CE) can be categorized as *aham* poetry. One of the major texts of Tamil, the *Kural* of Tiruvalluvar, includes love poetry under the section on love, *Kamattuppal*. Love is celebrated in all its worldly forms in these poems: clandestine, forbidden, permissive, formal, and domestic. The underlying theme in all these texts is the satisfaction of the heart or soul. A similar sentiment is later found in the devotional poetry of **bhakti** saints who used the imagery of love to convey the unity of divine and human souls.

From these simple beginnings of narrating the union of lovers and admitting love openly in its various phases, love evolved into a topic of philosophical, scientific, and literary enquiry. Love was presented as one of the major spheres of a male's life. Hence, the literature on love and sex describes the trials and tribulations of a male in obtaining and sustaining love in premarital, marital, and extramarital relations.

Premarital or extramarital love forms the central theme of a number of texts. In this type of literature, the heroine is described as young, innocent, and susceptible. The hero is responsible for courtship, and creating and sustaining love. Feminine love or charms are described in detail while masculine beauty is sparsely described. Bana's *Kadambari* (400 CE) describes youthful and tender love, confined not only to the present life but also to a series of other lives (Layne 1991). Bhavabhuti's *Malatimadhava* (800) describes the intense and passionate love of Madhava for Malati. The descriptions of their love illustrate the tenets of **Kama Sutra** of Vatsyayana.

Unlike premarital love, married love is said to be bondage for men. Married women as heroines are subdued but more strong willed than the heroines of premarital love poetry. Nonetheless, wedded love is praised. Bhavabhuti's *Uttararamacarita* (800 CE) incorporates an ideal picture of conjugal love. Married love can remain unspoiled when stimulated by constant courtship as seen in the descriptions of Rama and Sîta in this text. Carudatta's *Mriccakatika* (400) depicts the sad but dignified wife of Carudatta with gentleness and generosity. Married love is depicted as belonging to the home. While the married love of a woman is depicted as generous, forgiving, and kind, that of a man is depicted as restricted and not always bound by the conventions of marriage.

Extramarital love with a courtesan forms part of numerous Sanskrit narratives. *Kamasutra* describes three types of courtesans: *Ekaparigraha* are the courtesans who live exclusively with one man. *Anekaparigraha* are courtesans who form relations with more than one man. The *Aparigraha* practices her profession without attachment to any man. Although the love of courtesans is considered to be unloyal and fleeting, exceptions to this are also commonly found in medieval Indian literature. Vasantasena, the rich courtesan of *Mriccakatika*, is depicted as falling in love with Carudatta. Temporary **marriage** alliances with courtesans are noted in texts. These alliances are formed for a year and the man does not retain the right of love or the company of the courtesan after that period.

The quest for love and ultimate unity surpassed the human sphere. Another special feature, which developed during the medieval period, was the divine love concept of the *bhakti* saints. The *bhakti* saints imagined the divine (god) as the male lover and devotee as the female lover irrespective of the actual gender, although most *bhakti* saints were male. Love became both profane and sacred, encompassing the secular and religious lives of the people. The *Gitagovinda* of **Jayadeva** is foremost among the texts of this genre. As noted in the premarital and marital forms of love above, the love of the (female souled) devotee for the god is as the love of a woman that is loyal, pleasing, generous, and self-surrendering. *See also Ananga Ranga*; Kalidasa.

Further Reading: De, Sushil Kumar. *Ancient Indian Erotics and Erotic Literature*. Kolkata, India: Firma K.L. Mukhopadhyay, 1959; Devadhar, Chintaman Ramachandra. *Amaruśatakam with Sringaradīpika of Vemabhpâla*. Poona: Oriental Book Agency, 1959; Jha, Damodar, ed. *Vetalapancavimsati, with "Prakash" Hindi Commentary*. Varanasi, India: Chowkamba Vidyabhavan, 1968; Kale, Moreswar Ramachandra. *Uttararamacarita of Bhavabhuti*. Mumbai, India: Gopal Narayan, 1934; Layne, Gwendolyn. *Kadambari of Banabhatta: A Classic Sanskrit Story of Magical Transformations*. New York: Garland Publications, 1991; Penzer, N. M. *The Ocean of Story Being C.H. Tawney's Translation of Somadeva's Kathasaritsagara*. New Delhi: Motilal Banarsidass, 1968; Prentiss, Karen Pechilis. *The Embodiment of Bhakti*. New York: Oxford University Press, 1999; Ramanujan, A. K. *Poems of Love and War from Eight Anthologies and Ten Long Poems of*

Classical Tamil. New York: Columbia University Press, 1985; Ray, Hrudananda. *Śankara as a Romantic Philosopher*. Cuttack, India: Akash Publications, 1991; Sundaram, P. S., trans. *The Kural of Tiruvalluvar*. London: Penguin Books, 1991.

Lavanya Vemsani

HINDUISM. Although the term Hinduism came to be used by European scholars and administrators in the nineteenth century, it was from ancient times an ideological framework in the Indian subcontinent. The followers of this religion came to be known as the Hindus. Love and sex had a special place in the religion with a prescribed agenda for harmonious life. But, as in other religions, there had been deviant behaviors also.

Hinduism prescribed *varnashramadharma* (four stages) of life along with *purushartha* (four goals) of life. The four stages of life are: *brahmacharya* (**celibacy**), *grihasthya* (household life), *vanaprastha* (hermitic life), and *sanyasa* (ascetic life). Of the four goals of life, *moksha* (liberation or enlightenment) from this mundane world is considered inclusive and superior to the other three: *dharma* (duty or moral harmony), *artha* (wealth or fame), and *kama* (sensual or emotional pleasure). Love and sex were taboo for the life of celibates, hermits, and ascetics. *Kama* was permitted only in the life of a householder. The two important functions of **marriage** were *prajaa* (progeny for family) and *rati* (sensual and emotional pleasure). Kama was the physical union of man and woman. Sex within marriage is the prescribed norm in Hinduism in all ages, which gives societal harmony. For individuals, a balanced life is possible by channeling sexual energy within marriage.

This ideal frame of reference as defined by Hindu religious texts was not adhered to in medieval **India**. People deviated from the sanctioned agenda and found their own ways. "Third gender" sex, **adultery**, and **prostitution** were found among groups and individuals in Hindu society. In tantric ritual, where the woman personified the goddess Shakti and the man embodied the god Shiva, sexual intercourse between man and woman was general practice. In the Konarak temple in Orissa and the **Khajuraho temple complex** in Madhya Pradesh, sculptures of couples in sexual positions, group sex, and tantric postures celebrated carnal pleasure in its fullest ecstasy.

The Hindu sastras regarded sexual intercourse with a *ganika* (prostitute) as *adharma* (antireligious). But in the Middle Ages, there were zones earmarked for this activity in urban centers in India. The sexual life of the royal and elite was not limited to spouses, but found expression in dalliance with concubines and courtesans. The **harem** of a king was full of women, who were not legally married wives. **Polygamy** was restricted to the elite section of society. Therefore, India in Middle Ages was not a puritan society, and life of some persons did not go as per the dharmic sanctions.

Temple prostitution revolving round the **devadasi** system was common in many parts of India. Although the *devadasis* (temple dancers) were wedded to God only, immorality had crept into the system. The brahmins, who were upholders of dharmic traditions, might have indulged in sexual intercourse with the devadasis. But Hinduism did not formalize the devadasi system as such.

In the field of literature also, sexual relations were not within the parameters prescribed by Hinduism. Love poems in vernacular languages espoused *parakiya priti* (love outside marriage) and delineated the passionate love of **Krishna** with Radha in all its details in colorful language. Women were portrayed as persons having their own feelings, emotions, and desires to be united with their beloveds. The erotic longings between women were known. These women were referred as *svarini*. They were known for their independent spirit, and did not confine themselves to homes or desire a husband. Transgendered males who dressed as women were known as *hijras* and identified themselves as a separate third sex. Many had undergone ritual **castration** and engaged in sex with men. The *hijras* participated in rituals associated with marriage and the birth of a new child. In spite of religious sanctions, they became a part of Hindu society in the Middle Ages. Hinduism attempted to build a harmonious society within its prescribed norms. Sexual minorities did not reflect the trend of society. *See also* Bhakti; Hindu Literature; Sakthism.

Further Reading: Anand, Margo. *The Art of Sexual Ecstasy*. Los Angeles: Jeremy P. Tarcher, 1989; Babras, Vijaya G. *The Position of Women during the Yadava Period: 1000 AD to 1350 AD*. Bombay, India: Himalaya Publishing House, 1996; Klostermaier, Klaus K. *A Survey of Hinduism*. New York: State University of New York Press, 1994; Meyer, Johann H. *Sexual Life in Ancient India*. New York: Barnes and Noble, 1953; Nanda, Serena. *Neither Man nor Woman: The Hijras of India*. Belmont, CA: Wadsworth, 1990; Sharma, Tripat. *Women in Ancient India, from 320 AD to c. 1200 AD*. New Delhi: Ess Publications, 1987; Vanita, Ruth, ed. *Queering India: Same-Sex Love and Eroticism in Indian Culture and Society*. New York: Routledge, 2002.

Patit Paban Mishra

HOMOSEXUALITY, FEMALE. Female homosexuality is as scarcely documented in the Middle Ages as at any other time in history, compared to male homosexuality. There was not even a vernacular term known to have been used for female homosexuality. While the word "**sodomy**" was largely used to identify male homosexual activity (although sometimes covering any unusual use of sperm, like **masturbation**, oral sex, anal intercourse, etc.), the term "lesbianism" had not entered the vernacular, and "homosexuality" was to be first documented only in 1869. Female homosexual identity and practice were not clearly and uniformly defined even in medical, legal, theological, or literary discourse. Personal records of female homosexual experience are more scarce than those of male homosexuality.

Medieval Christian doctrine considered unnatural any sexual activity for purposes other than to conceive a child, which was required to take place within the **marriage** and only in what is called the "missionary position." Carnal pleasure was considered sinful, even between husband and wife. However, female homosexuality was less discussed by early-medieval theologians than other topics related to sexuality, and it was also judged less harshly. Although it was classified as "fornication," it is less clearly defined than other sinful sexual behavior and is many times abstractly associated with heresy, Satanism, sorcery, and others. The ninth-century theologian Hincmar of Rheims wrote about women who used "diabolical instruments to excite desire." The seventh-century *Penitential* of Theodore prescribed only a three-year penance for "a woman who practices vice with another woman," which was less than the penance for male homosexuality.

The theological discussions of female homosexuality were generally based on Saint Paul's criticism, in the New Testament, of the sinfulness of Roman women who engaged in acts "against nature" (Romans 1:26). The French theologian **Peter Abelard** (1079–1142), the canon of the Notre-Dame cathedral in Paris who secretly married Heloise, who was about twenty-two years younger than him, wrote in his *Commentary on St. Paul* that relations between women are "against nature, that is, against the order of nature, which created women's genitals for the use of men and not so women could cohabit with women." The irony was that Abelard got castrated by Heloise's uncle later on and Heloise became a nun to prove her devotion.

The German **Albertus Magnus** (c. 1193–1280) and his Italian pupil **Thomas Aquinas** (1225–1273) set the linguistic norm by including female homosexuality in the "sodomy" category. In *Summa Theologica*, Aquinas places sodomy second only to **bestiality**, which is considered the worst of all the sins of the flesh. Nevertheless, female homosexual interaction is believed to have been relatively common even in the Middle Ages. It was actually in the convents that the lesbians escaped the constraints of society and were able to follow their inclinations, although secretly and under very severe constraints. It is said that **Augustine** (354–420) warned his sister about the temptations of the monastic lifestyle when she chose to become a nun. Church leaders themselves were quite aware of this situation and hence imposed very strict regulations on convent life. For example, nuns were not allowed to sleep together or to enter each other's cell at night, and were required to sleep clothed, with lamps lit at all times, and not to lock their doors at night, and also not to form friendships within the convent. However, records of close relationships between nuns have survived. From the twelfth century, there are the anonymous verse letters written in Latin by one Bavarian nun to another, and also the writings of **Hildegard of Bingen** (1098–1179), a German abbess, mystic author, and composer, expressing her affection for another woman, Richardis von Stade. Although physical involvement is not mentioned in any of these texts, it might be read as implied in the context of medieval mysticism, where the spiritual and the physical tend to overlap.

Medieval literature largely reflects the views of the church on female homosexuality. Étienne de Fougères, bishop of Rennes, mentions female couples in his *Livre de Manières* (*Book of Manners*), written between 1174 and 1178, only to point them out as "against the laws of nature" and deserving to be beaten, stoned, or killed. There are also the medieval **romance**s that frequently include women dressed as men and getting romantically involved with other women, but leading to ambiguous denouements that do not really allow for female homoeroticism. For example, in *Huon de Bordeaux*, a thirteenth-century French romance, the Virgin Mary intervenes and transforms the cross-dressed woman into a man.

Early in the Middle Ages, secular law did not provide language to distinguish between male and female homosexuality, nor did it provide excessively harsh punishments. The situation changed in the thirteenth century, when lesbianism began to be viewed as a capital offence. The earliest legal text to make such a distinction is the French *Livre de Jostice et de Plet* (*Book of Justice and Complaints*), from about 1270, which in paragraph 23 lists the penalties for female sodomy: dismemberment for the first two offences and burning at the stake for the third. In Italy, Cino da Pistoia (1270–1336), poet and friend of **Dante Alighieri**, offered an interpretation of *lex foedissimam* (Roman sex law) in his *Commentaria* on Emperor Justinian's criminal code, as including "women who exercise their **lust** on other women and pursue them like men." This might have been taken into account by Bartolomeus of Saliceto in 1400 when he prescribed the death penalty for the defilement of a woman by another woman. In Germany, in 1507, the *Constitutio criminali* of Bamberg, Bavaria, decreed burning at the stake as proper punishment for women "who have lain together." By 1532 the death penalty became the legal norm for lesbianism throughout the later Roman empire when it was included in the criminal code of Emperor Charles V (*Constitutio criminalis carolina*).

In the medical field there is mention of drugs used to cure women's desire for other women (the earliest was found in an Arabic text). Also, genital mutilation as treatment for female homosexuality became common practice with its postulation by William of Saliceto in his *Summa conservationis* (1285) and would continue to be used for this purpose throughout the nineteenth century. *See also* Bieris da Romans.

Further Reading: Sautman, Canadé, amd Pamela Sheingorn. *Same Sex Love and Desire among Women in the Middle Ages.* New York: Palgrave, 2001.

Georgia Tres

HOMOSEXUALITY, MALE. The term "homosexuality," despite legitimate criticism, such as of John Boswell (1980, p. 41ff.), commonly designates both preference for as well as the actual act of erotic contact exclusively with a member of the same sex or gender identity. As far as components of sex and gender are subject to constant historical and psychosocial changes, the concept of homosexuality undergoes the same processes. Therefore, Michel Foucault has argued that talking about homosexuality necessarily would include a concept of heterosexuality, that same-sex experiences of a modern Western male were incommensurable with those of other cultures or times. This basic sociologic debate between constructionalism and essentialism took place primarily in the United States and the Netherlands. The first viewpoint is orthodox to authors such as Alan Bray or Barry D. Adam, the latter to Guido Ruggiero or John Boswell. During the last decade the opinion seems to prevail that a strict either-or dichotomy may lead nowhere. Still the problem in terminology remains: There was no such term as "homosexual" known in the Middle Ages.

The rising Christianity of late antiquity, with its general tendency toward downgrading the body in favor of transcendent values, formed the term "sodomy" in reference to the sinful biblical cities of Sodom and Gomorrah. This term was applied to a variety of sexual practices commonly regarded as being unnatural (*peccatum contra naturam*)—**bestiality**, necrophilia, and heterosexual intercourse in unaccepted manners such as anal and oral sex. Yet the condition of being a sodomite was not seen as innate but as an acquired habit or a temporary mistake resulting in full responsibility of the delinquent. In addition, there are only a few significant sources on the self-perception of those involved in acts of same-sex sexuality. Hence, most studies of medieval homosexuality rather focus on charting social responses and the social framework of the phenomenon, deemed both a deadly sin and a serious legal crime deserving severe punishments. This was true for Roman Catholic and Byzantine Christianity, and to a lesser extent for the Islamic world. Cultures of the Far East seem to have been more open toward a social acceptance of male homosexuality in those times. In **Japan**, for instance, legal restrictions cannot be traced prior to the Tokugawa government in 1629.

Islam considered homosexual practices (*liwat*) as acts of **adultery** (*zina*), which was a major moral and religious crime. However, numerous literary sources report on homoerotic relationships mostly between older and younger men. On the other hand, is it hard to disguise topical narratives within the sources since it seemed improper for Islamic poets to display female bodies in any erotic context. In legal practice, the strict rules of evidence actually prevented many trials against *luti* (i.e., men performing *liwat*). The earlier Byzantine chroniclers such as Procopius, Theophanes, and Johannes Malalas reveal brutal excesses against homosexuals. The Code of Justinian created the framework for the later trials against sodomites, while the Macedonian and Isaurian codifications provided the death penalty for adult sodomites. Justinian himself then added two Novells to the *Corpus Iuris Civilis*, with a demonising yet rather admonishing character. Besides the two passages from the Digests none of those penal laws found their way into the Basilics. Later **Byzantium** knows no surviving example of carrying out any of the strict penalties against homosexuals. The Eastern church fathers, such as

Gregory of Nyssa or Basilius, even compared male homosexuality to acts of adultery, incurring a fifteen-year excommunication.

The criminalization of sodomites in Western Christianity seems to have developed even more diversely. The Milano Codifications of 342 had threatened sodomites with harsh penalties (*poena exquisitae*) on life and body. But throughout the early Middle Ages, sexual deviation was mostly coped with in the sphere of **confession** and penance, of which the *libri poenitalis* and the *Decretum* of Burchard of Worms (1025) provide rich evidence. With the papal reforms of the eleventh and twelfth centuries, more severe persecution of sexual vices was pushed forward, formulated by **Peter Damian** in the *Liber Gomorrhianus*. The Third Lateran Council in 1179 imposed excommunication on laymen, and degradation combined with compulsory commitment to a monastery on clerics performing homosexual acts (X 5.31.4). It is hard to spot the point when sodomy reentered lay jurisdiction. The reception of **Roman law** brought the relevant passages from the Digests and Justinian's Novells into western European penal law, which still remained only a segment in the course of antisodomite legislation. Primarily, German and Italian town laws declared specific statutes against certain acts of sexual deviation, a process that is especially well explored in Venice. Most prescribed penalties ranging from fines to penalties of honor. The death penalty (mostly by beheading) was seldom imposed, although from the thirteenth century on sodomy had developed into a death-worthy offence in **canon law** (X 5.1.1–27; X 5.7.1–16) and certain town laws. In 1532 Charles V's *Constitutio Criminals Carolina* (§116) codified the death penalty by burning for the Holy Roman empire.

Accusations of homosexuality were employed from antiquity through the Middle Ages against targets including Magnus VII and Popes John XXII and Boniface VIII. Religious groups such as the Cathars who denied the strict connection of sexuality to reproduction were collectively suspected of homosexual misdeeds. The papal letter *Vox in rama* (1233) established the nexus between sexual deviation and heresy for centuries, which was widely spread by the vernacular sermons of itinerant preachers such as Giordano of Pisa, Geiler of Keysersberg, **Bernardino of Siena**, **Vicente Ferrer**, and Berthold of Regensburg. *See also* Abu Nuwas; Alain of Lille; Anal and Intercrural Sex; Pederasty; Sodomy.

Further Reading: Boswell, John. *Christianity, Social Tolerance and Homosexuality: Gay People in Western Europe from the Beginning of the Christian Era to the Fourteenth Century*. Chicago: University of Chicago Press, 1980; Dalla, Danilo. "Ubi Venus mutatur." *Omosessualità e diritto nel mondo romano*. Milano: Giuffrè, 1987; Hergemöller, Bernd-Ulrich, ed. *Sodom und Gomorrha. Zur Alltagswirklichkeit und Verfolgung Homosexueller im Mittelalter*. Hamburg: Männerschwarm Skript Verlag, 2000; Richards, Jefferey. *Sex, Dissidence and Damnation. Minority Groups in the Middle Ages*. London: Routledge, 1994; Ruggiero, Guido. *The Boundaries of Eros. Sex Crime and Sexuality in Renaissance Venice*. New York: Oxford University Press, 1987.

Hiram Kümper

HOURIS. In **Islam**, houris are charming, eternally youthful maidens who reward male believers in paradise. With their chastity intact after renewal, they wait in paradise for men who die as martyrs. Seventy-two wide-eyed beauties with ponderous and rounded breasts would entertain true Muslims in the grapevines as wives. The houris, untouched by man or *jinn*, would wait upon the believers reclining on beautiful carpets. Each one of the male faithful would have the pleasure of not one, but two wives or Hur al-Ayn in this house of paradise, surmounted by a dome of costly gems and having 80,000 servants. *Surah* 56 of the Qur'an states that the Muslims, who were guarding against evil, would be in a cozy place in paradise, wearing fine silks. They would get married to houris. The promised paradise also offered young boys, white as pearls. The *hadiths* or sayings of the Prophet described sensual pleasure in paradise for the true believers killed in battle. In this respect, Islam differed from Christianity, which found no place for sex in heaven. However, many scholars believe that the description in the Islamic texts of a sensual life in paradise is allegorical.

The Islamic belief in houris glorified the beauty of the maidens of paradise. But it also gave a special status to the female believers, who would be queens in paradise and have houris for their servants. This was the reward of Allah for women faithful. The houris had an advice for the mundane wives of the believers: not to annoy their husbands and thereby invite the wrath of Allah. These husbands were in the earth temporarily and would soon join the heavenly beauties. The Shiites believed that Fatima, Muhammad's daughter, was a houri and her husband Ali would have her only as wife.

This afterlife full of pleasure and sensual bliss had a striking similarity with the Persian ideas of paradise. Ancient Persian traditions speak of female spirits (*hur* in Pahlavi) enchanting the hearts of men. There is a similar concept in **Hinduism**: beautiful maidens or *Apsaras* residing in paradise or *swarga*.

Further Reading: Awde, Nicholas, ed. and trans. *Women in Islam: An Anthology from the Qur'an and Hadiths*. New York: St. Martin's Press, 2000; Stowasser, Barbara. *Women in the Qur'an, Traditions, and Interpretation*. New York: Oxford University Press, 1994.

Patit Paban Mishra

I

IBN DAWUD AL-ZAHIR, MUHAMMAD (d. 909). Ibn Dawud was a Zahiri jurist and compiler of poetry. Nothing is known of his life in detail, except a little about his Zahirism, a movement focusing on the "outer" (zahir) meaning of the Holy Book. He was the son of Dawud b. 'Ali, founder of the Zahiri legal school in Baghdad, and took over the movement upon the death of his father. Around him gathered not only Zahiri jurists, but also a group of scholars and grammarians of various denominations. He also wrote or transmitted many Zahiri works. However, his claim to fame is the *Kitab al-zahra* (*Book of the Flower* or *Book of Venus*). The *Zahra* is an anthology of poetry that has been interpreted as the Arab codification of **courtly love**, although it is difficult to comprehend its composition, its deeper purposes, and its guiding inspiration.

The book is dedicated to a friend whose identity remains unknown. A number of poems are ascribed to "a contemporary"; later writers assumed that Ibn Dawud himself was their author. The book consists of two parts: The first part is a collection of love poetry, a peculiarity that is explained by the fact that Ibn Dawud wished it to resemble a Qasida, the dominant form of pre-Islamic poetry, which centers in an elegy on past love. The second part is an anthology proper, which is devoted to different genres of poetry (elegy, wisdom, panegyric, satire, wine song, etc.) or to different poetical motifs. Both parts are arranged in chapters, each originally containing about a hundred verses or lines of poetry. The chapters are destined to illustrate different maxims, all of which are put into rhymed prose (the elegant style of a jurist) but are of varying importance. The first ten chapters are kind of an ethic of love, followed by the misfortunes that befall lovers like calumniators, slanderers, and "exile," but also by obstacles of a more permanent and serious nature, and by a classification of situations reminiscent of the Nasib as the love section of the Qasida. At the end of the first part, ethical values return to the foreground, in particular the virtue of keeping one's love hidden.

Ibn Dawud is the first to mention a Hadith, transmitted on the authority of his father, which focuses attention on the love-secret: "He who loves, remains chaste, does not tell his love, and dies, dies as a martyr." This Hadith aroused opposition especially among the Hanbalis, as it defended al-Nazar al-mubah (the lawfulness of glancing at young people and/or women) and Kitman (the obligation to refrain from speaking of one's love). This opposition is meaningful. Hanbali scripturalism, as can be inferred from **Ibn Qayyim al-Jawziyya**'s preoccupation with love, in spite of itself attributed to the passions a sort of therapeutic action and even tended to approve of the pure love of God. The Zahiri Ibn Dawud, however, being no less a scripturalist than the Hanbalis, had nothing of that sort in mind. He approved of any sort of passion as long as the lover refrains from speaking of his love, even to the person he loves. As this has some resemblance with the self-restraint of the **troubadours** and of the *Minnesinger* in the medieval West, this type of love has been classified as "courtly."

Further Reading: Giffen, Lois Anita. *Theory of Profane Love among the Arabs: The Development of the Genre.* New York: New York University Press, 1971; Raven, W. "Ibn Dawud al-Isbahani and His Kitab al-Zahra." PhD diss., Leiden, Amsterdam: Leiden University, 1989; Vadet, J.-C. *L'esprit courtois en Orient dans les cinq premiers siÈcles de l'hÈgire.* Damascus, 1956.

Susanne Enderwitz

IBN GABIROL, SOLOMON (c. 1022–c. 1070). Solomon ben Yehuda ibn Gabirol, the greatest Iberian Hebrew liturgical poet and an important Neo-Platonic philosopher, wrote during the golden age of Jewish poetry in Islamic Spain. He was born in Malaga, Andalusia, and was orphaned while young. Ibn Gabirol studied literature, philosophy, and science in Hebrew and Arabic with Yekutiel ibn Hasan in Saragossa (Zaragosa). By the time he was sixteen, he displayed such poetic skill that he was viewed as a prodigy. He wrote hundreds of poems and twenty books. Ibn Gabirol's religious poetry has been used in synagogue worship. Some liturgical poems are still in use in Sephardic worship. Some of his poetry was influenced by Neo-Platonism and expresses love for God. However, the love is intellectual and not emotionally devotional.

Gabirol did not speak directly of sex. His few discussions of love are expressions of a mystical desire for union with the ineffable. In both love poems and liturgical poems he uses "erotic" (for the times) images in the manner of the *Song of Solomon*. Ibn Gabirol praises God's faithful love (*hesed*). Human love for God centers on the Shema, "Hear O Israel ... you shall love the Lord your God with your whole mind." His emphasis on love is liturgical or Platonic. His poetic treatment of friendship stresses the importance of this form of love.

Gabirol's social poems are sometimes mistakenly called "secular." They are social poems because they deal with daily life, but they do not treat life as lived profanely apart from God. The themes of the social poems include friendship, life, or loneliness. Some are wine songs, love songs, spring poems, rain poems, or flower portraits. Some praise ibn Gabirol's patrons, others are satirical attacks, or dirges. The wine songs and love poems followed Arabic models, but were written in Hebrew.

Ibn Gabirol wrote on philosophy in some poems and in the *Fountain of Life* (Latin *Fons Vitae*). It was preserved for centuries under the name of Avincebron (or Avencebrol). It was heavily influenced by Neo-Platonist thought, including that of Plotinus, and influenced Christian scholasticism in the Middle Ages, Benedict Spinoza and the Kabballists. It was identified as the work of ibn Gabirol only in 1846. His other works include a collection of proverbs, *Mukhtar al-jawahir* (*Choice of Pearls*), an ethical treatise, *Kitab islah al-akhlaq* (*The Improvement of the Moral Qualities*), and *Keter Malkut* (*The Crown of the Kingdom*).

Ibn Gabirol seems to have been afflicted with a serious skin disease that kept him in seclusion, and he was unable to requite his youthful love. It may have contributed to his death in 1070 at Valencia.

Further Reading: Cole, Peter, trans. *Selected Poems of Solomon Ibn Gabirol.* Princeton, NJ: Princeton University Press, 2000; Loewe, Raphael. *Ibn Gabirol.* London: Peter Halban Publisher, 1989.

Andrew J. Waskey

IBN HAZM, ABU MUHAMMAD ALI (994–1064). Abu Muhammad ibn Hazm al-Andaluci was a versatile genius who notably contributed to jurisprudence, theology, literature, calligraphy, and history in the Islamic world. He was born into an aristocratic family of Cordoba, Spain, on November 7, 994, and was educated in Arabic philosophy and poetry. Like his father, Ibn Hazm was connected with the Umayyad caliph's court. His stormy political life resulted in being imprisoned thrice and being frequently banished from Cordoba. He served as the grand *Wazir* caliph Abdul Rahman IV (1018–1024). He engaged in scholarship from the age of thirty-two. Ibn Hazm took extreme positions in interpreting Islamic texts like hadiths and criticized vehemently scholars with whom he differed. For this, he was exiled and his books burnt.

Ibn Hazm is credited with about 400 works on varied disciplines, including *al-Akhlaq wa al-Siyar fi Mudawat al-Nufus* (Morals and Right Conduct in the Healing of Souls), *Tawq al-Hamama fi al-Ulfa wa al-Ullaf* (The Ring of the Dove: Love and Lovers), *Maratib al-'Ulum* (The Categories of the Sciences), and *al-Mujalla* (The Brilliant Treatise). A master of Arabic, his talent in prose and poetry was evident in the *Tawq al-hamamah*, a book including love poetry in praise of both men and women; numerous anecdotes of Ibn Hazm's contemporaries, male and female, free and slave; and instructions on the art and practices of love. Although it included sexually explicit and pedestrian verses, nevertheless, the *Tawq al-hamamah* analyzed the concept of love esoterically. For Ibn Hazm, the pinnacle of love was the love of God, and human affection was love at the nadir. Influenced by Plato, he believed that human love was an amalgamation of incomplete beings. Love would become fragile if a lover perceived appearance only. True love would occur if one went beyond appearance into the deeper realm. The *Tawq al-hamamah* was also a treatise on psychology and metaphysics with deeper meanings. The last part of Ibn Hazm's life was devoted toward managing his family estate, writing, and teaching. He died on August 15, 1064, at Manta Lisham, near Sevilla. *See also* Courtly Love.

Further Reading: Chejne, A. *Ibn Hazm*. Chicago: Kazi Publications, 1982; Fletcher, Richard. *Moorish Spain*. Berkeley: University of California Press, 1992; Ibn Hazm, Ali ibn Ahmad. *The Ring of the Dove: A Treatise on the Art and Practice of Arab Love*. Translated by A. J. Arberry. New York: AMS Press, 1981; Irwin, Robert, ed. *Night & Horses & the Desert: An Anthology of Classical Arabic Literature*. New York: Overlook Press, 2000.

Patit Paban Mishra

IBN QAYYIM AL-JAWZIYYA (1292–1350). A theologian and jurist in Damascus, Ibn Qayyim was a member of the Hanbali school, which offered strict interpretation of Islamic law. His father being the custodian (qayyim) of the Jawziyya school in Damascus, he became known as Ibn Qayyim. His doctrinal and literary output was considerable and includes Qur'anic exegesis, hadith, jurisprudence, rhetoric, poltics, and others. He is still very highly esteemed not only among the neo-Hanbali Wahhabiyya of Saudi Arabia, but also among the modernist-reformist Salafiyya in Egypt and in many circles of North African **Islam**.

Although he was of rather humble origin, Ibn Qayyim's education was particularly wide and sound. His father, who had received a firsthand knowledge of the Hanbali school of law, became his first teacher. After absorbing a training in Hanbalism and developing a predilection for **Sufism**, at the age of twenty-one Ibn Qayyim joined the circle of the renowened Hanbali teacher Ahmad Ibn Taymiyya (d. 1328). He helped to popularize Ibn Taymiyya's work, while retaining his own personality. Unlike his master, he was much more strongly influenced by Sufism. Much less of a polemicist than his master, he made himself known as a preacher and trained a number of famous scholars such as the historian Ibn Kathir (d. 1373), the jurist Ibn Rajab (d. 1397), and the traditionist Ibn Hajar al-'Askalani (d. 1449). His career was modest, as it was impeded by members of the ruling Mamluk circles who looked suspiciously upon the neo-Hanbalism of Ibn Taymiyya. In 1326 Ibn Qayyim was imprisoned in the citadel of Damascus, at the same time as his master, and only released after the latter's death in 1328. In 1331–1332 he made the pilgrimage to Mecca, together with a considerable number of other jurists and traditionists. When Ibn Qayyim died, he left behind him the justified reputation of a writer of great talent.

Apart from his juridical, doctrinal, and political works in the narrower sense, some of his more literary works deserve to be mentioned in greater detail. In *Rawdat al-muhibbin*, Ibn Qayyim gives the Hanbali doctrine of sacred and profane love its most eloquent and definite presentation. Although much of his interest in general is directed toward love in all of its forms, he clearly gives preference to the love of God, the love of His word, and the virtues of a pious human. The *Akhbar al-nisa'* is an anecdotic book in ten chapters that describe women and their qualities, passionate love, jealousy, and fidelity. However, it is now held to have been wrongly attributed to him. In his *Fawa'id*, he devotes himself to the uniqueness and inimitability of the Qur'an, and analyzes rhetoric and related topics. His *Madarij al-salikin*, a commentary on the famous spiritual guide *Manazil al-sa'irin* of al-Ansari al-Harawi (d. 1089), can be considered the masterpiece of Hanbali mystic literature. It seems that he also composed a large treatise on the Sufi "hearing" (sama'), in which he dealt with spiritual music, song, and poetry. In the work of Ibn Qayyim al-Jawziyya we find a remarkable amalgam of juridical sobriety with a deep sense for human emotions; a profound interest in the relations between love, longing, and pain; and even a tendency toward the pure love of God.

Further Reading: Bell, Joseph Norment. *Love Theory in Later Hanbalite Islam.* Albany: State University of New York Press, 1979; Giffen, Lois Anita. *Theory of Profane Love among the Arabs: The Development of the Genre.* New York: New York University Press, 1971; Kilpatrick, H. "Some late 'Abbasid and Mamluk Books about Women: A Literary Historical Approach." *Arabica* 42 (1995): 56–78.

Susanne Enderwitz

IBN RUSHD (Averroes) (1126–1198). Known in the West as Averroes, Abu al-Walid Muhammad ibn Ahmad ibn Muhammad ibn Rushd was one of the most important philosopher-physicians of Moorish Spain (al-Andalus). He was born at Cordoba in 1126 and served as an Islamic judge (qadi) in both Seville and Cordoba.

Ibn Rushd's commentaries on Aristotle were translated into Latin, winning him a reputation as "The Commentator." His *Destruction of the Destruction*, a defense of philosophy against theologians (1179), failed to save philosophic study from the antiphilosophic movements in the Islamic world. His writiings as a physician were numerous. He wrote *General Medicine* (*al-Kulliyat fi'l Tabb*, 1162–1169), translated into Latin as *Colliget*. Other medical works include *On Fever, On Humours, On Theriac,* and a long list of summaries of Galen's medical treatises. He also wrote a commentary on **Ibn Sina**'s medical poem *al-Urjuzah* (1179–1180).

In the *Colliget* Ibn Rushd discusses problems of male and female sterility. He reported, but somewhat skeptically, that the beginning of sterility lay in a bad complexion. Whether a bad complexion was due to a material or nonmaterial cause he was unable to say. Following Galen's teachings, Ibn Rushd said the function of semen is to generate. It is cast into the womb, which holds it closely in the uterus. The uterus has a retentive function as a hollow organ. It exercises its retentive function when the semen is planted so that it rests and is closed for the duration of the pregnancy. It then exercises its eliminative function. If a woman's womb has an ailment it can lead to expulsion of the sperm because excessive heat or cold had made it no longer viable.

Male sterility is caused by a decline in the ability of the testicles to absorb food from the blood. If the testicles are too hot the sperm may burst, but if too cool then the sperm will be undercooked. In discussing the health of the male genitalia, Ibn Rushd noted that if a man's testicles are cold, then he would be sluggish in coitus. If the testicles were both cold and dry then he would be impotent. Physical weakness or a distorted form can rob the penis of its expulsive power. In addition, the penis will be unable to ejaculate when the cord that sustains the erection is cut.

On questions of detecting **virginity**, Ibn Rushd reports that the vulva of a virgin is wrinkled. The size of the vaginal opening is an indicator of sexual experience. The smaller the opening the lesser the experience, so if a woman is tight and hard to penetrate it is a sign of virginity. If easy, then she is likely to be experienced. Ibn Rushd died in exile at Marrakesh in 1198. *See also* Medicine.

Further Reading: Besteiro, J. M. Forneas, and C. Alvarez de Morales. *Kitab al-Kulliyyat fi l-tibb*. Madrid: Escuela de Estudios Arabes de Granada, 1987; Fakhry, Majid. *Ibn Rushd (Averroes): His Life, Works and Influence*. Oxford: Oneworld, 2001.

Andrew J. Waskey

IBN SINA (Avicenna) (980–1037). Avicenna is the Latinized name of Abu 'Ali al-Husayn ibn 'Abd Allah ibn Sina, who was born in 980 in Afshana near Bukhara (now in Uzbekistan) to a Persian family. Growing up in the monarchial courts of the region, he acquired the skills of a courtier and mastered the Qur'an, Islamic law and logic, metaphysics, and **medicine**. While a young man he became the court physician to the Samanids. In 1022 Ibn Sina moved to Isfahan, where he joined the court of 'Ala ad-Dawlah. While in Isfahan he finished several major books including the encyclopedic *Kitab ash-shifa* (*Book of Healing*) and the *Qanun fi at-tibb* (*Canon of Medicine*). In all, he composed around 200 works including the first Persian commentary on Aristotle's philosophy.

In the *Canon of Medicine* Ibn Sina discussed numerous aspects of human sexuality. He thought the female orgasm was vital since this caused a woman to emit her seed. He stated that the hair around the vulva should be rubbed because it plays a major role in female arousal. It is one of three motions or rubbings that occur in coitus and that delight women. The second motion is that arising from the rubbing or flow of a woman's lubrication. The third motion that produces delight is the motion of the man's sperm. By this he seems to mean the man's climax during coitus. The man should also use his face and eyes to captivate the woman. Ibn Sina's medical opinion was that marital sex gave both husband and wife healthy pleasure. However, excessive sexual intercourse may produce numerous undesirable side effects. These include weakness, trembling, nervousness, ringing in the ears, protruding eyeballs, abdominal pain, hemorrhaging, and other symptoms.

Ibn Sina also wrote *Kitab an-najat* (*The Book of Salvation*) and *Kitab al-isharat wa at-tanbihat* (*The Book of Directives and Remarks*). He described the mystic's spiritual journey from the beginnings of faith to the final state of direct uninterrupted vision of God. His philosophy was strongly influenced by the Neoplatonism of al-Farabi. Philosophy explicated the ends toward which love moves each aspect of the cosmos in order to fulfill its potential. Love's role was to energize the cosmos and direct it to an end. Ibn Sina wrote an *Risala fi-l-'ishq* (*Epistle on Love*) using allegorical language to analogously describe the unseen. Ibn Sina died in 1037 while on a military campaign with 'Ala ad-Dawlah, the ruler of Isfahan. His health had been undermined by excessive drinking and sexual indulgence.

Further Reading: Fakhry, Majid. *A History of Islamic Philosophy*. New York: Columbia University Press, 1983; Heath, Peter. *Allegory and Philosophy in Avicenna (Ibn Sina)*. Philadelphia: University of Pennsylvania Press, 1992.

Andrew J. Waskey

ILLEGITIMACY. Illegitimacy, or bastardy, is the condition of a child born of parents who are not married. The concept was almost unknown before the spread of Christianity in western Europe in the early Middle Ages. The combination of church influence and a move to an individualistic society, in which inheritance rights were increasingly important, created a culture whose people valued monogamous unions and nuclear families.

In societies that practiced **polygamy** and/or **concubinage**, children produced by relationships outside of **marriage** carried no stigma and were not barred from inheriting property. Roman and Greek societies were the first to make a powerful move toward monogamy in the early Middle Ages. This was largely an attempt to break down extended kinship groups so that one family could not control wealth or power. By law, if not completely in practice, Romans recognized only monogamous unions, and children born outside of marriage could inherit nothing and retained the social status of the mother. The Roman church adopted these practices and supported them with interpretation of scripture. It was not as difficult to impose monogamy on Western cultures as it would have been in the East. In Western societies, polygamy was practiced to a lesser degree and not as frequently as it was in Asian and Muslim societies.

Illegitimacy in the Middle Ages was fairly well documented among the upper classes, and especially among royalty. Because its importance was mainly in the area of inheritance, it was not well recorded among the lower classes. In Europe, as in Rome, bastards were forbidden by law to inherit property. There were ways around this, however. Since legitimacy was related to the validity of a marriage, the church held the power to determine the legitimacy of a child. Rights of inheritance were left to secular courts. There were loopholes through which the secular courts would grant ownership of property even though the supplicant may have been deemed illegitimate by the church.

Although the church railed against sexual relations outside marriage throughout this period, illegitimacy did not carry as much social stigma as it did in later generations. Royal bastards were often recognized and loved as well or better than legitimate children. William I (c. 1028–1087), who conquered England in 1066, was often called William the Bastard even in official documents. William was the illegitimate son of Duke Robert I of Normandy and, after the duke's death, his family eventually recognized William as the heir. He went on to capture the throne of England on the basis of his assertion that Edward the Confessor, a distant cousin, had promised him the succession.

Among the poor, the church may have had more influence in the lack of acceptance of bastard children and their mothers. The church was so sexually repressive, especially after the thirteenth century, that unwed mothers might have faced unbearable shame within the village. Some left to places where they were not known, to bear their children. Some bore their children in secret, and the child was raised as a sibling to the mother. There have been attempts to investigate infant deaths and abandonment in order to determine the extent to which they represent bastard children. It has so far proved impossible to document. It is thought that some infants were killed or abandoned at birth and then pronounced stillborn. There are conflicting reports, however, about the numbers and types of infant remains found, and it is unlikely that we will ever know the truth.

The leaders of the Catholic Church itself were not immune from the temptations that led to bastardy. Many bishops raised their sons as nephews in their households and helped them rise within the aristocracy. Nepotism (favoritism of relatives by those in power), is derived from the Latin word for nephew and has its roots in this practice. Several popes were also known to have married or kept concubines and fathered children. The church reforms of the later Middle Ages appear to have had some effect, as there was a marked decrease in this activity during the thirteenth century.

Further Reading: Duby, Georges, ed. *A History of Private Life: Revelations of the Medieval World*. Cambridge, MA: Harvard University Press, 1988; Hanawalt, Barbara A. *The Ties That Bound: Peasant Families in Medieval England*. New York: Oxford University Press, 1986.

Jennifer Della'Zanna

IMPOTENCE. Impotence means the incapability of a man or a woman to have intercourse. This could arise, for example, from male erectile dysfunction, **castration**, lack of testicles, or vaginal constriction. Both men and women could alternatively suffer from frigidity, a lack of sexual desire and capacity. During the Middle Ages impotence was more than a mere medical problem as it could affect the validity of **marriage**.

All four main Islamic law schools allowed wives to obtain an annulment for their husbands' impotence, although Muhammed's views on **divorce** in such cases may have been more restrictive. The law schools insisted that a year had to elapse between marriage and annulment. Moreover, petition had to be made without delay. The schools disagreed on whether annulments were only possible before consummation and whether husbands could be granted annulments for vaginal blockage in their wives. Impotent men could licitly acquire magical healing amulets as a cure. In **India**, impotence was also an acceptable reason for women to divorce their husbands.

Conjugal intercourse was a significant aspect of Jewish matrimony as the **Jews** considered having children the main aim of marriage. Indeed, consummation was necessary for the validity of a Jewish marriage. Both spouses had a duty to grant each other the conjugal sexual rights, and persistent refusal was a ground for divorce. If a man was unable to provide his wife with her conjugal sexual rights because of weakness, illness, or impotence, and the inability persisted after a six-month convalescence period, the wife was entitled to a divorce. While Byzantine law permitted divorce for male impotence, the Orthodox Slavs had no such provision, consummation not being a precondition for valid matrimony.

Medieval Catholic marriage doctrine gave the most attention to impotence. The early medieval practice wavered between granting a divorce for impotence and forcing the spouses to remain together like brother and sister. In the twelfth century, impotence was perceived as an impediment to marriage but only if it prevented initial physical consummation. Impotence after consummation lacked legal relevance, and the conjugal bond remained intact. Medieval Catholic **canon law** distinguished between relative and absolute impotence, the former preventing intercourse with a particular partner—caused, for example, by sorcery—and the latter with everyone. Impotence could also be temporary or absolute.

Classical canon law knew three principal means of proving impotence: seven oath-helpers confirming the plaintiff's oath, physical examination, and triennial trial cohabitation. Physical examination, the paramount of these, involved knowledgeable laymen, honest and experienced matrons or expert witnesses (physicians, surgeons, or **midwives**), testifying of their findings in court. In addition, ecclesiastical courts heard witnesses attesting to repeated efforts to consummate. The impotent spouse was usually denied the right to remarry after the annulment.

The church remained skeptical of relative and temporary impotence caused by sorcery, even though former lovers or prospective suitors could wish to impede the consummation of the marriage by evil spells, tying knots, or putting hard beans in the conjugal bed or at the entrance. Unless the impotence caused by sorcery was cured by exorcism or countermagic, ecclesiastical courts occasionally annulled such unconsummated unions.

The medical profession devised remedies for impotence. Western, Islamic, and Jewish scholarly treatises dealing with this issue observed that grief, anxiety, exertion, or latent homosexuality could undermine erections and cause impotence. Signs of impotence were described; for example, penile failure to shrink in cold water and absence of erection. Lack of bodily heat due to cold and dry melancholic temperament could occasion deficient sexual desire and impotency. This was treated with enemata, hot oils, ointments, or warm and spicy foods. Operations could also be performed on too narrow women.

Chinese, Japanese, and Indian **medicine** dealt with the preservation of vitality and potency. Chinese sexual handbooks frequently dealt with preserving the male capacity and avoiding impotence: the "deer horn potion," for instance, healed infirmity and erectile failure. Cures for deficient potency were also known in other cultures, for example, the Incas used for this purpose the dried body of a minuscule hummingbird (*causarca*). *See also* Magic.

Further Reading: Brundage, James A. *Law, Sex, and Christian Society in Medieval Europe.* Chicago: University of Chicago Press, 1987; Gulik, R. H. van. *Sexual Life in Ancient China. A Sexual Survey of Chinese Sex and Society from ca. 1500 BC till 1644 AD.* Leiden: Brill, 1961; Jacquart, Danielle, and Claude Thomasset. *Sexuality and Medicine in the Middle Ages.* Cambridge: Polity Press, 1988; Murata, Sachiko. "Temporary Marriage in Islamic Law." See Al-Serat: A Journal of Islamic Studies Web site: http://al-islam.org/al-serat/muta/; Rider, Catherine. "Between Theory and Practice: Medieval Canonists on Magic and Impotence." In *Boundaries of the Law. Geography, Gender and Jurisdiction in Medieval and Early Modern Europe*, edited by Anthony Musson, 53–66. Aldershot: Ashgate, 2005.

Mia Korpiola

INCEST. In the Middle Ages, incest was one of the most common sexual offences, after fornication and **adultery**. However, its definition was much broader than it is today—it covered not only relationships of **consanguinity**, but also of affinity, which included even extramarital relations. From the eighth century on, ecclesiastical and legal interdictions were also placed on spiritual relationships fostered by baptism and confirmation, which meant that godparents and godchildren, not to mention the performing priests, became unacceptable kindred for **marriage** or intercourse. Eventually, godparents were even prohibited to marry each other. It appears that incest was either more common among the nobility than among peasants, presumably for economical and political reasons, or possibly just more likely to be recorded, because the strict regulations that were gradually developed would have prevented the marriage or sexual activity of most people living in small and remote villages.

In the early Middle Ages, condemnation of incest became increasingly strict. The Roman tradition and the Bible did not offer very much argument against incest. Until the fourth century, marrying a first cousin was legal according to the Roman code. First cousins of the same generation were not excluded from marriage or intercourse in the Old Testament either. There is no documentation showing that the church councils that met in Gaul in the fourth and fifth centuries were particularly concerned about marriage between relatives.

The Christian concern with incest started increasing in the sixth and seventh centuries, particularly on the Byzantine side. Joannes Jejunator (John the Faster), a sixth-century patriarch of Constantinople, wrote a penitential in which he distinguished between a great number of varieties of incest, although without being very particular about the heterosexual or homosexual nature of the relationships: between sisters, with a cousin, with the daughter of a cousin, with the wife of one's son, with the wife of one's brother, with one's mother-in-law, with the sister of one's mother-in-law, with a stepmother, with the concubine of one's father, with one's mother, with one's goddaughters, with a man in the company of one's wife, and so on.

It became law in 721, when Pope Gregory II forbid that marrying the godmother of one's child or the mother of a child to whom one was a godfather. A story written by an anonymous Frankish clergyman in 727 illustrates how the new legislation was taken advantage of by Fredegund, the concubine of King Chilperic. She persuaded Queen Audovera, in the king's absence, to serve as the godmother of her newborn daughter, which disqualified the queen from continuing as the king's wife. In 802 Charlemagne gave an ordinance that forbade any form of clemency for those who had defiled themselves through incest. In 732 Pope Gregory III extended the definition of forbidden kinship to the seventh degree (*generatio*). This view lasted until 1215, when the Fourth Lateran Council reduced the limit to the fourth degree.

A unified and specific antikin marriage policy began to be implemented from the eleventh century on, under ecclesiastical initiative, which helped increase the power of the church. Marriage between relatives within the four degrees of kinship of either blood or marriage (consanguinity or affinity) was only allowed with the consent of the pope himself. For Gratian, a twelfth-century canon lawyer from Bologna, incest, along with **sodomy** (in the larger sense), constituted as serious a crime as murder, forgery, arson, sacrilege, and heresy. In his *Decretum*, known also as the *Concordance of Discordant Canons* and written around 1140, he attempted to solve the apparent contradictions from canons of previous centuries. He used **Roman law**, the Bible, papal bulls, the acts of church councils and synods, and others to compose this analytical textbook that eventually allowed **canon law** to be taught in universities throughout the remainder of the Middle Ages. It would come to constitute the first of the six legal texts known as the *Corpus Iuris Canonici*, the Christian version of the *Corpus Iuris Civilis*, the collection of Roman law written during the reign of Justinian I. It should be mentioned that in it Gratian considers all sexual pleasures to be a satanic instrument.

The church was also concerned with the practice of incest among the clergy itself, which was perceived as an even more sinister threat than the fornication commonly practiced, to the extent that in some places the number of children born out of wedlock exceeded the number of those born in wedlock (in Germany the word *Pfaffenkind*, meaning parson's child, was used as a synonym for bastard). According to court records of those times, it appears that the incest cases involving clerics outnumbered those of laymen by up to fifty to one in some locations. In 1208, Cardinal Guala, the papal legate in France, ruled that the mothers and other relatives of the clerics could not live in the same house with them, a regulation that was continuously reinforced thereafter.

Nevertheless, sexual relations between people falling under the church's definition of incest were quite common as reflected by the literature of the times. For example, in **Giovanni Boccaccio**'s *Decameron* (1353), in the stories of the seventh day, under Dioneo's rule, there are two cases of sexual intercourse between spiritual relatives: in the third story Friar Rinaldo sleeps with the mother of his godchild, and in the tenth story Tingoccio also has sex with the mother of his godchild, but then he dies and afterward returns from the dead and tells his brother that the act did not count as a sin "down there." Incest's lack of consequence mirrors the treatment in the *Decameron* of other capital offences like fornication and adultery, whereby they go unpunished in most cases.

Further Reading: Bullough, Vern L., and James A. Brundage, eds. *Handbook of Medieval Sexuality*. New York: Garland Publishing, 1996; Jong, Mayke de. "To the Limits of Kinship: Anti-Incest Legislation in the Early Medieval West (500–900)." In *From Sappho to de Sade: Moments in the History of Sexuality*, edited by Jan Bremmer, 36–59. London: Routledge, 1989.

Georgia Tres

INDIA. India was one of the largest and most densely populated human communities in the medieval period. Its sexual culture was characterized by a strong emphasis on married heterosexual sex leading to procreation, while tolerating a variety of other practices.

HETEROSEXUAL LOVE AND MARRIAGE. **Marriage** and heterosexual intercourse leading to procreation were considered obligatory for nearly all Indians. Legal codes required husbands to make love to their wives frequently during their fertile periods. (The importance of procreation led to the public condemnation of **contraception** and **abortion**, although female infanticide was widely practiced, particularly during food shortages.) The principal intended audience of Indian **sex manuals** such as the ***Kama Sutra*** was married couples, although the works mentioned other contexts for sex as well. Later works in this tradition, some of the world's richest in the discussion of sexuality, include Kokkola's twelfth-century *Ratirahasya (Secrets of Love)*, Jyotirisvara's thirteenth- or fourteenth-century *Panca Sayaka (Five Arrows of the God of Love)*, and the ***Ananga Ranga***.

The average age of marriage seems to have declined during this period, and eventually India developed a system whereby girls were married as children, sometimes small children. Consuumation was usually delayed until after menarche, however, and sex manuals or *kamashastras* emphasized the importance of the husband's gentleness and consideration in introducing his wife to sex. Monogamy was the dominant marriage pattern, although **polygamy** was common among India's many kings and the social and economic elite. (Indian rulers maintained large **harems**, particularly after contacts with the Islamic world intensified in the eleventh century.) Polyandry was also practiced in particular regions such as the foothills of the Himalayas. Marriages were commonly arranged between families and followed strict laws of caste, which determined that persons could not marry outside their particular group. (Although cross-caste marriages were considered inappropriate at best, in legend they could be conceptualized as continuations of relationships established in previous lives.) Married women moved to their husband's homes, where they were subject to the control of the husband's mother, a very powerful figure in an Indian household.

Indian wives were expected to exhibit a high degree of chastity and seclusion. This extended to widows, who were forbidden to remarry and were expected to devote themselves to prayer and asceticism with the goal of being married to their husbands again in a subsequent rebirth. This was true even of widows whose husbands had died when they were children and whose marriages had never been consuumated. The practice of widows committing suicide by jumping into fire, shortly following their husbands' deaths, known as *sati*, was rare but not unknown in this period. Indian men were encouraged to be monogamous, but not required to do so—concubinage was practiced among the elite, and both urban **prostitution** and the institution of **devadasis**—prostitutes associated with Hindu temples—flourished.

India also possessed a rich romantic literature, reaching back to the love stories at the heart of the ancient epics the *Mahabharata* and the *Ramayana*, the stories of which were told and retold in many forms. This legacy was added to by medieval writers such as **Kalidasa**.

HOMOSEXUALITY AND "THIRD GENDER" ROLES. The importance given to procreation led to pronounced social stigmatization of barren women and impotent men, some of whom were viewed as members of "third genders," neither male nor female. The third-gender role became institutionalized with the establishment of the *hijra*, or cross-dressing males, as a distinct social group. Same-sex sex was stigmatized in Indian culture—male homosexuality was held to lead to **impotence**—and some forms were punished with fines or penances in Indian legal codes. However, punishments were not severe. There was an active culture of male prostitution and sexual exploitation of boy slaves, particularly in India's royal courts and large cities.

The recipient in male homosexual sex was particularly stigmatized, although Hindu mythology sometimes portrayed gods in this role. Medical treatises suggested that men who received semen from other men in sex had been formed by insufficient parental semen. Some medical writers also suggested that two women could make love and have a child, but the child would be boneless because there was no semen in its composition.

INDIAN RELIGION AND SEXUALITY. Indian religion was unique in the tight bonds between eroticism and devotion. Hindu temples frequently incorporated erotic art, with the most famous being the detailed sculptures of the **Khajuraho temple complex**, the **Kailasanath temple** at Ellora, and the Sun Temple at Konark. Some temples included textiles with pictures recounting the erotic adventures of heroes and apsaras, divine women resembling the Muslim houris. Legends of the Hindu gods and heroes included sexuality, and **Hindu literature** included descriptions of divine lovemaking, such as that of Shiva and his wife Parvati. The relationship between gods and their devotees was also conceptualized as erotic, particularly with the rise of the **bhakti** movement and the cult of **Krishna**. This eroticism was sometimes transgendered—there are legends of male devotees of Krishna

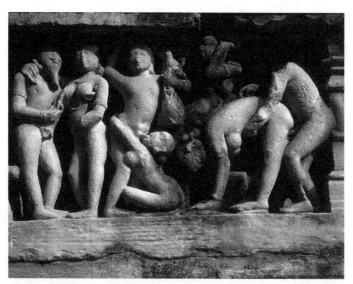

Erotic relief from the Laksmana temple in Khajuraho, India, 11th century. © The Art Archive/Dagli Orti.

being rewarded for their devotion with rebirth as milkmaids or *gopis*, Krishna's female lovers. The link between eroticism and divinity was also found in Indian **Tantric Buddhism**.

With the decline and eventual disappearance of Indian **Buddhism**, beginning in the eleventh century, celibate religious institutions vanished from most of India outside the small Christian and **Jain** communities. However, celibacy still retained a place as an attribute of many Indian ascetics and holy men and women, as well as recommended for people in the later stages of life and for all widows. The coming of **Islam** to India in the later medieval period introduced the sexual concepts associated with **Sharia** law and other Islamic traditions, both Sunni and Shia, and also led to the creation of new cultural forms with both Indian and Islamic aspects. This was particularly marked in Indian **Sufism**, which took many erotic forms of expressing religious devotion from the *bhakti* movement. *See also Cakramsamvara Tantra*; Jayadeva; Prithviraj III; Sakthism.

Further Reading: Vanita, Ruth, and Saleem Kidwai, eds. *Same-Sex Love in India: Readings from Literature and History*. New York: St. Martin's Press, 2000; Zysk, Kenneth G. *Conjugal Love in India: Ratisastra and Ratiramana: Text, Translation, and Notes*. Leiden: Brill, 2002.

William E. Burns

INTERCONFESSIONAL SEX AND LOVE. In many medieval societies, sexual relations between members of different faith groups were strongly discouraged and subject to harsh penalties, including confiscation of the involved parties' property and even physical mutilation or execution. At the same time, literary celebrations of interconfessional love persisted within the very cultures that officially condemned such relationships as contrary to divine and secular law.

In the Christian tradition, profound anxiety about interconfessional sex as a source of ritual impurity and a threat to the faith of Christians involved took the form of banning sex and **marriage** between Christians and non-Christians. As early as the fourth century, the church forbade its members to have sex with **Jews** under penalty of excommunication. Contemporary **Roman law** invoked the death penalty for the same offence, and periodic restatements of this decree appeared in the secular law codes of European kingdoms throughout the Middle Ages. For medieval Europeans sex between Christians and Jews or Muslims was believed to render the Christian's body and soul impure and unfit for social or sexual intercourse with coreligionists. Worse yet, such relationships might ultimately encourage Christians to become apostates in order to marry their non-Christian lovers.

The Crusades directed against the Islamic world began in 1095, and subsequent Christian settlement in the Levant resulted in an outpouring of Christian legislation to discourage interconfessional sex. As early as the First Crusade, Christian clerics insisted that setbacks suffered by the crusading armies were due to God's displeasure with Christian knights who had taken Muslim mistresses. Though laws instituted in the twelfth-century crusader kingdoms mandated that Christian or Muslim men engaging in interfaith sex would be castrated and their female partners' noses cut off, marriage between Christian colonists and Muslims who had converted to Christianity was permitted. In post-Reconquest Iberia, where large numbers of unconverted Muslims lived under Christian rule, miscegenation fears encouraged legislation, providing for the execution of Muslim men and the enslavement of Muslim women found guilty of having sex with Christians. Iberian law further dictated that Christian prostitutes who knowingly accepted Muslim or Jewish clients be burned at the stake.

An examination of the great **canon law** collections of the twelfth and thirteenth centuries suggests the Latin church became increasingly concerned in this period with regulating casual interaction between Christians and non-Christians that might lead to sexual relations. Since contact with Muslims was not a matter of concern for most European Christians, such legislation largely focused on separating Christians from Jews, the most visible religious minority in Latin Christendom. By the early thirteenth century, canon law prohibited Christians and Jews from living, eating, or bathing together, and required both Jews and Muslims living in Christian lands to wear distinguishing signs on their clothing. The motivation behind these prohibitions, as the Fourth Lateran Council of 1215 explicitly stated, was to prevent Christians from "accidentally" engaging in sex with non-Christians. Christians who ignored such prohibitions were equated with those who had committed **sodomy** or **bestiality**, and as such subjected to mutilation or execution. The fourteenth-century jurist Oldradus de Ponte claimed to have seen a Christian man castrated at the papal palace in Avignon for knowingly sleeping with a Jewish woman.

Though it is difficult to determine how widespread interconfessional sex really was, since the parties involved naturally desired to conceal their actions, it seems likely that the medieval fear of miscegenation greatly exceeded its practice. **Judaism**, Christianity, and **Islam** unanimously condemned extramarital sex in general, and within the Jewish and Christian traditions marriage—the only acceptable outlet for sexual desire—could only take place between coreligionists. Concern about interconfessional sex seems to have been less acute in medieval Islamic societies, where, although Christians and Jews were required to wear distinctive clothing or headgear that marked their status as *dhimmis*, or subject peoples, they mingled with the Muslim majority population in markets, baths, and private houses more freely than did their counterparts in Latin Christendom. While Shiites were more concerned with maintaining social distance from *dhimmis*, medieval Sunni authorities permitted Muslim men to marry Christian or Jewish women, with the proviso that the *dhimmi* wives agreed to respect Muslim ritual purity laws. Marriage between Muslim women and *dhimmi* men was more problematic, however, since men ruled over their wives and could therefore pressure them to abandon Islam.

While the secular and ecclesiastical authorities of European Christendom were engaged in preventing interconfessional relationships, however, tales of love affairs between Christians, Muslims, and Jews—often culminating in conversion and marriage—circulated throughout Europe and the Islamic world in chronicles, poetry, and even sermon collections. In this literary fantasy world, Christian crusaders won the love of Muslim princesses, beautiful Jewish women bestowed their favors on their Christian neighbors, and Muslim emirs took lovely Christian ladies as their consorts.

In the majority of such fantasies, the conversion of one of the parties involved was the inevitable climax. In the thirteenth century, the monk Caesarius of Heisterbach told of a Christian cleric who seduced a young Jewish girl, but atoned for his transgression by abandoning his church career and convincing the object of his affection to accept baptism so they could marry. Muslim princesses in European **romance** invariably betrayed their fathers or husbands in order to save their handsome crusader-lovers, and were subsequently miraculously "whitened" by the water of the baptismal font. Christian writers who romanticized interreligious affairs betrayed their fears of miscegenation by imagining the children of such unions were born deformed, covered in hair, or even as grotesque lumps. Such anxiety-ridden fantasies existed in the Islamic tradition as well; a tale from the ***Thousand and One Nights*** tells of a

Muslim tormented by **lust** for a beautiful Christian woman, resisting her charms with great difficulty until he is able to convince her to convert and marry him. The persistence of this conversion motif attests to an ongoing concern about the spiritual dangers of such relationships, and to a deeper association of interconfessional sex with physical pollution. *See also Aucassin and Nicolette.*

Further Reading: Brundage, James A. "Intermarriage between Christians and Jews in Medieval Canon Law." *Jewish History* 3 (1988): 25–40; de Weever, Jacqueline. *Sheba's Daughters: Whitening and Demonizing the Saracen Women in Medieval French Epic.* New York: Garland, 1998; Kruger, Steven F. "Conversion and Medieval Sexual, Religious, and Racial Categories." In *Constructing Medieval Sexuality*, edited by Karma Lochrie, Peggy McCracken, and James A. Schultz, 158–79. Minneapolis: University of Minnesota Press, 1997; Nirenberg, David. *Communities of Violence: The Persecution of Minorities in the Middle Ages.* Princeton, NJ: Princeton University Press, 1996.

Katherine Allen Smith

INTERCRURAL SEX. *See* Anal and Intercrural Sex

ISLAM. The religion of Islam was founded by Muhammad in the Arabian peninsula. Seventh-century Bedouin Arab culture and society determined many of its precepts, including strict norms in the realm of sex and sexuality. The Islamic religious text, the Qur'an, hadith (compendium of tradition of Muhammad), and sunna (the normative custom of Muhammad and his companions) are sources for information about sex and sexuality in Islam. As the religion spread from Arabia, it varied from place to place, time to time, and class to class. Islam condemns **lust**, **adultery**, and deviant behavior. Its agenda for sex and sexuality emphasizes maintaining a harmonious family life. But human nature does not work within a prescribed parameter.

Leading a chaste life without clandestine sexual liaisons is prescribed, and promiscuity condemned, in the Qur'an. The purpose of the sacred institution of **marriage** is the union between *muhsin* (chaste man) and *muhsinat* (chaste woman). The rights of husband and wife flow from this basic premise. Described as garments of one another, man and woman nurture each other. A husband sleeps with wife "skin to skin" and performs a task ordained by God. The sexual union is not an ordinary act, but an act of *sadaqa* (form of worship) for each partner. The couple may enjoy their sexual bliss in any manner they prefer, except anal intercourse and sex during **menstruation**. Five practices that are to be followed are **circumcision**, shaving the pubic region, clipping nails, trimming the moustache short, and shaving armpit hair. The Qur'an asks the husband to treat the wife with kindness and honor, and maintain her properly. The wife is to be loyal and honest. She should neither refuse her husband sexual intercourse nor entertain other men any time. She should make herself presentable, desirable, and cooperative. If the husband is returning after a long journey, the wife is to comb her hair and shave her pubic hair before sexual union. The husband on his part should not fall upon her like an animal and should do enough foreplay like kissing and caressing, which are like messengers between the couple. The man reaching inzal (orgasm) should wait for the wife's, and a simultaneous orgasm will be ecstatic for her. If a man is aroused sexually by the sight of a voluptuous woman, he should hurry home and have sex with his wife to release passion. The husband's demand for sex sometimes becomes more important than the woman's right of denying.

Like other patriarchal religions, Islam favors the power of men over women. The Qur'an says that men are in charge of women, and Allah has made "one of them to excel" the other. Muslim men could enjoy *sexual* freedom outside marriage by having concubines and through the institution of **mut'a** (temporary marriage). While a woman can have only one husband, a man can have as many as four wives. However, the Qur'an tells men to marry only one if equality and justice cannot be given to all the wives. The easy process of **divorce**, with the husband uttering *talaq* three times, began from the time of second Khalifa, Hazrat Umar (634–644), as the Islamic conquests led to an influx of captured women. A new spouse could be acquired by divorcing an old one. The quick process of divorce was initiated, in keeping with the extraordinary situation of the early Islamic wars, but persisting far beyond that period. Islam gives license to Muslim men to have *surriyah* (concubines) if the women are not Muslim. (Muslim women are forbidden to marry or have relations with non-Muslim men.) A man can possess any number of concubines taken captive in war or purchased. Sex outside wedlock is *haram* (illegitimate), but it becomes legitimate for a warrior to enjoy a captured woman. When Muhammad was given three women by the people of Taif, the last major city in Arabia to resist Islam in 631, he presented them to his father-in-law and sons-in-law. Sexual intercourse is permitted with the concubine, and a man can have *al azl* (coitus interruptus) so as not to beget children.

It is believed that the **houris** (celestial damsels) wait for the believers after death. A martyred *mujahid* (Islamic warrior) is promised a life of sensual pleasure and enjoyment in *jannat* (paradise). He could have the best in both worlds: captured women after the war in mundane world and beautiful virgins in *jannat* if dead. Sex was the bait for the warriors of medieval times to go for wars against the unconquered territories. However, the Qur'an views seriously sexual intercourse outside wedlock, or *zina*. Loss of **virginity** before marriage and adultery with neighbor's wife are grave sins. There is *hadd* (punishment) of 100 lashes each according to Islamic jurisprudence for consensual premarital intercourse. Punishment by stoning to death is reserved for a married man or woman committing adultery. The penalty is irrevocable once decided.

Punishment is also meted out to persons indulging in same-sex acts, either male or female. This deviant behavior is against God's wishes and capital punishment might be inflicted for **sodomy**. God's wrath is on men and women who try to resemble the opposite sex, persons committing **bestiality**, and men performing homoerotic acts. However, the Qur'an endorses some nontraditional gender identities, allowing the *mukhannath* (effeminate) **eunuchs**—those without the "defining skill of males" (24.31)—to work in the female quarters. They are indifferent to women's bodies and can see a woman naked. Although penetration of the anus in sodomy is a sin, there are some instances where **pederasty** was tolerated in Islamic society. Along with *houris*, there are *ghilmaan* (boys) as white as pearls, waiting upon the martyrs in *jannat*. In spite of Islam's rigid code of sexual conduct, sexuality was expressed in different ways in the medieval period of Islamic civilization. The **Thousand and One Nights** with its tales of infidelity and amorous affairs, or Nefzawi's *The Perfumed Garden*, a treatise describing sexual pleasures, did not adhere to the strict regime of Islam. **Abu Nuwas** (750–810) wrote couplets on homosexuality, and **Ibn Hazm, Abu Muhammad Ali** (994–1064) dealt with the art of love, writing homoerotic poems. The princess **Wallada bint al-Mustakfi** (1011–1091) was against the Islamic conventions and celebrated her love openly. **Nizami** (1141–1203), **Rumi** (1207–1273), and **Hafiz** (1327–1391) wrote passionate love poems. *See also* Interconfessional Sex and Love; Islamic Society; Sharia.

Further Reading: Abdalati, Hammudah. *Islam in Focus*. Kuala Lumpur, Malaysia: Islamic Book Trust, 2001; Ali, Abdullah Yusuf, trans. *The Holy Qur'an*. Indianapolis, IN: American Trust Publications, 1977; Awde, Nicholas, ed. and trans. *Women in Islam: An Anthology from the Qur'an* and *Hadiths*. New York: St. Martin's Press, 2000; Badawi, Jamal. *Gender Equity in Islam: Basic Principles*. Indianapolis, IN: American Trust Publications, 1995; Bano, Afsar. *Status of Women in Islamic Socity*. Vols. 1 and 2. New Delhi: Anmol Publicatons, 2003; Hambly, Gavin. *Women in the Medieval Islamic World: Power, Patronage, and Piety*. New York: St. Martin's Press, 1998; Hunt, Mary, Patricia B. Jung, and Radhika Balakrishnan, eds. *Good Sex: Feminist Perspectives from the World's Religions*. New Brunswick, NJ: Rutgers University Press, 2001; Speaker-Yuan, Margaret. *Women in Islam*. Detroit, MI: Greenhaven Press, 2005; Stowasser, Barbara. *Women in the Qur'an, Traditions, and Interpretation*. New York: Oxford University Press, 1994.

Patit Paban Mishra

ISLAMIC SOCIETY. The medieval period, which coincides with the classical period of Islamic society, was a major time of development and transition. **Islam** at this stage was continually evolving and developed its principal schools of legal interpretation, sects, and institutions.

Islam emerged out of Arabia as a religion and a major social and political force in the seventh century. From the seventh through the ninth centuries, Islamic society was dominated by the Arabs, who ruled their empire from Damascus and later from Baghdad. Their empire stretched from Spain and North **Africa** to **India**. At the end of the ninth century, Arab domination diminished and Persian and Turkish dynasties emerged. With time, Islamic literatures in languages other than Arabic also emerged. The area and peoples encompassed by Islam were tremendous and very diverse. Traditional customs and local practices varied greatly. These were also governed by class and rank. For the most part, this essay will concentrate on sex and love among the elite, as this segment of society is best documented. It is very important to note the past heritages of Muslims as past practices affected societies. A society's conversion to Islam was not unanimous and simultaneous but rather a process that took centuries.

PRE-ISLAMIC ARABIA. During the *Jahiliyya* or pre-Islamic period most people in the Arabian peninsula were pagan, although there were large Jewish and Christian minorities. A rich oral tradition of poetry survived from this period. Besides the theme of bravery and excellence in combat, this literature was full of **romance** and love. The poems are full of boastings of sexual prowess and conquests. But the concept of *hubb al-Udhri* (Udhrite or chaste love) was also born in this period. This important theme is encapsulated in the story of Layla and Majnun, a story later adopted by the Sufi Islamic mystics.

ISLAMIC LAW. Islamic jurisprudence offers a vast amount of legal material governing **marriage**, divorce, birth, and inheritance as well as guidelines on how to conduct oneself in all activities of life. Additionally, Islamic literature in the form of medical treatises, material medica, belles letters, erotica, and popular literature provides information on sexual practices, **contraception**, and **abortion**.

MARRIAGE. In contrast to the other Abrahamic monotheistic religions—**Judaism** and Christianity—Islam allows a man to marry a maximum of four women at any one time. It also allows for an unlimited number of concubines. While this was allowed, it admonished men not to marry more women than they could do justice to—not only sexually, but also economically, for all wives had to be provided for equally.

In medieval Islamic society, romantic courtships followed by marriage were not the norm. Islamic society revolved around the family and the community. It was the family that was foremost, not the individual. For this reason, marriages for love were extremely rare. Women were segregated and cloistered inside the home, and contact with males from outside their immediate family was rare. Love and marriage were for the good of the family. Marriages were usually arranged by the family, for economic and political reasons. Children were sometimes betrothed at an early age, and their marriages consummated when they reached puberty. First-cousin marriages were especially prized.

SEXUAL MORALITY IN ISLAMIC SOCIETY. The following elements contributed to the sexual morality of medieval Islamic societies: (a) marriage was polygamous, (b) sex was not confined to marriage but extended to concubines, (c) marriage was not viewed as necessarily permanent, (d) marital intercourse needed no justification for procreation because it was based on the right to sexual fulfillment for both partners, and (e) contraception was permitted and abortion tolerated.

Three types of sexual relations were considered legitimate by Islamic law: (1) with a wife who was a free woman, (2) with a wife who was a slave of someone else, and (3) with his own female slave. A man could marry a free woman or a slave, but he could only have sexual relations with his own slave as a concubine, not as a wife. All forms of sexual union within these limits were deemed licit.

Contraception was widely practiced, especially in the case of intercourse between master and slave girl, to prevent unwanted pregnancies. However, many Islamic jurists held that sexual intercourse between a free woman and her husband could not be practiced without the consent of the woman. The main reason for this was the woman's right to complete sexual satisfaction, and it was believed that coitus interruptus, the most commonly practiced method, diminished the woman's pleasure. Intravaginal suppositories and tampons were some of the other methods practiced.

A woman's consent to contraception was necessary because of her right to have children. Birth control was also practiced to protect the woman from the dangers of **childbirth**, to preserve her beauty, and for economic reasons. In the case of concubines, the practice was a kind of protection of property, because if she gave birth to her master's child, she could not be sold. The majority of jurists allowed abortion anytime within the first four months of conception. It was believed that after 120 days the fetus received its soul. Some jurists allowed abortion without a husband's permission, while others insisted upon it.

Many jurists allowed **masturbation**. Their reasoning was that it would satisfy **lust** in the absence of a legitimate partner. It was especially licit for the prisoner, traveler, or lonely people. Women alone without a husband were allowed to masturbate. It was also allowed during Ramadan, the Muslim month of fasting, because of the belief that unless accumulated semen was released, it would cause damage to the body. Those jurists who believed that masturbation was abhorrent still permitted it when performed by the hand of a man's wife or concubine.

Within medieval Islamic courtly societies, many servants and retainers were trained to entertain. Talented female and male slaves were trained to sing and dance along with other skills. They entertained at court and the higher circles of society and brought a high price when sold at market. Courtly dalliances between courtesans and members of the court and visitors were common. Secret liaisons within courtly circles were not unheard of, but the cloistering of women made this extremely difficult.

Prostitution was common in large cities but was illegal. The laws against it were enforced to varying degrees. Within Shia Islam, there was a provision for temporary marriages, known as *mut'a* **marriage**, which allowed for marriages to be contracted for as short a time as a few hours. While these marriages were condemned in Sunni Islam, they provided an outlet for sexual fulfillment within an Islamic context, which laid out the conditions and responsibilities between both parties.

Homosexuality was not permitted in Islam. However, it was widely practiced, especially among the Persians and the Turks. Within courtly and elite circles, though, there were parameters. Homosexual relations were most commonly practiced between adult elites and prepubescent boys. Sexual relations typically ended when the boy reached puberty and was able to grow a beard. In one early Persian work of the "Mirror for Princes" genre, written in the eleventh century by a Persian king for his son, the king advises his son to sleep with boys in the winter and with girls in the summer.

In the ninth century, Persian poetry and literature began to emerge. A large body of it has been translated into English and other European languages. Much court love poetry describes the beauty of the "beloved," and in many cases the "beloved" is a handsome boy. Due to Western taboos against homosexuality and the ambiguities of the Persian language, some translations make the male beloved a female one. (There are no gender-identifying pronouns in Persian. The third person could designate a male or a female.) References to lesbianism are found, most commonly between wives and concubines, confined to the harem. **Eunuchs** stood guard over the ruler's women, but they were also assigned to princes to protect them from sexual predators. Homosexual activity, outside the environment of the circles of power, was performed in secrecy.

A large body of literature exists around the theme of romantic love, in both poetry and prose. Within Persian and then later Turkish poetry, these works take the form of epic poems of thousands of verses. Famous lovers such as Layla and Majnun, Khusraw and Shirin, and Joseph and Potiphar's wife are portrayed in a number of settings, both secular and mystical. The theme of mystical love between man and God is a rich genre full of allegory.

NON-MUSLIM COMMUNITIES IN THE ISLAMIC EMPIRE. The Islamic empire included a broad spectrum of religious groups, including Jews and Christians, as well as ethnic groups. While Islam preached equality, there were hierarchies of class and ethnic divisions. Initially, the Arabs dominated the other ethnic and religious groups. Many converted to Islam but still others kept their faith and customs. Most noticeable in contrast to Islam was a strict adherence to monogamy and a prohibition on divorce. These other communities kept their traditions and customs, but intermarriage was allowed. Muslim men were allowed to marry "people of the Book," **Jews** or Christians. For example, the prophet Muhammad married Maryam, a Christian woman. However, Muslim women were not allowed to marry outside of Islam.

Before the Muslim conquests, the Persian empire under the Sassanian dynasty reigned from the border of **Byzantium** to India and **China**. While this empire encompassed many religions including **Buddhism**, Manichaeism, **Hinduism**, and Shamanism, Zoroastrianism was the predominant state religion. Within Zoroastrianism, incestuous relations were permitted. It was acceptable to marry one's mother, sister, or daughter. Additionally, the literature talks of the Mazdakism or Khurramdiniyya, who held women as common property.

Medieval Islamic society had a healthy and well-developed attitude toward love and sex that was based on an ethical system that respected and protected the rights of all parties. However, different customs and practices abounded from region to region and between ethnic groups, but more importantly between the different classes of society. At the lower levels of society, ignorance, superstition, and folk practices deviated from the theoretical. Glimpses of this segment of medieval Islamic society may be found in such works as the ***Thousand and One Nights***. *See also* Genital Contact in Islamic Law; Sharia.

Further Reading: Kai Ka'us ibn Iskandar. *A Mirror for Princes*. New York: E. P. Dutton, 1951; Musallam, B. F. *Sex and Society in Islam: Birth Control before the Nineteenth Century*. Cambridge: Cambridge University Press, 1986; Nafzawi, Muhammad ibn Muhammad. *The Perfumed Garden of Sheykh Nefzawi*. Translated by Sir Richard Burton. New York: Castle Books, 1964.

Mark David Luce

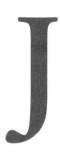

J

JAHIZ, ABU UTHMAN AMR B. BAHR AL- (c. 776–868). Abu Uthman Amr b. Bahr al-Jahiz, a famous, prolific, and diverse Arab prose writer of the early Abbasid age, owed his sobriquet "the goggle-eyed" to a malformation of the eyes, which gave rise to numerous comments on his ugliness. He was born in Basra to a family probably of Abbyssinian origin, as his grandfather is said to have been a black cameleer and a mawla (freedman) of the Kinana tribe. He received his early education in Basra rather informally in the teaching circles around the Friday mosque and at the Mirbad, the stopping place of caravans, where scholars met in order to learn from the Bedouins as the genuine sources of Arab language, poetry, and tribal lore. In time al-Jahiz became a pupil of the Mu'tazili (rational) theologian Ibrahim al-Nazzam and composed his first treatise on the question of the imamate, which gained the favor of the caliph al-Ma'mun.

From now on (after 815), he spent most of his time in the new capital of Baghdad, although he never became a courtier. For a short period, he served as a scribe, as a teacher, and in the chancery, but he held no official post and took on no regular income. However, he seems to have received considerable sums for the dedications of his books, and we know that he was given an allowance by the Diwan. Most probably, he acted as a semi-official publicist who propagated the claims of the ruling dynasty, which had adopted Mu'tazili thought as the official doctrine of the state. In this, influential men like the vizier Ibn al-Zayyat, the chief Kadi Ahmad b. Abi Du'ad and his son, and the courtier al-Fath b. Khaqan successively acted as his patrons. But he never lost contact with his hometown, and in his old age, at a time when he suffered from hemiplegia and Bagdhad turned out to be less congenial, he retired to Basra to live out the rest of his long life.

The list of al-Jahiz's writings is impressive; when duplications are discounted, somewhat over 190 remain, both large-scale works and short treatises, of which 75 survive in whole or in part. The range of his subjects is impressive, ranging between theological works and the typical Jahizian **Adab literature**, a medieval Arabic mixture of entertainment and teaching, for which he was celebrated. He unsystematically composed a number of anthologies, like the *Kitab al-hayawan* (*Book of Animals*), the *Kitab al-bayan wa l-tabyin* (*On Arabic Rhetoric*), and the *Kitab al-bukhala'* (*Book of Misers*). His treatment of avarice belongs to a whole number of books, treatises, and epistles in which al-Jahiz—sometimes to their glory and sometimes to their expense—depicted different ethnic groups (Africans, Turks), social classes (merchants, scribes), and professional entertainers (singers, slave girls). The *Risalat al-qiyan* (*Epistle on*

Singing-Girls), explaining the dangers of falling prey to the professional entertainers, stands out for its remarkable shrewdness. On the other hand, the *Kitab fi l-'ishq* (*Book of Love*) categorizes different forms or stages of human love, including amour fou or passionate love. Last but not least, al-Jahiz wrote a *Kitab mufakharat al-jawari wa l-ghilman* (*The Respective Merit of Girls and Boys*), which, dealing with the delicate subject of heterosexual and homosexual love, borders on the obscene.

Further Reading: Jahiz, Abu Uthman Amr b. Bahr al-. *The Epistle on Singing-Girls by Jahiz.* Edited and translated by A.F.L. Beeston. Warminster: Aris and Phillips, 1980; Jahiz, Abu Uthman Amr b. Bahr al-. *Nine Essays of al-Jahiz.* Translated by William M. Hutchins. New York: Peter Lang, 1989; Pellat, Charles. *The Life and Works of Jahiz: Translations of Selected Texts.* Translated from the French by D. M. Hawke. Berkeley: University of California Press, 1969.

Susanne Enderwitz

JAINISM. Jainism is an ancient Indian religion established around 500 BCE by Vardhamana Mahavira. *Brahmacarya* (**celibacy** or abstention from sex) is one of the five vows of Jainism. However, descriptions of love and sex abound in Jain narrative literature.

Premarital love is full of wonder and surprise. This type of love is the focus of an early Jain text, the *Vasudevahindi* (300–400 CE) of Acarya Sanghadasagani Vacaka, and its sequel, the *Vasudevahindi Majjimakhando* (700) of Dharmadasagani Mahattara. The stories in these books, set in a religious milieu, reveal interesting aspects of love and sex in Jainism. Love is placed in the sphere of women's activities, and lovers interact both on earth and in an imaginary world of love, the world of Vidyadharas (*Vidyadharaloka*). Vidyadharas are semi-divine beings living on the Himalayas in their own world. The Jain texts describe them as followers of Jainism who travel by air in their aerial chariots to visit Jain holy sites. They possess magical arts and help humans in need and occasionally form relations with humans through **marriage**.

The sequence of these love stories—the desire of the leading lady, her efforts, use of magical arts, help from other female friends, help from Vidyadharas, or travel to the Vidyadhara world—clearly portray women as seekers and perpetrators of love. Love is a passion and pleasure not only of humans but also of beings from other worlds. Love requires special skills (*vidyas*) and surpasses the human sphere or earthly limits.

Marital love or family love is an important aspect of the women's sphere, and it is a worldly possession and bondage for men. Escape from it is both desirable and a religious duty in didactic literature. In Jain literature, women cling to their love and urge men to stay in the relationships, while men leave to join the ascetic order.

Adventurous love is the pleasure and passion of women as well as men. The adventurous love of hero and heroines is laden with numerous perils, trials, and tribulations, concluding in union of the lovers. The *Kuvalayamala* (1200) of Udyotanasuri is a classic tale of adventurous love.

Extramarital love is equated with **lust** and condemned. Love and sex with prostitutes and married women is variously narrated in Jain texts. The *Nammaysundarikatha* (1130) of Mahendrasuri describes prostitutes and their sexual life. The *Kathakosa* (1052) of Jinesvarasuri narrates stories of extramarital love. The superiority of love over the other *dharmas* is extensively discussed in the eighth-century *Smaraiccakaha* of Haribhadrasuri.

The passion of love in Jainism is the focus of numerous anthologies of love stories, some of which are noted above. This indicates the status of love as an important subject in Jain religion.

Further Reading: Bhyani, H. C., ed. *Vasudevahindi Majjimakhando.* Lalbhai Dalpatbhai Series 99. Ahmedabad, India: Lalbhai Dalpatbhai Institute of Indology, 1979; Jacobi, Hermann, ed. *Samaraiccakaha.* Kolkata, India: Asiatic Society of Bengal, 1926; Jain, Jagadish Chandra. *The Vasudevahindi: An Authentic Jain Version of the Brhatkath.* Lalbhai Dalpatbhai Series 59. Ahmedabad, India: Lalbhai Dalpatbhai Institute of Indology, 1977; Jaini, Padmanabh S. *The Jaina Path of Purification.* Berkeley: University of California Press, 1979; Muni, Jinavijya, ed. *Kathakosa Prakarana of Jinesvara Suri.* Singhi Jain Grantha Mala 11. Mumbai, India: Bharatiya Vidya Bhavan, 1949; Trivedi, Prathibha, ed. *Sri Mahendra Suri Viracita Nammayasundari Kaha.* Mumbai, India: Bharatiya Vidya Bhavan, 1960; Upadhye, A. N. *Kuvalayamala Katha Samksepa.* Mumbai, India: Bharatiya Vidya Bhavan, 1961.

Lavanya Vemsani

JAPAN. Japanese civilization began to emerge from obscurity during the medieval period. Its sexual and romantic culture blended indigenous with imported elements, including Mahayana **Buddhism** and Confucianism.

The best-documented social element of early medieval Japan was the court and aristocracy of the so-called Heian period, from 794 to 1185. The customs of the Heian aristocracy included the **seclusion of women**, arranged **marriages**, **concubinage**, and **polygamy**. Taking multiple wives was important for the creation and maintenance of alliances at the Heian court, and there is some evidence that at the highest levels of aristocracy, men with only one wife were looked down upon. (However, even emperors and the most powerful political leaders did not have the massive **eunuch**-staffed **harems** of contemporary Chinese and Islamic rulers.) Much of Heian literature, the first substantial body of world literature primarily written by women, is focused on the jealousies between wives and concubines over access to men and the advancement of their children.

The literature of Heian court women such as **Murasaki Shikibu** and **Sei Shonagon** gives a somewhat misleading picture of the lives even of aristocratic women, as women at court were much less secluded than other aristocratic women. Many provincial upper-class women lived their lives behind screens, with little contact with men other than fathers, brothers, husbands, and sons. Having many love affairs, as Shonagon depicts herself doing, was simply not an option for the majority of Japanese elite women. (Even court women were required to retreat into seclusion during their menstrual periods.)

The physical separation of men and women made letter-writing a particularly important way of initiating relationships among the Heian aristocracy. Calligraphy was extremely important for both men and women, and even the selection of paper and inks could carry an erotic charge. Like conversation, aristocratic flirtation in letters often relied on a shared familiarity with classical Chinese romantic poetry, which had a great influence in Japan. Chinese literature did much to shape the Japanese treatment of love and sex in general. **Zhang Zhuo**'s *Dwelling of Playful Goddesses* was particularly popular in Japan, far more than in its native **China**.

The standard of female beauty among the Heian aristocracy, which influenced subsequent eras in Japan, was based on Chinese styles. The ideal Heian woman was plump, with a narrow waist and large breasts. However, her most important physical feature was not her body, which under most circumstances would be concealed under several layers of clothing (unlike their Chinese contemporaries, Heians had little interest in the nude), but her hair, which was expected to be very long, ideally reaching the ground on which she was standing. The Buddhist tonsure gained particular meaning for nuns as a renunciation of worldliness, given that their hair would not ever grow back to its original length. Teeth were blackened, a practice universal among the Heians that would later be restricted to married women.

Marriage among the aristocracy of the Heian period (we know very little about the lives of ordinary Japanese people at the time) was often matrilocal, particularly in its early stages. The narrowness of the Heian elite and the importance of marriage for maintaining political alliances meant that marriages between close kin, first cousins, aunts and nephews, and uncles and neices were relatively common. The marriage would often follow three overnight visits by the man and be symbolized by the joint eating of rice cakes. Sex was viewed as necessary for health, and it was believed that a woman too long virgin was vulnerable to demonic possession. It was not uncommon for young men to marry a woman several years before the two lived together under one roof. In the meantime, the girl would continue to dwell with her parents, and the man would visit at night.

JAPANESE RELIGION. Japanese religion in the medieval period combined a growing multitude of Buddhist sects, many imported from China or Korea, with the indigenous religion of Shinto. Buddhism was introduced from China in a monastic form in the seventh century, and its patronage by the imperial family and many high aristocrats, male and female, led to the founding of many houses of monks and nuns. In the following centuries, the role of nuns was steadily marginalized, although Japan, unlike several other Buddhist countries, never eliminated women's religious orders entirely. One of the principal problems faced by nuns, and other Japanese women in religious life, was the strong Shinto belief, which extended to Buddhism, of the defiling and impure qualities of menstrual blood as well as blood shed in childbirth. This led to women, including young girls and postmenopausal women, being barred from an increasing number of temples and religious sites in the early modern period.

Buddhist monasteries were often alleged to be nests of homosexuality or other practices in violation of the monks' supposed celibacy. The founder of the Shingon tradition of esoteric Buddhism in Japan, Kukai, would also be credited by later legend with being the first to introduce sex between men from China to Japan. The later medieval period saw the creation of a literary genre known as Chiba Monotagari, "acolyte's tales," which focused on the love affairs between boys and older monks and used these stories to form Buddhist ideas about the transitoriness of love and the world. Japanese male homosexuality in this period was based more on relationships between younger and older men rather than on men adopting female gender roles. Sexual misconduct was also a charge made against fringe Buddhist sects, most notably the **Tachikawa-ryu**, which was accused by its enemies of practicing sexual rituals.

The later medieval period saw the introduction of Amidism, a form of Buddhism based on the worship of the Buddha Amida, who promised his worshippers rebirth in the "Western Paradise." Part of the strength of Amidism was its departure from the monastic model. Shinran (1173–1262), the founder of the Jodo Shin or the True Pure Land sect, the most popular Amidist group, explicitly renounced the monastic culture, including **celibacy**. Jodo Shin priests married and founded hereditary lines of temple priests, giving the sect an unprecedented level of penetration and institutional continuity. Other Buddhist sects would follow this pattern.

RISE OF THE WARRIOR CLASS. Over the course of the eleventh and twelfth centuries, the imperial court slowly declined as a power center, and provincial warriors began to be real leaders of politics and, increasingly, culture. Influenced by Confucianism, the warrior leaders and their followers, the "samurai," shifted to a different model of marriage, largely shunning polygamy in favor of a combination of monogamous marriage and concubinage. They also shifted from matrilocal to patrilocal households.

The shift away from the Heian court culture to the military culture of the provincial samurai led to a rise in male homosexuality among the elite, often involving **anal or intercrural sex**. This practice, although sometimes ridiculed, was not widely condemned or outlawed. The economic development of Japan at the time also led to the formation of new urban centers, with brothels and **prostitution**.

Further Reading: McCullough, William H. "Japanese Marriage Institutions in the Heian Period." *Harvard Journal of Asiatic Studies* 27 (1967): 103–67; Morris, Ivan. *The World of the Shining Prince: Court Life in Ancient Japan*. New York: Alfred A. Knopf, 1964; Totman, Conrad. *Japan before Perry*. Berkeley: University of California Press, 1981.

William E. Burns

JAYADEVA (1147–1170). Jayadeva is the author of the *Gita Govindam*, a much-acclaimed Sanskrit poem dealing with the divine love between Lord **Krishna** and Radha. Jayadeva was born in the Kenduli village of Khurda district in the state of Orissa, **India**, the son of Bhojadeva and Ramadevi. Most of his life was spent in the temple of Lord Jagannatha of Puri, where he wrote the *Gita Govindam* and his wife Padmavati danced before the statues of the gods. Emphasizing salvation through **bhakti** or personal devotion to God, the epic became a source of inspiration for Vaishnavism, devotional music, dance, and paintings. A new era began in the classical Odissi dance form and music, and the impact of the *Gita Govindam* spread throughout India. The poem is recited in the festival held annually in Bengal and Orissa in his commemoration.

An erudite scholar of ancient Indian texts, Jayadeva became the spiritual preceptor and court poet of the king of Bengal, Lakshmana Sena. To Jayadeva, Krishna of the *Gita Govindam* was the Supreme Lord Vishnu himself, and the latter had taken one of the *dasa avatars* (ten incarnations) to be born in this mortal world as Krishna. The poem begins with an invocation of the Lord with the ten incarnations. The lyrical description of passionate love between Krishna and Radha is the union of *jeeva atma* (human soul) with *param atma* (the supreme Lord). The unbridled eroticism the two display is the desire of the human soul to merge with God. Eroticism was not taboo in ancient and medieval Indian texts, but an expression of contentment of life. The emotional and passionate longing of the couple has been lyrically delineated by the poet, touching the reader's heart. Jayadeva expresses the lover's passion in a celebrated stanza, where Krishna wants Radha's tender feet to embellish his head so the venom of Kamadeva, the God of Love, would be dispelled. In another stanza, Krishna drinks the sweet nectar from Radha's face.

Connoisseurs of poetry have praised the *Gita Govindam* for its lyricism, emotion, passion, and philosophical content. Jayadeva also wrote *Ratimanjari* (garland of sexual union) and *Chandralok* (light of moon). The sweet couplets of the *Gita Govindam* are still recited by many in eastern India.

Further Reading: Chandra, Moti. *Gita Govinda*. Lalit Kala Series Portfolio No. 3. New Delhi: Lalit Kala Akademi, 1972; Miller, Barbara Stoler. *Gita Govinda of Jayadeva: Love Song of the Dark Lord*. New Delhi: Motilal Banarsidass, 1996; Pathy, Dinanath, et al., eds. *Jayadeva and Gitagovinda in the Traditions of Orissa*. New Delhi: Harman Publishing, 1995.

Patit Paban Mishra

JEANNE D'ARC. *See* Joan of Arc

JEROME, EUSEBIUS HIERONYMUS (347–420). Jerome was born in Stridon, Dalmatia, to Christian parents. Well educated in Latin literature and Christian theology, Jerome later mastered Hebrew and Greek, becoming a prolific translator of biblical commentaries. He compiled the Vulgate, a translation of the Bible from Hebrew and Greek into Latin. He lived during the flowering of the Eastern Christian monastic movement and was an early and vocal supporter of the ascetic lifestyle in the Western Roman empire.

For most of his life, Jerome was preoccupied with the body, sex, and religion. His fascination with asceticism and the Christian hermits living in the Syrian desert enticed him to Syria, where he lived from 374 to 379. However, he quickly became disillusioned with the Syrian monks, who were not embracing the strict standards of behavior that Jerome thought they should. Upon returning to Rome, Jerome became an outspoken proponent of **virginity**, a theme appearing often in his writings, especially letters and biographies of saints. He found a ready audience among wealthy female Christians who often invited him to speak in their homes. Among this group Jerome met Paula, who became his lifelong friend and companion. His hasty departure in 386 from Rome to the more hospitable climate of Bethlehem was strongly influenced by opposition to his teachings. At Bethlehem, Paula provided the financial support Jerome needed to build and maintain a monastery and a convent.

Jerome was often involved in controversies, the most noted and long lasting of which concerned the third-century theologian Origen of Alexandria. Origen's works were often suspect due to their excessive use of allegorical biblical interpretation. Jerome admired Origen during much of his early life, translating several of his works into Latin. Doubts of Origen's orthodoxy eventually drove Jerome to change his views and condemn Origen. This condemnation marked the final break between Jerome and his childhood friend Rufinus, who continued to champion Origen's teachings.

In his *Letter to Eustochium*, *Adversus Jovinianum* and his work against the heretic Helvidius, Jerome argued that **marriage** was second to virginity. Virginity was man's state before the Fall, and marriage came with the advent of sin. Marriage drew the mind away from study and contemplation of God, while virginity enabled people to pursue higher truths. In his correspondence with his former circle in Rome, Jerome urged wives and husbands to adopt **celibacy** and to raise their daughters to remain virgins. Though he considered marriage as inferior, he recognized it as a way to avoid fornication. It was, however, to be temperate. He warned men against loving their wives too much, calling them adulterers to God. As for widows who wanted to remarry, Jerome stated that this would be slightly better than **prostitution**. *See also* Catholicism.

Further Reading: Campenhausen, Hans von. *Men Who Shaped the Western Church*. New York: Harper and Row, 1964; Kelly, J.N.D. *Jerome: His Life, Writings and Controversies*. London: Duckworth, 1975; Steinmann, Jean. *Saint Jerome and His Times*. Translated by Ronald Mathews. Notre Dame, IN: Fides Publishing, 1959.

Lisa R. Holliday

JEWS. Medieval **Judaism** sanctioned sex and love between men and women only within the context of **marriage**. Marriage was both a legal, contractual agreement between a bridegroom and his bride and a holy covenant between man and woman where God serves as an intermediary. In fact, the purpose of marriage was to fulfill the will of God. The term that designates marriage, *kiddushin*, literally means "sanctification," pointing to the reverence Jewish culture accorded this institution. All sins were forgiven at the time of marriage. Furthermore, men were required to marry in order to satisfy the commandment to "be fruitful and multiply" (Genesis 1:28).

The covenant initially consisted of two distinct ceremonies. It began with betrothal or *kiddushin*, usually the reading of the marriage contract (*ketubah*), and ended with the nuptials or *nissuim*. Betrothal could also be contracted through money, deed, or sexual intercourse. The blessings constituting the marriage ceremony were to be recited in front of a quorum of ten adult Jewish men. Technically as much as a year could elapse between the two ceremonies, but during the eleventh century the ceremonies were commonly held together as they are today.

Jewish marriage laws primarily protected the woman, and the *ketubah* dictated the obligations of the bridegroom to his bride. The *ketubah* guarantees a woman economic security in the case of **divorce**, abandonment, or the death of her husband. This is especially important because according to Jewish law only a man can initiate a divorce. The Hebrew Bible only references a man divorcing his wife (Deuteronomy 24:1), but Rabbenu Gershom ben Yehuda (965–1028) decreed that a woman must give her consent. A Jewish court can compel a man to grant his wife a divorce under certain circumstances such as the refusal to have sex, infidelity, beating, lack of provisions, or disease. As specified in the *ketubah*, it is the Jewish wife who had a right to sex, food, and clothing; however, total refusal to have sex with her husband was also grounds for divorce. The marriage documents, written in Aramaic, began to be elaborately illuminated during the tenth or eleventh century.

Many marriages were performed in a synagogue, some in open-air services, but the *huppa*, or marriage canopy, came into use during the Middle Ages. This open canopy symbolized the couple's future home and their openness to the Jewish community in which they will live. They ranged from simple prayer shawls held over the couple to ornate structures made especially for the occasion.

At the conclusion of the marriage ceremony, the groom breaks a glass. This has been interpreted as a reminder of the destruction of the Temple (70 CE) and as an attempt to ward off evil spirits. In the Middle Ages, some men smashed the glass against the north wall because it is the direction from which people felt evil spirits came. This is the same reason church bells are rung at Christian weddings and ships are christened with breaking glass.

Judaism prohibits marriages in cases of **consanguinity**, affinity through one's own marriage, or lack of an official divorce agreement (*get*) ending a previous marriage. Of course, Jews were also forbidden to marry non-Jews. On certain days and festivals, such as Shabbat and the High Holy Days, marriages were forbidden. These proscribed days are still observed.

Torah and Talmudic law permit a man to marry more than one woman, but **polygamy** was never common among Jews. The Talmud itself is based on monogamy. Rabbenu **Gershom ben Judah** officially forbade polygamy among Ashkenazic Jews although evidence indicates this decree to be largely a matter of history as opposed to actual practice. The Islamic influence may account for the few recorded polygamous Sephardic Jewish marriages.

In the Middle Ages, girls were betrothed as early as twelve, much earlier than in Talmudic times (eighteen years). One reason for this may be the relatively elevated economic position of Jews within Europe. Another explanation is that the fear of political persecution leading to the confiscation of funds led fathers to arrange marriages earlier while their dowries were secure. Men also married younger although early rabbinic code states eighteen as the normal age for a man; twenty was deemed late. At the time, child marriages were more prevalent on all fronts.

Matchmakers or *shadchan* moved between Jewish communities in order to appropriately pair Jewish men and women. *Shadchan* achieved legal status in the twelfth century. They were considered agents and fees provided upon the arrangement of marriage. Most *shadchan* were men.

The Spanish Hebrew poet and philosopher **Judah Halevi** (1075–1141) idealized the love between a man and his wife. Some of his poems eventually became part of the Hebrew liturgy. Family represents an intimate and romanticized unit. This is as close a parallel as we can see in medieval Jewism literature to the **courtly love** so central to medieval Christian poetry.

Sex is sanctioned within Judaism for procreation and furthering intimacy between husband and wife. **Moses Maimonides** (1135–1204), the foremost medieval Jewish philosopher, considered nonmarital sex as equivalent to **prostitution**. Jewish law and medieval practice with regards to sex strive to enforce moderation, respect, and love between a man and his wife. Sex is only permissible within marriage, and homosexual relationships have always been prohibited ("Do not lie with a man as one lies with a woman," Leviticus 18:22). Interestingly, the Torah does not explicitly forbid female homosexuality, and the Talmud is practically silent on the matter. Sexual contact (as opposed to intercourse) is also prohibited outside of marriage. Homosexuality, **adultery**, and **incest** are all punishable by death (Leviticus 20:13), although medieval rabbis were reluctant to impose the death penalty, favoring communal discipline. *See also* Ibn Gabirol, Solomon; Interconfessional Sex and Love.

Further Reading: Abrahams, Israel. *Jewish Life in the Middle Ages*. Philadelphia: Jewish Publication Society of America, 1896; Epstein, Louis M. *Sex Laws and Customs in Judaism*. New York: Bloch Publishing, 1948; Winkler, Gershom. *Sacred Secrets: The Sanctity of Sex in Jewish Law and Lore*. Northvale, NJ: Jason Aronson, 1998.

Deborah Thalheimer Long

JOAN, POPE. *See* Pope Joan

JOAN OF ARC (Jeanne d'Arc) (1412–1431). Joan of Arc was a mystic woman, heroine and leader of the French army in the Hundred Years War. She was born in the village of Domremy in 1412. After having had supernatural revelations, she wanted to meet the heir to the French throne, persuading him to be crowned king of France with the name of Charles VII and to entrust her with the leadership of the French army, which was opposing the English invasion of France. After a series of victories, and a defeat near Paris, where she was injured, Burgundians captured Joan in Compiègne and entrusted her to the English, who tried her as a witch and a heretic. Joan was condemned to the stake, where she was burned in 1431 in the public square of Rouen. Eventually, she was rehabilitated, thanks to a process instigated by Pope Callistus III in 1455–1456, and canonized in 1920, to be proclaimed Patron Saint of France in 1944 by Pope Pius XII.

Many novels and movies have been made based on her story. Many historians have written about Joan's sexuality, with differing conclusions. That Joan wore men's clothing has made scholars to infer that she was consciously or unconsciously a transvestite, bisexual, a lesbian, or even asexual. The twentieth-century lesbian writer Vita Sackville-West, in her book *Saint Joan of Arc*, claimed Joan was a lesbian. Some scholars emphasize Jean d'Aulon's statement that he overheard some women say that they never saw Joan menstruate. In 1981 the endocrinologist Robert B. Greenblatt diagnosed a rare genetic anomaly that could have affected Joan's sexuality. Others want to see in Joan the ancestor of modern feminism. The historical Joan was always proud to be a woman and a virgin. She called herself "Jeanne, la Pucelle," or Joan, the Maid, because she wanted to emphasize this fact. She was never interested in having sex with men. Her drive and passion were directed solely toward accomplishing her God-given goal, her sexuality sublimated in her love for God. *See also* Transgenderism and Cross-Dressing; Virgin Martyrs.

Further Reading: Pernoud, Regine. *Joan of Arc by Herself and Her Witnesses*. Translated from the French by Edward Hyams. New York: Stein and Day, 1982.

Elvio Ciferri

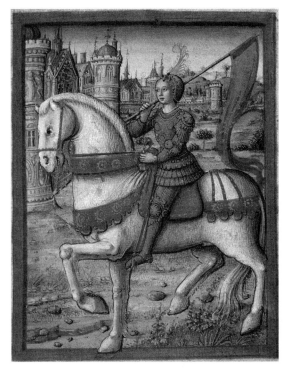

Portrait from *La Vie des Femmes Celebres* (Life of Famous Women), by Antoine du Four, 1505. © The Art Archive/Musée Thomas Dobrée Nantes/Dagli Orti.

JUDAISM. The prescriptive aspects of Judaism relating to sex and love are found in the Torah (the Pentateuch) and in the Talmud, the recorded interpretations and discussions among Jewish scholars in various locations from roughly 200 to 500 CE. The medieval Jewish legal interpreters and codifiers continue to promulgate the general views of those rabbis cited in the Talmud. According to rabbinic interpretation, the first positive commandment in the Hebrew Bible is "to be fruitful and multiply" (Genesis 1:28), making sex and procreation a central element in Jewish theology. Jewish law considers having a child each of both sexes the minimum necessary to fulfill that commandment. Sex and procreation were only permitted within the covenant of **marriage**, and wedded life was considered the most natural and exalted state. Divorce was not easily accomplished, but the commandment to be fruitful and multiply was considered so important that a man was permitted to divorce his wife provided that she had been barren for a decade.

Yet Jewish theology denied that procreation is the only reason for sex. Torah explains that God created woman because "it is not good for man to be alone" (Genesis 2:18). Companionship, love, and intimacy were the primary reasons for the creation of the two sexes. Sex and sexual pleasure were considered divine, and although a complex religious code governed sexual activity, Judaism did not deny or forbid sexual gratification provided it occured within the boundaries established by the Torah and the Talmud. Jewish law and commentary strived to establish a legal code of sexual morality based on moderation, respect, and love within the covenant of marriage.

Most laws thus derive from both the desire to establish a warm, committed relationship between husband and wife and the desire to increase the population of **Jews**. Absolute fidelity is required of both husband and wife. Under no circumstances, even when in danger of death, is a Jew permitted to commit **adultery**, idolatry, or murder; death is considered preferable. Judaism sanctions sex within marriage only on a mutually consensual basis. It is considered the woman's right to be satisfied sexually, a right explicitly stated in the marriage contract. This represents a vast divergence from the medieval Islamic tradition, as does the Jewish insistence on monogamy. Jewish law considers sex an expression of intimacy between a man and his wife, and it should only occur out of respect for one another and within the boundaries established by the purity laws.

Judaism prohibits a man from having sex with his wife during her menstrual period and for seven days following it, a time considered ritually impure. During this time, all physical contact between husband and wife is forbidden. This separation and the complex laws that govern it are referred to as *niddah*. Following the "unclean days" a woman is required to immerse herself in a *mikvah*, a ritual bath in natural spring or river water. The separation and abstention that surround **menstruation** may increase the probability of conception when Jewish couples are permitted sexual intercourse. *Niddah* also ensures a moderation of sexual activity and perhaps helps to build a desire between married couples.

There is no evidence of post-Talmudic **prostitution** in Jewish culture until the fourteenth century. Offences of sexual immorality such as the adultery of a married woman and her lover are technically punishable by death although medieval rabbis were reluctant to impose capital punishment. Although Jewish law does consider the act of sex a result of the evil impulse or the *yetzer ha-ra*, it is not a base or evil action. The evil impulse also accounts for several natural desires, such as hunger and thirst. Sexual desire is a base passion in and of itself, but it can and should be properly channeled to serve higher purposes, such as procreation and intimacy between husband and wife. The need to intelligently moderate sex (*niddah*) and avert temptation accounts for much of the Jewish ethical code and practice concerning physical contact, dress, and chaperones. These laws are intended to avert improper sexual urges.

Nahmanides (1194–1270), a preeminent Spanish Talmudist, considered sex in observance with Jewish law to be holy and pure. He decreed that sex is natural and that nothing corporeal is unholy unless intended or used in impure ways. At the same time Pope Innocent III declared that sex is shameful and wicked. Christian theology offered "spiritual marriages" and looked upon sex and sexual gratification with disdain. In direct opposition to the priestly class, rabbis were compelled to marry and expected to present a model home life. **Celibacy** is even prohibited according to interpretations of Genesis 1:28. For a Jew, marriage and the study of Torah are the paramount religious obligations. Medieval Christianity stressed the evil inherent in all sexual desire, advocating celibacy or spiritual marriages. **Thomas Aquinas** (c. 1225–1274), following **Augustine** (354–430) on celibacy, taught that the sexual act itself transmits original sin. Contrary to medieval Christian thinking, for Jews, sex becomes a *mitzvah* or good deed when performed out of love between a husband and his wife at the proper moment. The ascetic, monastic aspect to medieval Christianity is completely absent from Judaism in the same period.

Love is central to Jewish marriage and sexual intercourse, but love is also prescribed toward God, neighbor, and stranger. Torah gives three positive commandments to love: love of God ("Love the Lord your God with all your heart and with all your soul and with all your strength," Deuteronomy 6:5), love of neighbor ("Love your neighbor as yourself," Leviticus 19:18), and love of stranger ("You are to love those who are aliens for you yourselves were aliens in Egypt," Deuteronomy 10:19). Nahmanides explained that loving a neighbor entails wishing for them as one does for oneself in terms of prosperity, honor, and wisdom. Loving a stranger was usually interpreted as a commandment to provide for them. Acting as if one loves both their neighbor and stranger practically encompassed the mandate to strive for the ideal consideration of and compassion toward all other humans. Love of God entailed following all of his prescriptives and studying Torah, both of which leads back to love—love of neighbor, stranger, and God. Therefore, love remained the center not only of sexual relations between Jews in the Middle Ages, but also of their religious lives in total.

Further Reading: Abrahams, Israel. *Jewish Life in the Middle Ages*. Philadelphia: Jewish Publication Society of America, 1896; Epstein, Louis M. *Sex Laws and Customs in Judaism*. New York: Bloch Publishing, 1948; Winkler, Gershom. *Sacred Secrets: The Sanctity of Sex in Jewish Law and Lore*. Northvale, NJ: Jason Aronson, 1998.

Deborah Thalheimer Long

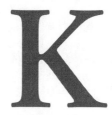

KAILASANATH TEMPLE AT ELLORA. The Kailasanath (or Kailasha) Temple is a rock-cave temple located in Ellora, **India**. It is approximately twenty-six kilometers north of Aurangabad. It is one of the thirty-four cave temples that were carved out of basalt on the face of an escarpment of the Deccan plateau over a 600-year period.

The Kailasanath Temple was built around the seventh century by King Krishna I of the Rashtrakuta dynasty. It is a huge monolithic structure in the South Indian style, carved from the top down by master craftsmen under royal patronage. It is estimated that 200,000 tons of rock were carved for the massive structure. Stories from the *Ramayana* and the *Mahabharata* are carved into the rocks. The temple was dedicated to Shiva and was named for his mountain home in the Himalayas, the snow-covered peak Kailasa. Shiva is one of the triumvirate of **Hinduism**, which includes Brahma (the creator) and Vishnu (the preserver). Shiva is the "destroyer" and was first worshipped in South India.

At the entrance to the temple is a symbolic river representing the three river goddesses. For Hindus a bath in a river is a ritual of purification. Inside the sanctuary are sexual symbols, the lingam and yoni. The lingam, Shiva's sign, is a phallic symbol, while the yoni represents a vagina. These sexual symbols represent energy. Shiva is a recreator god so the energy expended is used to re-create life. Shiva is often depicted along with his consort, Sati, presented as a voluptuous woman. However, she can take several forms reflecting different aspects of Shiva. Sati may be Parvati, reflecting gentleness; Durga, representing mystery; or Kali, representing ferocity. The sexual iconography in the temple was developed over a number of years. The increasing depiction of sexuality demonstrates the growth of Tantric beliefs. *See also* Phallic Worship.

Further Reading: Gupte, Ramesh Shankar, and B. D. Mahajan. *Ajanta, Ellora and Aurangabad Caves*. Mumbai, India: D.B. Taraporevala, 1962; Spink, Walter. *Ajanta to Ellora*. Mumbai, India: Marg Publications for the Center for South and Southeast Asian Studies, University of Michigan, 1967.

Andrew J. Waskey

KALIDASA. Kalidasa, one of the greatest and most accomplished Sanskrit writers on love and other topics, adorned the court of Chandragupta II (375–413), a ruler of the Gupta dynasty of **India**. Kalidasa was one of the "nine gems" of the king's court. He became famous for his wit and sarcasm as well as the vivid descriptions of nature, romantic love, passion, and the pangs of suffering for beloved found in his writings. Little is known about his early life from authentic sources. Most authorities agree that he lived during the middle of the fourth century. Legends depict him as a buffoon, but one who was blessed by Goddess Saraswati (Goddess of Learning) to be able to pen excellent dramas and epics. According to legend, the goddess blessed him with a famous saying, *Ttvam Ev Aham* ("You are none other than me").

Kalidasa's famous dramas are *Abhijnanasakuntalam*, *Malavikagnimitram*, and *Vikramorvasiyam*. His magnum opus, *Abhijnanasakuntalam*, has been translated into English and German. In this, the king Dushyanta falls in love with the beautiful Shakuntala while in hunting expedition in forest. They marry and the king gives her a ring, but Shakuntala is cursed by a sage, because of which Dushyanta is unable to remember her. After many travails the lovers finally unite. The hero of *Malavikagnimitram* is King Agnimitra, a historical figure who falls in love with a commoner Malavika. Malavika is imprisoned by the queen but is revealed as a true princess, and the lovers are reunited. In *Vikramorvasiyam* Kalidasa depicts the passionate love affair between King Pururavas and the exquisitely beautiful Urvashi, a celestial nymph. While performing in heaven, she falters after pronouncing the name of her lover. She is asked to leave the heaven, and after much suffering meets her lover in the mortal world.

Kalidasa also wrote lyrics and epic poems. *Meghaduutam* (Cloud Messenger) is one of the finest pieces of world literature. A yaksha, an attendant of Kubera, the God of Wealth, is exiled for dereliction of duty. He has left behind his beautiful wife and suffers in her absence. He sends messages to his wife through moving clouds after the rainy season, expressing his deep love for her. Passion, erotic sentiments, and the desire to unite with the beloved are fully expressed in this poem. The *Ritusamhara* (Seasonal Cycle) describes the six seasons of the year. It is replete with deep emotion, love, and the erotic sentiments pertaining to different seasons. The epic *Kumarasambhava* describes the love between God Shiva and Parvati, the daughter of Himalaya, their **marriage**, and the birth of the war God, Kumara. The God of Love, Kamadeva, disturbs the meditation of Shiva, who burns Kamadeva to ashes. Afterward, Shiva himself is aroused by love, and his marriage with Parvati results in the birth of Kumara. Kalidasa never hesitated to describe the physical beauty of a woman. In Kumarasambhava, for instance, he describes the rain drop falling over Parvati, when she is meditating to get Shiva, as moving down her eyelids, lips, breasts, triple fold, and finally vanishing in her navel. Sometimes, he vividly portrays lovemaking scenes with all his imagination in an ornamental style as in Canto VIII. According to legend, Parvati cursed the poet for the too explicit description of these scenes, and he could not complete the epic. The *Raghuvamsha* is about the dynasty of Raghu, to which Rama belonged. Kalidas describes the events of the *Ramayana* of Valmiki in an elegant style.

Critics point out that Kalidasa had no interest in the contemporary problems of society. His forte as a Sanskrit poet was the description of love and other human sentiments.

Further Reading: Devadhar, C. R. *Meghaduta of Kalidasa*. New Delhi: Motilal Banarsidass, 1985; Kanitkar, Hemant. *Kalidas's Abhijnana Shakuntala*. Mumbai, India: Popular Prakashan, 1984; Nandgrikar, G. R., ed. *Meghdutam of Kalidas*. With English translation and notes. New Delhi: Asiatic Books, 2001; Singh, A. D. *Kaalidaasa: A Critical Study*. Columbia, MO: South Asia Books, 1977; Thapar, Romila. *Sakuntala: Text, Readings, Histories*. New Delhi: Kali for Women, 1999.

Patit Paban Mishra

KAMA SUTRA. The *Kama Sutra* is the world's oldest book on the pleasures of sensual living. The text cannot be attributed to any one single author. It was originally compiled in the third century by the sage Vatsyayana, who lived in northern **India**. Vatsyayana claimed to be a celibate monk, and that his work in compiling all of the sexual knowledge of ages past was for him a form of meditation and contemplation of the deity. Written in a rather complex form of Sanskrit, the *Kama Sutra* is the only surviving textual account of that period of ancient Indian history. In scholarly circles it has been widely consulted by scholars trying to understand the society and social mores of that period. The title of the text, *Kama Sutra*, literally means "a treatise on pleasure." Far more complex than a mere listing of contortionist sexual positions, the *Kama Sutra* makes a comprehensive manual of living for the good life. Although the central character is the citizenly man-about-town, the text was written to be read by, and provide detailed advice for, both men and women.

The basic tenet of the *Kama Sutra* is that for **marriage**s to be happy, both man and woman should be well versed in the arts of pleasure, both carnal and cerebral. Some people refer to the *Kama Sutra* as a marriage manual, but it is a far cry from the monogamous and dutiful tomes that Westerners produced as part of the proliferation of advice manuals in the Victorian era. One of the central figures of the *Kama Sutra* is the courtesan, who must also master and practice a variety of arts in learning how to please and coerce her man. What is especially unique about the *Kama Sutra* is that it maintains a special focus on creating pleasure for the woman. A man who fails to provide and bring about those pleasures is subject to a woman's recourse, that is, to seek pleasure elsewhere where she may find it.

As the original study of sexuality, the *Kama Sutra* became the fountainhead of all subsequent compilations, including the fifteenth-century **Ananga Ranga**, which is a revised version and builds upon Vatsyayana's basic tenets. Yet because of the complex and rather inaccessible style of Sanskrit in which it was written, the *Kama Sutra* for many centuries fell into obscurity. Scholars of Sanskrit and ancient India did not much consult it. It was not until the late nineteenth century that the *Kama Sutra* again began to gain its former prominence in the textual traditions of India. That resurgence came about after the 1870s, when Sir Richard Burton, the noted linguist and Arabic translator, was working with his collaborators, both Indian and British, on producing a translation of the *Ananga Ranga*. In pursuing the many references to Vatsyayana in the text, Burton led the pundits back to the *Kama Sutra* and an English translation was produced. Burton's persistence in publishing the *Kama Sutra* in the West, and the interest the text generated in both India and abroad, has led to a proliferation of translations and versions of the original masterpiece. *See also* Hinduism; Sex Manuals.

Further Reading: *The Kama Sutra and Ananga Ranga.* Translated by Sir Richard Francis Burton. New York: Barnes and Noble, 2006.

Anne Hardgrove

KHAJURAHO TEMPLE COMPLEX. The Khajuraho temple complex is situated in the state of Madhya Pradesh in central **India**. The structure was built in the Indo-Aryan Nagara style of architecture somewhere between 950 and 1050.

The temple complex was erected near a small village named Khajuraho during the reign of the Chandelas, Hindu Rajput kings. Only twenty-two of the eighty-five original temples remain. The temples are celebrated all over the globe for their unique architectural features and exquisite carvings. Unlike most Indian temple structures, the Khajuraho temples are not contained within an enclosure; instead, each temple stands on a high, solid masonry platform. The temple architecture is a living testimony to the complex commixture of thought, and represents a harmonious blending of various Indian religious traditions including Shaivism, Vaishnavism, and **Jainism**. The temples seamlessly blend architecture and sculpture, honoring religious sentiments and artistic genius. The temple structure looks graceful and elegant emanating deep-rooted tradition and value.

The three main components of a Khajuraho temple are its entrance (*ardhamandapa*), assembly hall (*mandapa*), and the sanctum sanctorum (*garbha griha*). Further, geospatially the temples have been divided into three parts, that is, western, eastern, and southern. Of the western group, the Kandariya Mahadev Temple has been considered the most beautiful of all. It is thirty-one meters tall and is full of spectacular, fine, and highly skilled scuplture work. The temple has sculptures of various deities, graceful maidens, dancers, and musicians. The depictions are varied, including very sensuous postures as well. Other temples in the same group are the Chaunsat Yogini, the only granite temple in Khajuraho, the Devi Jagadambe Temple, the Chitragupta Temple, and the Lakshmana Temple, all having fine ornate sculptures on their walls. The eastern group features Hindu and Jain temples. The three Hindu temples are the Brahma, Vamana, and Javari temples, and the most famous Jain temple, namely the Ghantai Temple, with its sculptured images of the sixteen dreams of the Jain founder Mahavira's mother. The southern group is most known for its splendid Chaturbhuj Temple. Its defining feature is the exquisitely carved idol of Vishnu in the inner sanctum.

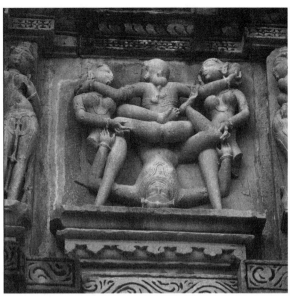
Erotic carvings celebrating the marriage of Gods Shiva and Parvati from the Kandariya Mahadev temple in Khajuraho, India. © The Art Archive/Stephanie Colasanti.

Though most of the temple structures of central India have simple interiors with no superfluous elements, Khajuraho temples are rich in very detailed sculpture. Other than numerous deities enshrined in wall niches, there are attendants, graceful maidens in various sensual images, dancers, musicians, and embracing couples. In one temple complex itself, over 650 figures are depicted. These compositions are symbols of great sensuality. Explicit sexual activity is also depicted, possibly illustrating the tantric rites that were part of the temple worship ritual. Some of the sexual postures are based on the tenets of **Kama Sutra**. The Khajuraho group of monuments has been listed as a UNESCO World Heritage site. *See also* Hinduism.

Further Reading: Brown, Percy. *Indian Architecture*. Mumbai, India: Taraporevala, 1959; Michell, George. *The Penguin Guide to the Monuments of India*. Vol. 1. London: Viking, 1989; Tadgell, Christopher. *The History of Architecture in India*. London: Phaidon Press, 1990.

Jitendra Uttam

KISS OF INFAMY. The *osculum infame* or kiss of infamy was a medieval Christian belief with ancient roots. Heretics and witches were believed to kiss the devil on the mouth, genitals, or anus or perform other degrading kisses at their meetings. This kind of kissing was a diabolical parody of the kiss of peace, and also referred to the use of

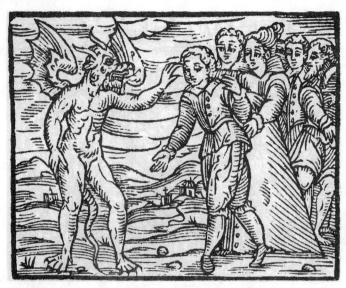

"The Kiss of Infamy," from R.P. Guaccius' *Compendium Maleficarum*, Milan, 1626. Courtesy of Dover Pictorial Archives.

kissing in feudal ceremonies of homage—by making this degrading kiss, the witch-initiate was accepting the devil as his or her lord.

A description of secret gatherings of heretics kissing a demonic black cat on the feet, under the tail, and on the genitals can be found in Walter Map's *On the Folly of Courtiers*, written about 1180. The scholastic philosopher and theologian William of Auvergne (c. 1180–1249) described demon-worshipping heretics as kissing cats and toads, really demons in animal form, on the mouth and buttocks. Similar claims appeared in Pope Gregory IX's bull *Vox in Rama* of 1233, which charged that Rhineland heretics of Cathar beliefs were kissing the devil in the form of a toad, goose, duck, black cat, or thin man on the mouth or anus as a prelude to a bisexual orgy. Obscene kisses were also exchanged between the leader of the heretical group and his followers.

The kiss of infamy played a prominent role in the **trial of the Templars**, who were charged with requiring their initiates to kiss the mouth, navel, and buttocks of the former. This claim, which broke from the previous emphasis on kissing the devil or demons, was connected to the charges of homosexuality made against the Templars. In the later Middle Ages, the kiss of infamy became more strongly associated with witches. Charges of kissing the devil or a demon show up fairly often in fifteenth-century witch trials. *See also* Witches and Witch-Hunting.

Further Reading: Russell, Jeffrey Burton. *Witchcraft in the Middle Ages*. Ithaca, NY: Cornell University Press, 1972.

William E. Burns

KRISHNA. In the Hindu tri-theistic pantheon (Brahma, Vishnu, and Shiva), Krishna is an avatar of Vishnu, the loving preserver. Krishna is first mentioned in the *Chandogya Upanishad*. He has a major role as a warrior in the *Mahabharata*, especially in the *Bhagavad Gita* section, where on the battlefield of Kurukshetra he is the charioteer of Arjuna and a preacher. However, most worship of Krishna in **Hinduism** has been as a divine lover.

The *Bhagavata Purana* ("ancient stories of the Lord") provides many of the details of Krishna's life and destiny. The details are important to the cult of Krishna as a **bhakti** way of salvation. The *Bhagavata Purana* tells that one day the wife of a king of Mathura was strolling in the woods when a demon lusted for her. He assumed her husband's form and had sex with her. She bore the demon's son who was named Kansa. Cruel from birth, Kansa grew up to dethrone his father. With his tyranny weighing very heavily on the earth, complaints reached Indra and the other gods, who approached Vishnu for help. Vishnu took a white hair and a black hair from his head. The white hair would be incarnated as Balarama and the black hair as Krishna. A voice prophesied that Devaki, wife of Vasudeva, would bear Krishna, who will slay the evil Kansa.

When Devaki gave birth to Krishna, her eighth child, he was immediately substituted for the new-born son of Yasoda, the wife of a herdsman named Nanda. When Kansa heard that Devaki's eighth child had been born he killed its substitute to stop the prophecy. Hidden within his earthly foster family, Krishna grew as a mischievous child, which endeared him to women.

As a young man he performed numerous heroic deeds and played tricks on the *gopis* (the wives of the cowherds), who were madly in love with Krishna although they were married. Once when the *gopis* were at the river bathing, Krishna stole their clothes and sat in a tree. He refused to return their clothes until each naked *gopi* came to claim them with hands lifted as a suppliant.

In one story, Krishna danced with the *gopis* while his friend, Balarama, played the flute. Krishna multiplied into so many forms that he seemed to be dancing with each individual *gopi* and each one believed that she alone possessed the hand of the true Krishna. Krishna's favorite *gopi* was Radha. Once she was afraid that her jealous husband might kill her. However, Krishna changed his form to fool him, so when the husband found them she appeared to be worshipping Kali.

Later, after Kansa learned of Krishna's existence, Krishna killed him. As further events unfolded Krishna fell in love with Rukmini. In order to win her he had to fight several battles. He killed a king who had 16,100 damsels locked away. Krishna wed them all at once and so multiplied himself that he had a wedding night with each simultaneously.

The cult of Krishna produced romantic poetry, music, and artistic expression of the details of Krishna's love life with Radha, Rukmini, and the *gopis*. The passion of women expressed in these works shows longing for an absent lover. The channeling of that love to Krishna was the way of salvation.

Further Reading: Archer, W. G. *The Loves of Krishna: In Indian Painting and Poetry.* 1957. Reprint, Mineola, NY: Dover Publications, 2004; Bhattacharya, S. K. *Krsna-cult in Indian Art.* New Delhi: M.D. Publications, 1996; Lal, Kanwar. *The Religion of Love.* New Delhi: Arts & Letters, 1971.

Andrew J. Waskey

KYTELER, ALICE (1280–c. 1325). The trial of the Irish noblewoman Alice Kyteler in 1324 was one of the first, along with the **trial of the Templars,** to link witchcraft and human-demon sex. The wealthy Kyteler, of Flemish descent, had survived three husbands and was currently married to a fourth. Some of the children of her husbands by their previous wives accused her and eleven others—four men and seven women of Ossory—of having bewitched her husbands and murdered them by sorcery, and of poisoning her current husband, Sir John Le Poer, who was in truth very ill. Bishop Richard Ledrede of Ossory, an Englishman currently conducting an aggressive antiheresy drive, condemned Kyteler as a heretic and a sorcerer.

Confessions obtained under torture showed that Kyteler had renounced Christ and the church, sacrificed to demons, and had a devil called Robert Artisson as a familiar. One of Kyteler's women attendants, Petronilla of Meath, confessed to having witnessed intercourse between Kyteler and Robert Artisson in the form of a black man. The charge of human-demon sex had little immediate precedent but would become prominent in the later witch-craze. Its appearance in Ireland, a place largely spared witch trials and witch hunts, at this early date remains mysterious, although Ledrede had studied in France during some early witch trials there and was a client of Pope John XXII, famous for his opposition to sorcery. Petronilla was flogged and burned at the stake for her role as a go-between. Kyteler fled to England, where her ultimate fate remains unknown. *See also* Witches and Witch-Hunting.

Further Reading: Cohn, Norman. *Europe's Inner Demons: The Demonization of Christians in Medieval Christendom.* Rev. ed. Chicago: University of Chicago Press, 2000; Williams, Bernadette. "'She Was Usually Placed with the Great Men and Leaders of the Land in the Public Assemblies'—Alice Kyteler: A Woman of Considerable Power." In *Women in Renaissance and Early Modern Europe,* edited by Christine Meek, 67–83. Dublin: Four Courts Press, 2000.

William E. Burns

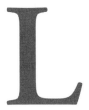

LENT. Lent (a period of forty days leading up to Easter) is traditionally a time of abstinence for Christians. While in most cases this means limiting meals and the types of food eaten, for medieval European Christians Lent was also a time when married couples were supposed to avoid sexual activity.

Several early Christian writers stated that married couples should abstain from sex for a part of the year, often taking 1 Corinthians 7:5 as a proof text: "Do not refuse one another except perhaps by agreement for a season, that you may devote yourselves to prayer." In the early sixth century, Caesarius of Arles specified that Lent was "a season" in which abstinence was required (as were major feast days). While it is not known whether Caesarius invented this rule or was merely the first to write down an account of a common practice, the prohibition against sex during Lent entered into the legal collections and pastoral handbooks of the early Middle Ages.

Between the seventh and eleventh centuries, the Lenten prohibition was gradually expanded. While fasting during Lent was suspended on Sundays, sexual abstinence was not, which meant that the period of prohibition could last as long as forty-seven days depending on the liturgical calendar of a given diocese. In addition to the weeks leading up to Easter (the Great Lent), there were two other periods of time (also called Lents) when general and sexual abstinence were required: Advent, which extended approximately twenty or forty days before Christmas depending on local practices; and a period ranging between seven and forty days before Pentecost. Between them, the three Lents could make marital sex a forbidden activity for up to one-third of the year.

Beginning in the twelfth century, a greater emphasis on the role of the "conjugal debt" in **marriage** led to some relaxing of the strictures against marital sex during Lent. The theory of conjugal debt holds that one partner in a marriage is obliged to provide sex should the other partner request it. Thus, if one partner in a marriage requested sex during Lent, the other partner was allowed, indeed required, to engage in the requested sexual activity. Ideally, neither partner would ask the other to break the Lenten prohibition, but if such an occasion arose, the burden of sin would only fall on the partner who asked for it. *See also* Catholicism.

Further Reading: Brundage, James. *Law, Sex, and Christian Society in Medieval Europe.* Chicago: University of Chicago Press, 1987; Payer, Pierre J. "Early Regulations Concerning Marital Sexual Relations." *Journal of Medieval History* 6 (1980): 353–76.

Stephen A. Allen

LESBIANISM. See Homosexuality, Female

LUST. Lust is an inordinate desire for the pleasure found in sexual intercourse. It is one of the seven cardinal sins set forth by Pope St. Gregory the Great (590–604) in his treatise *Magna Moralia*, an exposition of Job. Gregory's list includes, in order of increasing spiritual severity, the following: lust, gluttony, sadness (later sloth, utter apathy), avarice, wrath, envy, and pride. This is an authoritative compilation of the seven deadly sins, but it was not the first: St. John Cassian wrote *The Institutes* between 420 and 429, in which he included eight principal sins. Evagrius Ponticus, an Egyptian ascetic (346–399), also described a number of evil contemplations in *On Discrimination in Respect of Passions and Thoughts*.

Lust is the subject of many key passages in the Bible. According to the Ten Commandments (Exodus 20:17), a man must not covet his neighbor's wife. Job says that if a man lusts after another woman—his neighbor's woman—then let his own wife be taken by another. He compares lust to a fire burning up crops in a field (Ch. 31). In the Sermon on the Mount (Matthew 5:28), Jesus Christ states that lust is not only a sin of the flesh but also a sin of the mind: if a man looks at a woman and thinks lecherous thoughts, it is as if he has committed the action. Saint Paul teaches that it is the will of God that men learn to control their bodies and abstain from fornication (1 Thessalonians 4:3–5); Christian men and women must not rage with lust like the heathen. Paul also says that to marry is better than to burn—though being celibate is preferable (1 Corinthians 7:8–9).

Saint **Augustine** of Hippo succumbed to lust as an adolescent. In *The Confessions*, he describes his senses being obscured by concupiscence. He could no longer distinguish between pure love and the degradation of lust. Intemperance forced him into abominations, which he regrets throughout the work. Saint Augustine recounts how his spirit and flesh lusted against one another—drawing each other away from their intended aim. In *On Christian Doctrine*, he further develops the idea that chaste love is proper because it moves the soul toward God, whereas lust compels an individual to think only of himself. All things, including the love for a person, should be *used*, not *enjoyed*. Hence, the love between man and woman must be used to seek God, not enjoyed in the transitory world. Lust is said to pervert the mind because it inverts the rational hierarchy—God, others, self. For this reason, lust is a mortal sin. However, according to Augustine's *On the Good of Marriage*, occasional incontinence, the inability to contain or control one's passions with reason, is not damnable in wedlock so long as it does not interfere with a dedication to God. Rather, it helps preserve fidelity and thus is only a venial sin.

Saint **Bernard of Clairvaux** adds to the understanding of lust through his development of the four degrees of love in *On Loving God*. He shows how the relationship between human beings and God mirrors the way a couple grows in relationship with each other. First, a man loves only himself. Second, he loves another, God or woman, for the sake of himself. Third, the individual learns to love another for the other's sake, and, finally, man may come to love himself through his love for God. In fact, his love for a woman may help lead him to God, but the first and second degrees are characterized entirely by lust. The purpose of the work is to demonstrate how a person moves beyond concupiscence to achieve something greater.

Theological conceptions of lust are treated significantly in vernacular literature. In *Erec and Enide* (c. 1170), Chrétien de Troyes makes Erec yield to lust with the advent of his **marriage** to Enide. This proves to undermine their entire purpose as a couple. **Dante Alighieri** constructs the second circle of hell in *The Divine Comedy* as an enclosure for the lustful. The souls are caught in a never-ending whirlwind, just as in life they were

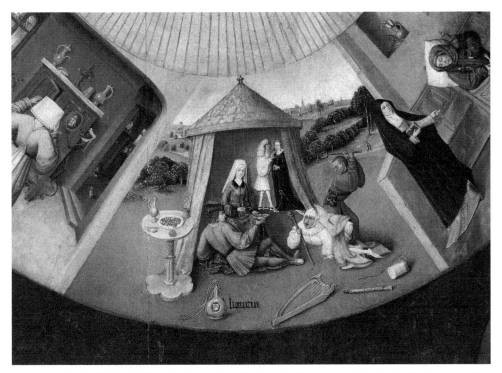

"Lust." A detail of *The Table of the Seven Deadly Sins*, by Hieronymus Bosch. © Erich Lessing/Art Resource, NY.

driven by their uncontrollable passions. It is a punishment to fit the sin. **Geoffrey Chaucer**'s Wife of Bath in *The Canterbury Tales* personifies lust. She is crafted not only to exhibit the evils of the sin but also to show how a person can become entrapped by such a lifestyle.

Further Reading: Augustine of Hippo. *On Christian Doctrine*. Translated by D. W. Robertson Jr. Upper Saddle River, NJ: Prentice Hall, 1997; Bernard of Clairvaux. *On Loving God*. Translated by Emero Stiegman. Kalamazoo, MI: Cistercian Publications, 1995; Newhauser, Richard, ed. *In the Garden of Evil: The Vices and Culture in the Middle Ages*. Toronto, ON: Pontifical Institute of Mediaeval Studies Press, 2005.

K. Sarah-Jane Murray and Hannah Zdansky

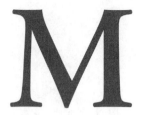

MAGIC. Belief in magic was an integral part of all cultures of the medieval world, across socioeconomic barriers and gender lines, across continents and religions. Practitioners of magic were both revered and feared, sometimes at the same time. As the era drew to a close and the renaissance began, scientific discoveries were able to convince many, at least on an intellectual level, that magic did not rule their lives. Urban areas came to this realization earlier than the rural areas, and some of the rural areas held on to their beliefs far into the renaissance period and beyond. In fact, even today many believe that the power of magic in our lives cannot be denied.

Tribal societies of the early Middle Ages based their magic on the powers of nature. Magical forces were held responsible for any inexplicable event. Natural objects and animals were imbued with their own spirits, and these spirits could be controlled with spells or incantations performed by those trained in the art. Magic was sometimes seen as a force unto itself and sometimes as an integral part of the religion of the time, with gods and goddesses protecting and dwelling within certain trees or wells or sacred grounds. Magic often overlapped with early medical practices, as the mixtures and applications of herbal treatments were also seen as magical by people of this time.

Sexual magic is usually associated with Eastern magic, but almost all societies believed that the fluids secreted during sex had magical properties. Hindu and Buddhist magicians believed that sexual energy could be channeled into the mind, taking one to a higher spiritual plane. Tantric yoga is one of the products of such beliefs.

HERBALISM AND MAGIC. Wise women and men, or witches, of the time were responsible for almost all health care in early medieval villages. Because they had knowledge about ways in which plants, minerals, and other ingredients could be combined to effect cures, they were thought to have an unnatural power over natural elements. If someone had a problem they thought only magic could cure, and consulted the local herbalist. Young women consulted them for love philtres. Married women may have asked for help with a wandering husband, either with another love potion or punishment, such as a dose of southernwood to cause **impotence**. Men could seek advice from the wise women if they had such a problem, and they might receive dragon's blood herb. Both **contraception** and fertility were issues then, and there were magical herbs, actions, and incantations that could be tried. Of course, many of the remedies of the time were either ineffective or went horribly wrong, in which case the wise woman was condemned as a sorceress who had purposely harmed her patient.

Recipes for love potions and **aphrodisiacs** still exist from ancient and medieval times, but the names of some plants have changed and are no longer recognizable.

However, there are several that are still common today. Caraway, mallow, and lovage, for example, were important ingredients in love potions. In a related potion, anointing oneself with chicory combined with oil was thought to make one popular. Cloves, garlic, mandrake, marigold, mustard, nettle, radish, saffron, sage, and valerian were considered aphrodisiacs. Mustard and valerian were specifically for women, supposedly able to make even virtuous women lustful. There were also herbs to calm sexual desires; some were rue, cowbane, hops, and coriander. These were quite commonly grown in monasteries. Interestingly enough, some scholars believed that coriander might also have increased potency.

The most popular magic has always been the love spell. Sometimes a witch will use a combination of an incantation and a charm to be worn, or an herbal concoction that had been made during a propitious astrological period. Charms were a form of sympathetic magic, which is the belief that objects are linked by a magical bond and one object (or person) can be influenced by its linked artifact. Ritual magic, the type of magic that relies on ceremonies with prescribed chants and actions, was considered a very powerful way of achieving the desires of one's heart—although this form was highly associated with black magic.

RELIGION AND MAGIC. The Jewish community acknowledged the existence of magic in their lives, but they condemned its practice. Black magic, or sorcery, was associated mainly with women, and the practice of sorcery was inevitably tied to sexual vices, to which women were more susceptible because they were morally weaker. Since the Jewish people were a nomadic group, much of their folklore and magic was adopted from the areas in which they settled. Islamic peoples were similarly influenced by magic, as evidenced by the fact that there are warnings about it in the Qur'an, the holy book of **Islam**. According to Mohammed (570–632), all magic was bad, but could be used to ward off the evil eye or counter other evil.

Because most of the world was polytheistic, polygamous, and tolerant of homosexuality, many societies were familiar with sexual practices within the context of religion. Temple prostitutes, both male and female, were a widespread phenomenon. In Celtic religion, Beltane was the festival associated with the beginning of summer and had famously sexual overtones. The maypole was a phallic symbol around which maidens danced. Young people often stayed out all night to welcome the first dawn of summer, and many of the girls returned the next morning without their maidenheads.

Of all the world religions, none had such negative impact on the practice of magic as Western **Catholicism**. When a new religion is introduced to an area, it must push out the existing one in order to take hold of the majority of the population. This means debunking old mythology and either condemning or subsuming existing practices. From the early to late Middle Ages, there were two important evolutions within Christianity as it relates to magic. The first was the conversion of old pagan practices into Christian ones. The holiday of Easter coincides with the pagan festival of Eostre or Ostara, a celebration of spring and fertility. In fact, many religions' holidays centered around the agricultural year, so Christianity picked up those times as religious celebrations and renamed them to suit the situation. In western Europe, they also tore down the temples of the existing religions and built churches there instead. In effect, they made it easy for pagans to convert, because they could celebrate at their regular times and go to their regular places of worship. This step succeeded in changing the popular religion, but it did not stop belief in, or practice of, magic. Whereas magic had been part of the old religion, now it was a separate entity and eventually became a thorn in the side of the Catholic Church.

The second evolution was an increasingly puritanical viewpoint and demonization of sex. In the beginning of the Middle Ages, when the church was trying to convert the populace to Christianity, they were content to change the usual magical practices to include Christian elements. For instance, one belief was that if a wife held consecrated host in her mouth while her husband kissed her, he would continue to love her. As the centuries passed, the church turned to sexual asceticism. At the beginning of the period, there were some married clergy with families, and some even kept concubines. The Second Lateran Council in 1139 decreed that any priests with wives or concubines be deprived of their offices, and it admonished clergy to set a good example for their followers. During this time it was preached that magic was an illusion, that it did not really exist. Eventually, practicing magic was counted as heresy (because it was a belief in something that did not exist) and also came to be considered proof that the practitioner worshipped the devil. With the help of such books as *Malleus Maleficarum* (Witches' Hammer) in the late fifteenth century, the identity of witches became mainly feminine. They were depicted as sexual playmates of the devil and guilty of many deviant sexual behaviors. This set the stage for brutal witch hunts at the end of the period, which had little to do with the practice of magic and more to do with the sexual deviance of which they were accused.

While there were certainly different kinds of magic in the world during the Middle Ages, they all had some startling similarities. Before the move toward monotheism in much of the world, religion and magic were inextricably linked as a belief system. The spirits of the world in which they lived could alternately rule or be ruled, depending on the situation. Much time and thought was given to learning to live with, and harness the powers of, the world of magic. It is impossible to consider the cultures of the Middle Ages without considering the influence of magic on all parts and stages of life. *See also* Witches and Witch-Hunting.

Further Reading: Jacobs, Joseph, and Ludwig Blau. "Magic." See Jewish Encyclopedia Web site: http://www.jewishencyclopedia.com/view.jsp?artid=45&letter=M; Jolly, Karen Louise, ed. "Magic in the Middle Ages: A Preliminary Discussion." See Online Reference Book for Medieval Studies (ORB) Web site: http://www.the-orb.net/encyclop/culture/magwitch/orbmagic.htm; Porta, John Baptist. "Natural Magick." See The Works and Life of John Baptist Porta Web site: http://homepages.tscnet.com/omard1/jportac9.html#bk9XV; Taylor, Gordon Rattray. *Sex in History*. New York: Harper & Row, 1973.

Jennifer Della'Zanna

MAIMONIDES, MOSES (1135–1204). Moses ben Maimon, better known by the Hellenized form of his last name as Maimonides, was born March 30, 1135, at Cordoba in Spain. Maimonides was also known by the acronym "Rambam" for Rabbi Moses ben Maimon, and in Arabic was Abu 'Imran Musa ibn Maymun ibn 'Ubayd Allah. He was the most important Jewish philosopher-physician and rabbinical jurist of the Middle Ages.

Maimonides was taught at home by his father Rabbi Maimon ben Joseph. In 1148, the Maimon family fled Almohad persecution. Moving at first to Spain, then to Fez in North **Africa**, they eventually settled down in Fostat near Cairo, where Maimonides began practicing **medicine** to support the family. His reputation as a skillful physician spread quickly and he was appointed physician to the sultan. He eventually became the *Nagid* (leader) of the Jewish community. He died in 1204, and was buried in Tiberias in the Holy Land.

Maimonides wrote many works on the problems of the Jewish community and his profession. They fit into three related categories: Jewish law and religion, philosophy, and medicine. His religious writings include a commentary on the *Mishna* (*Kitab al-Siraj*), and a rabbinical study of Jewish law, the *Mishne Torah* (*The Torah Reviewed*). Discussion of sex, love, and culture can be found in them in several places. As *Nagid* of the Jewish community in Egypt, Maimonides objected to using *muwashshah* (devotional love songs) during synagogue worship. He believed that the command to love the Lord is satisfied with study of the law because knowledge of God is the same as loving God. In the *Mishne Torah* Maimonides commented in numerous places on the love of God, on **marriage**s, **rape**, **circumcision**, illicit sexual relations, and sexual hygiene.

The Guide for the Perplexed (Arabic: *Dalalat al-ha'irin*; Hebrew: *More nevuhkim*) was Maimonides's chief philosophic work. It makes reference to sexual matters in numerous places. For example, it says the study of metaphysics is not for those with a high sex drive (discussed with a medical description of testicles) because it distracts from the calm needed for study. Maimonides also comments that those (**Jews**) who are agitated in their organ of generation should find distraction in the house of study. He argues that circumcision is a remedy for **lust** and not a medical corrective for a birth defect. Its effect is to weaken the member in order to reduce lust. (He cites Aristotle's *Ethics* and *Rhetoric* as supporting authority.) He also discusses marriages and illicit unions, as well as why bastards and those with crushed testicles or injured members were excluded from the Temple.

As a physician Maimonides taught in the local medical school and wrote several medical works on topics including poison, health rules, and hemorrhoids. His three-part work on sexual intercourse, *Fi al-Jama'ah*, was dedicated to Malik al-Mustafir, sultan of Hamat. *See also* Judaism.

Further Reading: Maimonides, Moses. *The Guide for the Perplexed*. Translated by M. Friedlander. 1881. Reprint, New York: Dover, 1956; Maimonides, Moses. *Maimonides "on Sexual Intercourse": Fi 'l-jima*. Brooklyn, NY: Rambash Publishing, 1961.

Andrew J. Waskey

MANICHEANS AND CATHARS. "Manichean" is a term applied by modern scholars to several groups of medieval Christian heretics. These heretics shared a philosophy and practiced values that were superficially similar to that of the third-century Manichees of whom **Augustine** had briefly been a follower.

The best known of these groups is commonly called Cathars, although they are also known by other names, including Patarenes (Italy, thirteenth century) and Bogomils (Balkan region). Most Manichean groups appear to have been governed by bishops. At their peak, the sects spread from western Europe to Constantinople. Western European Cathar groups are known from the France, Italy, the Rhineland, Flanders, and England, with the English population being the smallest. Eastern European groups were centered in the Balkans.

Despite some philosophical similarities, there were significant differences between Eastern and Western Manicheans. Perhaps the most important difference was the religious texts they used, which tended to match mainstream Christian texts in the region. For simplification of explanation, here all are called Cathars unless reference is made to a particular region.

Manicheanism differed from mainstream Christianity in its emphasis on the rival and opposing principles of good and evil (dualism). Dualism underpinned Cathar belief and helped structure thought on important matters like society, relationships, and sexuality. Good created the invisible and spiritual universe, evil the material world. The relative influence and power of each varied regionally.

Dualist philosophy had important implications for love, sexuality, and relationships. The division of the world into good and evil principles meant that a great deal of attention was paid to actively avoiding the evil principle: French Cathars admired those members who had given up everything related to sexual activity, including eating food that was linked to it (leaving a vegetarian diet and fish). This asceticism was balanced by a valuing of companionship, according to Inquisition records. It is because to these records that we know more about the interface between the dualist philosophy and the emotional and physical life of Cathars from the south of France than for any other region.

Cathars were known for avoiding Catholic rituals (including baptism with water) and organizational structures. An important difference between Cathars and Catholics in relationship terms were that, at a time when Catholics were beginning to shape **marriage** into a sacrament, Cathars still saw it as something less.

The highest level of practice was to take the Consolamentum. Once a person had taken it, he or she was able to administer it to others, and some Cathars are known to have traveled east in search of a genuine Consolamentum. After the Consolamentum had been taken, the strictest interpretation of belief and daily life applied, including denial of the body, avoidance of sexual intimacy, and marriage. Other prohibitions included the prohibition of lying and of taking oaths, of indulging the body in general, and of immodesty. Most Cathars did not go so far, however, and lived more like ordinary Catholics. While it is possible that the Bogomils were influential in developing Western belief and practice, there is no direct evidence, and scholars have inferred links through similarity of diet and ritual and religious doctrine.

The dualist beliefs were apparent first in the Balkan region from about the tenth century. The Bogomil practices appear to have continued until the thirteenth or fourteenth century and to have faded into mainstream belief naturally. The Bosnian church was not proscribed until 1459.

In the West, the most important centers of Cathar activity were the south of France and northern and central Italy. Catharism in northern France, Germany, and the Low Countries was largely over by the beginning of the thirteenth century. The Cathars of the south of France were violently suppressed by the Catholic Church and the French state in the first half of the thirteenth century (the Albigensian crusade). Some Cathars from the south of France were given refuge by their Italian counterparts; for instance, the Cathar bishop of Cremorna was offered asylum after the Montségur massacre of 1244. Repression of the Italian Cathars was strongest from the 1260s, due to changes in local politics. However, Cathar belief probably survived in Italy until the early fourteenth century. *See also* Catholicism; Celibacy.

Further Reading: Barber, Malcolm. *The Cathars: Dualist Heretics in Languedoc in the High Middle Ages.* New York: Longman, 2000; Lambert, Malcolm. *The Cathars.* Malden, MA: Blackwell, 1999; Lansing, Carol. *Power & Purity: Cathar Heresy in Medieval Italy.* New York: Oxford University Press, 1998.

Gillian Polack

MARCABRU (fl. 1130–1150). Marcabru was arguably the most important early **troubadour**. A central contributor to the concept of *fin'amor* (purified love), he argued, with poetic intensity, that true love was the result of *entier cuidar* (integrated thinking) while false love arose from a fragmented mind—one that separated reason from desire, carnality from spirituality, the moment from eternity. Unlike many troubadours, he condemned **adultery**. He chastised those who would reduce love to sexual opportunism and was an enemy of venality—the use of physical intimacy for financial gain. Thus he criticized women who judged lovers on the basis of social rank. The signs of true love, Marcabru felt, were "joy, humility, and measure." Approximately forty-five of his songs survive, four with music.

Though sharp-tongued, Marcabru was not self-righteous; he included himself in his criticism, acknowledging a battle within between true and false love. (See his song "Doas cuidas ai, compaigner"—"There are two ways of thinking, companions.") Nor are the songs prudish; at times the language is vivid, even coarse. Yet Marcabru felt passionately that our earthly, physical desires need to be in harmony with our deepest ethical selves—agreeing in advance with the twentieth-century American philosopher Eli Siegel who observed, "Love is proud need."

In Marcabru's poetry we find greater respect for the mind of woman than perhaps given by any other troubadour. Where many elevated women to the realm of "Platonic perfection," Marcabru called for something more revolutionary: simple equality. "For love grows where it recognizes its equal," he says in "Lo vers comenssa" ("The *vers* begins").

Far from being the misogynist he is sometimes declared, Marcabru honored women by seeing their capacity—just like men—for good and evil. So as he condemns venality, he praises wisdom. In the *pastorela* "L'autrier jost' una sebissa" ("The other day, by a row of hedges"), a lowly shepherdess bests an amorous knight through the keenness of her mind. When he flatters her, implying she belongs among the higher classes, she replies: "He who calls himself a knight would do better to work, like us peasants, six days every week."

In "A la fontana del vergier" ("By the fountain in the orchard"), Marcabru gives a deep and strikingly realistic portrait of the inner life of a woman in grief—here, a young woman of the nobility. Her lover has been taken off to fight in the distant crusades. She damns King Louis (VII) for it, and even tells Jesus this attempt to defend his honor has only caused her anguish. "I believe God may show me pity in the next world," she says, "but here He takes from me the one thing that brings me joy."

Though few biographical facts are certain, it appears Marcabru was born among the lower classes—perhaps illegitimately—and received some clerical education. Among thinkers who likely affected him was William of Saint Thierry, who, in *De natura et dignitate amoris*, makes a distinction between natural and unnatural love that foreshadows Marcabru's central poetic and ethical concern. The contemporary relevance of these concerns is evidenced by James Cowan's recent novel about Marcabru, *A Troubadour's Testament*.

Further Reading: Cowan, James. *A Troubadour's Testament*. Boston: Shambhala Publications, 1998; Gaunt, Simon, Ruth Harvey, and Linda Paterson. *Marcabru: A Critical Edition*. Cambridge: D.S. Brewer, 2000; Harvey, Ruth. *The Troubadour Marcabru and Love*. London: Westfield Publications, 1989.

Edward Green

MARGARET OF HENNEBERG (1254–1276). The Dutch countess Margaret of Henneberg is the subject of a legend whose earliest surviving mention dates back to the late fourteenth century. The legend is that she died after giving birth to 364 or 365 tiny children. The children, equally divided between male and female, died immediately after being baptized. Although one of the earliest references to the legend, in a chronicle called the Tabula of Egmond, simply states that she died after giving birth, other writers portrayed the incident as divine punishment. Countess Margaret supposedly charged a woman who had given birth to twins with unfaithfulness to her husband, based on the belief that twins must have different fathers. (The rank of the accused woman varies in different versions from the wife of a knight to a beggar. This theme is found elsewhere in medieval legend and literature as well, including the work of **Marie de France**.) The maligned woman supposedly prayed to God for vengeance and vindication, and was answered when the countess herself was the victim of a multiple **childbirth**.

The legend, commemorated with wooden plaques at the church at Loosduinen, where the countess died, persisted into the early modern period. Some modern obstetricians have suggested that the countess might actually have expelled a hyatidiform mole, a deformation of the placenta into a connected network of small cysts that could have been mistaken for tiny children.

Further Reading: Bondeson, Jan. *The Two-Headed Boy, and Other Medical Marvels*. Ithaca, NY: Cornell University Press, 2000.

William E. Burns

MARIANISM. Marianism means devotion to Mary, who was, according to Christian and Islamic scriptures, the virgin mother of Jesus Christ. At the Council of Ephesus in 431, she was proclaimed *Theotokos* (Bearer, Mother of God) as opposed to *Christotokos* (Mother of Christ, the man). This was a reaction against the Nestorian dogma, which insisted that Christ had two natures, human and divine, and that Mary as mother of Christ's human nature was not the mother of God. The honor or "service" due to her is described in theological terms as *hyperdulia*, a term unique to Latin **Catholicism**. This is more than *dulia*, the veneration of saints, but not the same as *latria*, which is reserved for God. (*Dulia* and *latria* are terms found in Orthodox theology as well as in Latin.) Most of the tenets of Marian devotion are patristic in origin—or might stem from pagan goddess-worship—but flourished impressively during the Middle Ages Eastern practice generally took the lead with regard to theology (especially in the eighth and fourteenth centuries), feast days (Mary's conception and assumption into heaven), hymns (such as the celebrated *Akathistos* hymn by Romanos the Singer, which inspired popular Latin hymns like the *Salve Regina* and *Stabat Mater*), the liturgy, and iconography (the earliest depictions of Mary in the Latin West, such as fol. 7v in the *Book of Kells*, c. 800, look like Byzantine or Coptic images). The founder of Marian doctrine in the Latin West was Ambrose of Milan (d. 397). There, the twelfth century in particular has been called a "Marian century."

Mary is the Blessed Virgin because she conceived without intercourse, through the action of the Holy Spirit. It was agreed, despite a particularly vigorous debate in the ninth century, that she remained "ever-virgin" (her hymen remained intact) even though she gave birth to a child. Mary is therefore the purest of women, the model for all consecrated virgins (Abbot Odilo of Cluny, d. 1049, expanded this to include male monks), and without equal since she was chosen and prepared by God for the supreme honor of giving birth to him. Humility is nevertheless one of her most celebrated virtues. She is the perfect mother, who tenderly loves her perfect son and suffers terribly with him when he is crucified. By bringing Christ into the world to redeem it—Ildephonsus of Toledo (d. 667) called her *cooperatrix* in her own redemption, and Ubertino of Casale (d. after 1325) used the term *socia* "associate"—Mary is a "second Eve" who compensates for the sin of the first. She was considered the woman of the prophecy in Genesis 3:15, whose offspring was supposed to crush the serpent's head.

Prefigured in other Old Testament images such as the burning bush (which was not consumed by the fire) and Aaron's rod (which flowered without moisture), she is called a lily among thorns, pure white wool (Alcuin of York, d. 804), or the chestnut, which is smooth although it comes out of a spiny husk (Eadmer of Canterbury, d. 1124). The related doctrine of the Immaculate Conception, according to which she was conceived by her mother, St. Anne, without original sin (as opposed to being purified by God at a later time), is of medieval origin. Its leading champions included Eadmer and the Franciscan John Duns Scotus (d. 1308), while others including St. **Bernard of Clairvaux** (d. 1153) and St. **Thomas Aquinas** (d. 1274) opposed it. Another medieval innovation is the Rosary or "Marian Psalter." This was popularized by Alanus de Rupe (d. 1475), who claimed it was an ancient practice, which the Virgin recommended in an apparition to St. Dominic (d. 1221). Alanus himself was called "the new bridegroom of the Blessed Virgin Mary" because she appeared to him in 1464 and placed a ring on his finger. The Franciscan preacher **Bernardino of Siena** (d. 1444) earlier had aspired to the same position, saying that he loved the Virgin Mary with all his heart and wanted to be her chaste betrothed. Her original bridegroom, of course, is Christ, who is said to have left her womb like the bridegroom coming forth from the bridal chamber (a reference to Psalms 19:5)—in other words, Mary is at once the mother and the spouse of God. The image of the Christ Child with his head upon her breast is polyvalent; increasingly, her relationship with Christ was understood in light of the sublimely erotic Old Testament book of the *Song of Songs*. Rupert of Deutz (d. 1130) was the first to interpret the whole of this book in relation to Mary; he was followed by Aelred of Rievaulx (d. 1167), Philip of Harveng (d. 1183), and many other writers, artists, and composers of music. (Musical settings of the *Song of Songs* were common in Marian masses of the fourteenth and fifteenth centuries.) Aelred and Philip both insisted that Mary was beautiful—she had pretty eyes and rosy cheeks—and that God was drawn to her because he recognized her inner beauty. Godfrey, abbot of Admont (d. 1165), even said the Trinity were Mary's "lovers" (*amatores*).

In the context of this mystical **marriage** with God, Mary, whose womb was sometimes referred to as Temple or Tabernacle, is a type of the church, which is also called the Bride of Christ. This idea underlay and found its ultimate expression in the great twelfth- and thirteenth-century *Notre-Dame* (Our Lady) cathedrals of Noyon, Senlis, Paris, Sens, Chartres, Bourges, Soissons, Le Mans, Coutances, Reims, Amiens, and Beauvais. (Mary also came to be associated with the color blue around this time.) The Venerable Bede (d. 735), an important witness for early medieval Marian devotion, followed St. Ambrose when he stated that Mary is a figure for the church because both conceived through the Holy Spirit while married to an earthly groom (St. Joseph; the pope). Other writers chose to think of Mary as the mother of the church—hence the mother of all Christian believers—or as "the neck" connecting Christ, the head, with the church, which is his body. This alludes to one of Mary's most important functions, that of *Mediatrix* between Christ and human beings. The title is Greek Orthodox in origin and first occurs in Latin in the retelling of the popular Theophilus legend (precursor to Faust) by Paul the Deacon (d. c. 799). Echoing the patriarch Germanus of Constantinople (d. 733), who called himself Mary's "slave" (*doulos*) and stated that no one could obtain either knowledge of God or redemption except through her, **Peter Damian** (d. 1072) devised the formula *ad Jesum per Mariam*, "to Jesus through Mary," emphasizing that she is the mother of the body of Christ consumed in the Eucharist. Saint Bernard of Clairvaux called her "the aqueduct" by which grace descends from God to human beings. Bernard himself was known as the Champion and

Singer of the Virgin; he recites her praise in **Dante Alighieri**'s *Paradiso*, canto 33. He and numerous others agreed that while one *could* pray directly to Christ, Mary was more likely to show mercy, and her intercession might in fact be indispensable. She was credited with many miracles, interventions, and apparitions.

Mary has abundant titles, such as St. **Jerome**'s *Stilla Maris* (Drop of the Ocean), which became *Stella Maris* (Star of the Sea), or *Mater Misericordiae* (Mother of Mercy), which she supposedly revealed to the Cluniacs. Among these, *Domina* (Lady), based on an old Syriac etymology, is very important. In the Middle Ages it had feudal connotations. Mary is the queen of the universe—in this sense she is God's partner—and the service she receives from monks and clerics is akin to that which a knight would offer his lady. Knights themselves were thought of as showing devotion to Mary. In the *Song of Roland* (c. 1090), the dying Roland prays to Mary as he tries to break his sword Durendal, whose pommel contains a fragment of her clothing; in the *Pseudo-Turpin Chronicle*, he delivers an eloquent justification of Mary's **virginity** to a Muslim opponent. King Arthur, according to Geoffrey of Monmouth's highly influential *History of the Kings of Britain* (1136), had a shield named Pridwen (white/fair form), on which Mary's portrait was painted, so Arthur would always be thinking about her. Gerald of Wales (*De prinicipis instructione*, c. 1193–1199) adds that Arthur used to look at this image in battle and kiss its feet with great devotion. *See also* Cantigas de Santa Maria.

Further Reading: Gambero, Luigi. *Mary and the Fathers of the Church: The Blessed Virgin Mary in Patristic Thought*. Translated by Thomas Buffer. San Francisco: Ignatius Press, 1999; Gambero, Luigi. *Mary in the Middle Ages: The Blessed Virgin Mary in the Thought of Medieval Latin Theologians*. Translated by Thomas Buffer. San Francisco: Ignatius Press, 2005; Graef, Hilda. *Mary: A History of Doctrine and Devotion*. Vol. 1, *From the Beginnings to the Eve of the Reformation*. New York: Sheed and Ward, 1963; Martin, John. *Roses, Fountains, and Gold: The Virgin Mary in History, Art, and Apparition*. San Francisco: Ignatius Press, 1998; O'Carroll, Michael. *Theotokos: A Theological Encyclopedia of the Blessed Virgin Mary*. Wilmington, DE: M. Glazier, 1983; O'Dwyer, Peter. *Mary: A History of Devotion in Ireland*. Dublin: Four Courts Press, 1988; Pelikan, Jaroslav. *Mary through the Centuries: Her Place in the History of Culture*. New Haven, CT: Yale University Press: 1998; Warner, Marina. *Alone of All Her Sex. The Myth and the Cult of the Virgin Mary*. 1976. Reprint, New York: Vintage, 1983.

Matthieu Boyd

MARIE DE FRANCE (fl. 1165–1215). Marie de France, the first French poetess, is most famous for her portrayal of the complexities of human love in the *Lays* (c. 1165). Very little is known about her, although it is generally believed that she lived in England during the second half of the twelfth century and maintained close ties to the court of King Henry II.

Marie's *Lays* consists of twelve short poems in octosyllabic verse, intended to be performed to music. In the prologue, Marie reveals that the stories are of ancient Celtic provenance. Women occupy a prominent role in all the *Lays*, which often focuses upon an illicit love affair. Thus the shortest tale, *Chevrefoil* (118 verses), depicts a brief encounter between legendary lovers **Tristan** and Iseut. Sometimes, Marie overtly condemns **adultery**: the heroine of *Équitan* is punished for betraying and plotting against her good and dutiful husband. Frequently, however, Marie draws attention to the unfair treatment of women in medieval society, who, unable to marry for love, are subjected to the whims of cruel and elderly husbands. Marie's heroines long for true love and their prayers are answered in the most unexpected ways. In *Guigemar* and *Yonec*, Marie's youthful heroines are locked up in towers by their jealous husbands.

Living in forced seclusion, both women are able nonetheless to maintain secret love affairs. In the first tale, a handsome knight, Guigemar, sails to the maiden's tower in a magical boat. In the second, the heroine engages in a sexual relationship with a supernatural figure, Muldumarec, who flies in through her bedroom window in the shape of a hawk. In both cases, the lovers triumph: Guigemar and his lady are married many years later; and although Muldumarec dies, Marie's heroine soon bears him a son, Yonec, after whom Marie's tale is named.

Marie's *Lays* is also imbued with Christian elements. *Eliduc*, the lengthiest with 1184 verses, contrasts the selfish love of the flesh with Christian love, or charity (*caritas*). The male protagonist, Eliduc, abandons his wife Guilliadun, a righteous and noble woman, for a younger maiden, Guildeluec. Yet Eliduc's wife, out of love for her husband, retires to a convent leaving him free to remarry. Many years later, Guildeluec follows Guilliadun's example and becomes a nun. Eliduc in turn becomes a monk. Thus, Marie's three protagonists (like **Peter Abelard and Heloise**) spend the rest of their lives in physical separation, but unified in their love of God. The lay of *Eliduc* possesses a profound theological dimension and illustrates, in accordance with the teachings of St. **Bernard of Clairvaux**, how a love born of the flesh can be turned toward God. In addition to the *Lays*, Marie composed *Fables*, a collection of 103 fables (c. 1167–1189) and the *Purgatory of Saint Patrick* (c. 1189).

Further Reading: Bloch, R. Howard. *The Anonymous Marie de France*. Chicago: University of Chicago Press, 2003; Burgess, Glyn S. *The Lais of Marie de France: Text and Context*. Athens: University of Georgia Press, 1987.

K. Sarah-Jane Murray

MARRIAGE. Although marriage in the Middle Ages had its roots in an exchange of property between families, under the influence of the Christian church it began to develop a more modern character. The early Christians viewed marriage as a monogamous and permanent relationship, founded on the mutual and free consent of persons who had reached the age of puberty, who were not closely related, and who felt some form of affection for each other.

THE ROOTS OF MEDIEVAL MARRIAGE. Marriage in the early medieval era was about wealth and status, not love. Marriage represented the merging of two families, as well as two farms or businesses. Because this union involved the exchange of family land and had an impact on both families' future prosperity, the decision of who to marry was considered too important to leave up to the bride and the groom. The significance of family involvement can be traced through marriage customs. Among the Germanic peoples, suitors were expected to pay a bride price (*pretium uxoris*) that began as a payment for the bride herself, but over time was transformed into the purchase of the family's rights over her. In some areas, for example among the Salic Franks, by the seventh century the bride price had grown into a bride gift, a symbolic payment to the bride's father, suggesting discomfort with the idea of treating women as property. In other areas, such as Anglo-Saxon England, the notion of a substantial payment given to the bride's parents continued until well into the eleventh century. Although the law codes represent the bride gift in monetary terms, in practice real property was turned over to the wife. The groom was also expected to provide his bride with a morning gift (*morgengabe*), a gift of real property awarded after the consummation of marriage. This grant was sizeable: in an attempt to curb the inflation of morning gifts, the Lombard code stipulated that it could not surpass a quarter of the husband's patrimony. In many southern European areas, the Roman practice of providing daughters with generous dowries also continued after the fall of Rome. As these ritual exchanges suggest, women were considered their husbands' property, and expected to play a subordinate role in marriage. One of the few exceptions to this rule can be found in Celtic Ireland. Because the early Irish defined marriage entirely in terms of a spouse's financial contribution, if a woman came into the marriage with more property than her husband, she was expected to play the dominant role. Their union occupied a special category known as "union on woman-contribution" (*lanamanas for bantinchur*), and husbands were incapable of making any legal contracts, or buying or selling goods or property. Since early medieval marriage was so tightly focused on the exchange of property, it was considered inappropriate to marry below one's status in society. This attitude was most characteristic of society's upper ranks, whose marriages were primarily diplomatic alliances between the wealthiest and the most powerful families of medieval Europe.

THE INFLUENCE OF CHRISTIANITY. The increasingly powerful Christian church presented a formidable challenge to traditional ideas of marriage. Influenced by the Pauline notion that marriage created a union of flesh, the early church tirelessly campaigned for the permanence of marriage. Among the Germanic peoples, the first changes in marital customs can be traced to the time of Charlemagne (742–814), king of the Franks. Not only did he outlaw **polygamy**, he also introduced legal prohibitions against **divorce**. This was only the first step in the Christianization of medieval marriages. Over the next few centuries, the church imposed its own ideas on marriage, drawing principally on the writings of St. **Augustine** of Hippo. Augustine's position on marriage was twofold. Foremost, he saw marriage as a remedy to sin: the conjugal union was the only licit relief from **lust**, and thus a protection against fornication. Moreover, the central goal of marital sex was procreation; thus, marriage provided the ideal Christian atmosphere for child rearing. This position on marriage starkly contrasted with secular marriages based on family status and inheritance. Because traditional notions of marriage were so deeply entrenched in medieval society, the church's battle against the secularism of marriage was not easily won.

MARRIAGE AS A SACRAMENT. During the High Middle Ages, marriage acquired a sacred character. Although canonists debated the spiritual nature of marriage as early as the twelfth century, it was not until the Fourth Lateran Council of 1215 that marriage was recognized officially as a sacrament. Because marriage was now considered a spiritual union, the church became the marital overseer, and was expected to be the final judge in all questions regarding the formation and dissolution of marriages. The sacred side of marriage evolved out of a high medieval debate over what constituted a valid marriage. This debate prompted a number of other changes in marital policy:

1. *Consent Theory*. The most fundamental change centered on the question of whose consent was necessary to create a valid marriage. Under Pope Alexander III (1159–1181), the church determined that an indissoluble marriage could be created in two ways: first, by an exchange of vows in the present tense (i.e., "I take you as my wife") between parties capable of matrimony; second, by an exchange of vows in the future tense (i.e., "I will take you as my wife") between parties capable of matrimony, followed by consummation (thus, the act confirms the intention). The church expected this new strategy of marital formation, in which only the consent of bride and groom were necessary, to include even the marriages of serfs. The church's stance on consent was a dramatic departure from traditional marriages, which valued the influence of both parents and feudal lords in the choice of marriage partners. Neither was content to be excluded from marriage formation, and studies demonstrate that both lords and parents

continued to play a critical role in spousal selection throughout the rest of the medieval period. Nevertheless, some couples did use **canon law** to escape these controls and assert their own choice in spousal selection; moreover, the church courts enforced marriages contracted by free consent of spouses, regardless of the wishes of parents and feudal lords. The imposition of the theory of consent by the Christian church distinguishes the history of European marriage from contemporary cultures; for example, in both medieval **Islam** and medieval **India**, arranged marriages, which placed little value on the opinions of the participants, were normal.

2. *The Marital Process.* If marriage was a sacrament, it was now incumbent upon the church to play a role in the formation of marriage. Accordingly, medieval parishioners were encouraged to have their marriages solemnized: meaning, the reading of the banns on three consecutive Sundays, an exchange of present consent at the church door in the presence of a priest, followed by a nuptial mass. Any marriage without solemnization (a clandestine marriage, also known as *handfasting*, or *trothplight*) was still considered valid, but the couple had sinned and were liable to be fined for failing to solemnize their union.

3. *Ages of Marriageability.* The Fourth Lateran Council also addressed the issue of ages at marriage. It determined that a girl might marry at twelve, a boy at fourteen. It should be noted that these were considered to be minimum, not maximum, ages of marriage. Although southern European women were often married at such young ages, in general, most medieval brides and grooms were much older. The council's pronouncement did have an important impact on the marriages of the upper ranks, however, where previously it had been usual to marry children as young as four to ensure good relations and future prosperity between families or nations.

4. *Incest.* The Fourth Lateran Council ended all debates on **incest**, reducing the prohibited degrees of **consanguinity** (relation by blood) and affinity (relation by sexual union) from seven to four degrees, counting back to the common ancestor. Spiritual ties generated through baptism or confirmation were also deemed to create lasting relationships, and fell under the same rules of incest. With such strenuous regulations regarding who one might marry, historians have often assumed that these rules were ignored. Incest did provide the grounds for some cases of marriage litigation in this period, however. It is also clear that couples too closely related regularly appealed to the pope for dispensations to marry (or, more usually, to stay married) despite an existing impediment.

5. *Marital Affection.* Canonists may also have had an important impact on the emotional relationship between couples in marriage by stressing the need for marital affection (*maritalis affectio*). Although this concept was never fully defined, and may sometimes have been understood simply as a healthy reciprocal sexual relationship, it is certainly possible that parishioners understood affection in a more meaningful way.

See also Bigamy; Concubinage; Domestic Violence; Wedding Rituals.

Further Reading: Brundage, James A. *Law, Sex, and Christian Society in Medieval Europe.* Chicago, IL: University of Chicago Press, 1987; Helmholz, R. H. *Marriage Litigation in Medieval England.* London: Cambridge University Press, 1974; McNamara, Jo-Ann, and Suzanne F. Wemple. "Marriage and Divorce in the Frankish Kingdom." In *The Chivalrous Society*, edited by Georges Duby, 112–22. Berkeley: University of California Press, 1977.

Sara M. Butler

MARY MAGDALENE, CULT OF. Mary Magdalene (of Magdala, a locality of Galilee) is a character in the Gospels, appearing as a reformed sinner. Her devotees were widely spread in the Middle Ages and always linked with the redemption of prostitutes. In Western Patristic tradition, beginning with Gregory the Great

(590–604), Mary Magdalene was the result of a fusion of different women, mentioned in Gospels: the anonymous sinner (Luke, 7, 36–50); Mary of Bethany, sister of Martha and Lazarus; Mary Magdalene, "freed by 7 demons," follower of Christ, the first witness of his Resurrection. Later, she was associated with the adulterer met by Jesus in Samaria, who saved her from stoning (John, 4). Finally, Odo of Cluny (878–942) described Magdalene as the model of a reformed sinner.

Her cult is very ancient in the East, while in the West testimonies were found from the tenth century in Vezelay in the south of France, where, since the eleventh century, pilgrimages were organized near the cave of Sainte-Beuve and the grave of the saint. According to a legend reported by various authors beginning during the tenth century, Mary Magdalene went to the cave to lead her life as a penitent. This legend reached the height of its popularity in the thirteenth century, thanks to the editing of James of Varazze in his work *Legenda Aurea*, which tells of Mary Magdalene being like the abandoned bride of the disciple John. A large basilica was built on her grave, which became the place of pilgrimage for her the followers of her cult.

The influence of the Mary Magdalene cult in the Middle Ages was huge: sacred art, literature, and religious life were all affected by it. In the Middle Ages, she was a protagonist of theatrical representations, where sometimes she is described as a beautiful and elegant woman who gives herself to the joys of sex (Passion d'Angers of J. Michel, 1486), other times like a girl who gave her body for enjoyment and not for money, converting only because she couldn't find a lover (Passion d'Arras of Mercadé, 1430).

From the thirteenth century, numerous religious houses were created in honour of the Magdalene, to welcome reformed prostitutes who desired to change their life. These houses were called "of the Magdalenes," because Magdalene was the adjective that identified ex-prostitutes who decided to redeem themselves, as by the example of the sinner of Gospels. Pope Innocent III, with his *Universis Christifidelibus* letter of 1198, exhorted all Christians to promote the redemption of prostitutes.

The abbey of Saint Antoine des Champs, for the will of Folco of Neuilly and of the bishop of Paris William of Alvernia, was perhaps the first to receive the approved subsidies from King Louis IX, to support 200 ex-prostitutes who wished to change their life. Other similar foundations were opened quickly in Marseille, Aix-en-Provence, and Avignon. In Toulouse the Franciscan theologian, Vitale du Four, opened a religious house for ex-prostitutes around 1307. Many institutions like these were created in France and subsequently in Italy and Spain, with the definitive approval of Pope Gregory XI in 1376. All were independent. In Germany, Rudolph of Worms founded in 1226 a religious order of "Magdalenes," recognized the next year by the pope. The building of convents in Treviri, Strasbourg, Wurzburg, Muhlhausen, Cologne, Ratisbon, Magdeburg, Brussells, and many other cities followed. Most of these houses were closed by the protestant reform and only one survives today. *See also* Catholicism; Prostitution.

Further Reading: Cuesta, Angel Martìnez. "Maddalene." In *Dizionario degli Istituti di Perfezione*, vol. 5, 801–12. Roma: Edizioni Paoline, 1978.

Elvio Ciferri

MASTURBATION. In antiquity the topic of masturbation was of interest only to satiric and erotic poets. Physicians hardly ever mentioned it. Medieval physicians also discussed it very little and only with regards to excessive practice. Hebrew did not even have a word for it. From a theological point of view, though, masturbation constituted a sin for Christians and Muslims, although it was not regarded as a major offence during the early Middle Ages. It became one later on.

The concerns of the Christian church with masturbation, seen as a "wasting of seed," as with all other aspects of sex, seems to have been determined in great part by the massive plague that decimated southern Europe in the sixth century. Until then, only the fifth-century abbot John Cassian had been concerned with the ethics of solitary sex. Possibly mainly out of concern with the population decline, the church's **penitentials** focused on seminal emission more than anything else. Early on, the required atonement was of only seven days of fasting for an involuntary seminal emission and twenty days if manually assisted. Masturbating in church demanded a thirty-day fast for a monk and fifty days for a bishop. However, if not solitarily performed, the penitence was much more severe. Flagellation and singing penitential psalms were added in the eleventh century. For monks it was self-flagellation, and for the laics it was performed by the parish priest. When experiencing involuntary nocturnal emissions, a man was expected to rise immediately and sing seven psalms, and then thirty more in the morning. *The Penitential of Cummean*, Frankish in origin and written around 650, raised the penance for masturbation to 100 days for the first offence and a year for repetitions. The penitential of Theodore, archbishop of Canterbury (668–690), prescribed three years for lesbianism and female masturbation.

Feminine masturbation was generally equated with lesbianism, and lesbian sexual activity was regarded as masturbation since sexuality was understood as essentially phallocentric. In the early eleventh century, around 1007, the bishop Burchard of Worms advised in his writing that women should be questioned closely during **confession** about such practices and prescribed a one-year penance for a woman who would use an engine or a mechanical instrument shaped like a penis in order to commit fornication upon herself in solitude.

It was later in the eleventh century that masturbation became a very serious offence—an unnatural act that was classified as a species of **sodomy**. **Peter Damian** (c. 1007–1072) accomplished that with *Liber Gomorrhianus* (*The Book of Gomorrah*), published around 1049. Damian was a reformist monk who eventually became cardinal and was declared doctor of the church. **Dante Alighieri** mentions him in the *Divina Commedia* and places him in the highest circles of the *Paradiso*. Damian's effort to incorporate masturbation to sodomy was part of the initial theological mobilization against the erotic culture of cloisters in all its aspects, which was to amplify into an aggressive revision of all the gray areas of clerical **celibacy**.

Masturbation was also associated with heresy and witchcraft. In the thirteenth century, Caesarius of Heisterbach, the prior of a Cistercian monastery, wrote a hagiographic text titled *Dialogus magnus visionum ad miraculorum*, which contains many sensational stories of miracles and is considered to be the second largest best-seller of the late Middle Ages. It was frequently quoted by priests in their sermons. In it he writes about incubi and succubi, lewd demons or goblins who sought intercourse with humans. Like many other church authorities, he claimed that the incubi not only took the male form and emitted semen, but they also collected the human semen released through masturbation and used it to create new bodies for themselves.

Even **Thomas Aquinas** (1225–1274), the angelic doctor, subscribed to this belief, arguing that the creation of new bodies for the demons took place when the incubi poured the semen into female repositories. Aquinas considered masturbation as one of the most serious sins of lechery (*luxuria*), even greater than **rape**. In *Summa Theologica*

(1265–1272) he divided the sin of lechery, or **lust**, a sin against reason, into six categories: the vice against nature, simple fornication, **incest**, **adultery**, seduction, and rape. He further divided the vice against nature into four categories: masturbation, zoophilia, homosexuality, and nongenerative heterosexual sex. According to this classification, masturbation is a sin against both nature and reason, while rape is a sin against reason alone. This hierarchy was repudiated by the Catholic Church fairly recently, in the encyclical *Aeterni Patris* (1879) of Pope Leo XIII (1810–1903).

Further Reading: Laqueur, Thomas W. *Solitary Sex: A Cultural History of Masturbation.* New York: Zone Books, 2003; Stengers, Jean, and Anne Van Neck. *Masturbation: The History of a Great Terror.* Translated by Kathryn A. Hoffmann. New York: Palgrave, 2001.

Georgia Tres

MEDB (fl. first century BCE). Medb, daughter of the High King of Ireland and warrior-queen of Connaught, is one of the most prominent mythico-historical figures of the Celtic world. She is renowned for her voracious sexual appetite and her role in the Cattle Raid of Cooley (*Táin Bó Cúailnge*). Her name means "she who intoxicates."

Medb entertained sexual relations with many men for her own pleasure and for political gains. Only the legendary hero Fergus mac Roich, who mated with the goddess of wild animals (Flidais), could satisfy her. Medb herself is often regarded as a deity. She is reputed to have been a close friend of Aongas Óg, God of Love, and is frequently conflated with both the sovereignty goddess of Tara (also named Medb) and Medb Lethberg, queen of Leinster. The female sovereignty goddess, representing the land, was central to the pagan rituals of Ireland. For a king to be properly instated, he had to perform intercourse with the goddess to ensure the fertility of his territory. This relationship symbolized the bond between the people and the land itself. By failing to maintain a proper union, a king's reign would be forfeit. Medb Lethberg married nine kings so as to guarantee the success of their rule. Likewise, it is said that no man could rule at Cruachan (modern-day Rathcrogan in Co. Roscommon) unless wedded to Medb of Connaught, who took at least five husbands during her alleged lifetime.

The famous Cattle Raid of Cooley began with a dispute between Medb and her third husband, Ailill mac Ross, who had the most property. According to Irish law, whoever owned the most in a **marriage** became the head, to which the other partner submitted. Ailill possessed authority because Medb's marvelous white bull abandoned her herd, not deigning to be owned by a woman, and relocated to his. In order to regain equality, Medb decided to acquire the twin of the beast, a brown bull belonging to Daire mac Fiachna, offering the knowledge of her inner thighs as payment. Daire agreed to the trade but later recanted. A lengthy battle then ensued, during which the young hero Cúchulainn single-handedly defeated Medb's troops. *See also* Pagan Europe.

Further Reading: Aldhouse-Green, Miranda J. *Celtic Goddesses: Warriors, Virgins and Mothers.* London: British Museum Press, 1995; O'Rahilly, Cecile, ed. *Táin Bó Cúailnge.* Dublin: Dublin Institute for Advanced Studies, 1976.

K. Sarah-Jane Murray and Hannah Zdansky

MEDICINE. The practice, philosophy, and tools of healing have been part of the social fabric of all cultures in the world ever since the beginning of time. Much of the evolution of medical art, from its reliance on **magic** and religion in ancient times to the science it is today, happened during the Middle Ages. Many diseases that frustrate us today were also problems for medieval practitioners. Treatment of sexual and reproductive problems for both men and women was big business then, as it is now.

BACKGROUND. Medicine in medieval Christian and Islamic societies was based on Greco-Roman tradition, including the works of Hippocrates (460–377 BCE) and Claudius Galen (c. 129–c. 216 CE). Much of Galen's work went unchallenged until the sixteenth century. Because of the lack of authoritative medical texts in medieval Latin Europe, medieval medicine is often seen as a mixture of herbal remedies, erroneous anatomical knowledge, and a good bit of magic. While some of that is true, there was movement in the practice of medicine during the Middle Ages that laid the foundation for later discoveries. Healing became less folk medicine and more science. Schools, hospitals, health boards, and licensing procedures were all developed in the Middle Ages and provided the framework within which later scholars could safely and confidently learn and practice medicine.

Much of the progress made in medicine during this period was due to the work done in **Islamic societies**. The Arabs were recipients of volumes of ancient Greco-Roman, Indian, and Persian works of medicine. During the ninth century, a caliphal library was established to house classic scientific and medical works, which were then translated into Arabic. It was the willingness of Arabs to incorporate wisdom from as many cultures as possible into their body of knowledge that allowed them to excel in the practice of medicine.

Arabic works dealing with sexuality from a medical perspective include a treatise on gynecology that originated in Muslim Spain; and Ibn al-Jazzar's (c. 900–980) voluminous work, one book of which deals with sexual diseases of both men and women. Sexual issues were also discussed in such encyclopedic compilations as **Ibn Sina**'s *Canon of Medicine*. Despite these works, there was little progress in the field of women's health in the Arab world, simply because it was taboo for a man to examine a woman's body except in cases of extreme emergency.

WESTERN EUROPE. At the beginning of the medieval era, in most of western Europe, healthcare was still a cottage industry. Women of the house provided the day-to-day care of a family's health. If a problem arose that she could not handle, the local healer was called. If the problem was too large for the healer, a physician was called if one was available. If none of these people could cure the patient, then they usually turned to faith.

Although the church started the first hospices and treated the poor free of charge, their moral teachings were often in conflict with the burgeoning science of medicine. Eventually, towns took over the task of providing hospitals and a healthcare system for even the poor, and clergy were edged out of medicine altogether. In the late medieval period, medical schools became plentiful, and medicine, which had been part of a philosophical education, became a specialized area of study. The most famous schools were in Paris, France, and Salerno, Italy.

The theory of humors (fluids), developed by Hippocrates, was in use at this time. Philosophers believed that everything in the universe, including our bodies, was made of four elements: air, fire, water, and earth. Blood was actually four different fluids, according to Hippocrates, and these were observed in the separation of what he had drawn from a body. Each of the layers was associated with an element, a humor, heat, and moisture. The first layer was blood, the sanguine humor, which was the element air and was hot and moist. The second was yellow bile, the choleric humor, which was the element fire and was hot and dry. The third layer was phlegm, the phlegmatic humor, which was the element water and was cold and moist. Finally, there was black bile, the melancholic humor, which was the element earth and was cold and dry.

MEDICINE

To be healthy, the four humors must be in balance. If they were not, the one out of balance was brought into balance, either by expelling some of it or adding to it. Depending on the problem, a trained physician could determine which humors were out of balance and prescribe appropriate treatment. Sometimes it was as simple as adjusting diet, and at other times it became more drastic. Inducing diarrhea or vomiting and increasing urine output were all used as treatments. In other cases, blood had to be released from the body, and there were several methods for doing so.

SEXUAL HEALTH. Physicians of the time believed that sex was essential to health, for both men and women. It was commonly believed that both men and women produced semen, and a build-up of seminal humors was dangerous. Sex, or **masturbation**, was often prescribed for a problem in which semen needed to be expelled from the body. Regular sexual relations were considered necessary for good health.

Menstruation was a problem for the medical community at the time. There are many medical treatises on starting or stopping the flow of an irregular menstrual cycle, which was probably a fairly common problem due to inadequate nutrition and lack of regular gynecological care. The belief was that bad humors were stored in the uterus until it was full, at which time the woman menstruated. If they did not regularly menstruate, it was believed the humors would accumulate until the woman died.

Love sickness was considered an actual illness, and it could be recognized by its symptoms of insomnia, anorexia, depression, jaundice, and sunken eyes. Until the end of the Middle Ages, this was primarily a man's disease and could be treated with a combination of herbs, a change in climate, wine, bathing, and sex with a prostitute. During most of the medieval period, this disease was thought to be caused by a spell cast by a woman. Toward the end of the period, love sickness was identified as a sexual disease and, since women were thought to be more sexually wanton than men, the disease was feminized.

FERTILITY AND CONTRACEPTION. Fertility control has been a concern for women and men for many thousands of years. There is a cave painting in France, thought to be 12,000–15,000 years old, which depicts a man using a condom during intercourse. In medieval times condoms were usually made of animal tissue such as sheep intestines. Various substances have also been used by women to block the entrance to the womb, including crushed roots, moss, and sponges soaked in vinegar, olive oil, alcohol, honey, and even animal dung. Of course, this often led to other medical problems due to infection. By the end of the fifteenth century, many contraceptive remedies were lost due to fear of being accused of witchcraft or heresy for using them. We do know, however, that pomegranate, pennyroyal, pine, and vitex (also known as chaste-tree) were used, and they have been found today to have contraceptive properties.

As it is today, producing children was more problematic for people of the Middle Ages than preventing them. What was known about the anatomy and functions of the human body mainly applied to men. Women's medicine was still very much a mystery. This is demonstrated by the fact that there were herbal remedies for hundreds of specific diseases during this time, but any gynecological treatments are described as simply "good for treating women's diseases."

Besides the belief that both men and women produced sperm, it was also believed that conception could only occur if the woman experienced pleasure during sex. This was fine for married women, but it added to the shame of a raped woman if she conceived. Many fertility aids of the time were more attributable to magic than medicine. One text, *De Secretis Mulierum (On the Secrets of Women)*, offered suggestions for the woman, such as eating hot foods, becoming inebriated and having a good massage, as well as falling asleep immediately after sex. The author of the text assures that these conditions will most certainly cause conception. *See also* Contraception; Ibn Rushd; al-Razi, Abu Bakr Muhammad ibn Zakariya; Sexually Transmitted Diseases; Sun Simiao.

Further Reading: Bos, G. "Ibn al-Jazzar on Women's Diseases and Their Treatment." See National Institute of Health PubMed Central Web site: http://www.pubmedcentral.nih.gov/articlerender.fcgi?artid=1036748; Heckel, N. M. "Sex, Society, and Medieval Women." See Robbins Library at the University of Rochester Web site: http://www.lib.rochester.edu/~camelot/medsex/text.htm; Livingston, Michael. "Misconceptions about Medieval Medicine: Humors, Leeches, Charms, and Prayers." See Strange Horizons Web site: http://www.strangehorizons.com/2003/20030317/medicine.shtml; Turner, B. "Muslims' Contributions to Medieval Medicine and Pharmacology." See Yale University Library Web site: http://www.library.yale.edu/~bturner/neareast/.

Jennifer Della'Zanna

MEISTERSINGER. With the fourteenth-century formation of guilds of *Meistersinger* (master singers), European vernacular song took on, for the first time, unmistakably urban and bourgeois coloring. Unlike their "courtly" German predecessors, the **Minnesinger**, Meistersinger saw themselves as sturdy artisans: poet-musicians who had their fellow townspeople as audience. Moreover, they typically worked professionally outside the world of music. The most famous among them, Hans Sachs, was a shoemaker in Nürnberg. It was Sachs whom Wagner immortalized in his 1868 opera, *Die Meistersinger*.

These guilds (*Gesellschaften*) functioned as did others of the time: there were masters, journeymen, and apprentices. They established strict rules concerning the proper use of melody and poetic meter, and also what subject matter and what style of public performance would be acceptable. So restrictive did these rules become that, as 1500 approached, the life was nearly sapped out of the art. It was only when a barber from Worms, named Hans Folz, persuaded the Nürnberg guild to permit more freedom to the art—including allowing new tunes to be created (for, earlier, the art largely was finding new words for old songs)—that a final flowering come to be. Sachs (1494–1576) worked in this later, more adventurous, period.

The subject matter of the songs ranged from religion to farce, from historical narrative to university subject matter. The idealization of women, so central to troubadour, trouvère, and Minnesinger literature, is here largely restricted to the adoration of the Virgin Mary. There are, however, many songs in praise of the virtues of **marriage**. Occasionally, the supernatural is called upon to assist: legends of "Chastity-Testing"—of a drinking horn that will not allow itself to be touched by the lips of a cuckold, or of a mantel that will not stay on the shoulders of an errant woman. Eroticism, per se, is exceedingly rare in Meistersinger literature.

Despite the implication of their name, "Meistersinger," these artists did not restrict themselves to songs. There were also long poems, in rhyming couplets, called *Spruchgedichte*, and plays, including *Fastnachtspiele*—carnival or "Shrovetide" dramas. These last ones, in particular, permitted somewhat racier subject matter: for example, **Boccaccio**'s tale of Lorenzo and Isabetta was told four times by Hans Sachs, including in a Fastnachtspiel. It is a story of a woman whose lover is murdered by her brothers. As Sachs tells it, the brothers hide under her bed at night to confirm their sister's illicit corporeal activity.

Musically, the preeminent song structure was *Barform*, in which each stanza (*Gesätz*) began with two melodically identical sections called *Stollen*—a term taken from carpentry, meaning "posts" or "props." These together comprise the "rising song," or *Aufgesang*. The stanza concludes with a section having a distinctly different melody. This is the *Abgesang,* the "downward" or "exiting" song.

Though guilds existed in many German cities—including Mainz, Strasbourg, and Augsburg—the Nürnberg Meistersingers were by far the most esteemed. Among them were Konrad Nachtigall, Lienhard Nunnenbeck, and Hans Winter. Some guilds survived into the nineteenth century; however, the movement largely went out of existence by the early 1600s.

Further Reading: Friedman, Clarence William. *Prefigurations in Meistergesang: Types from the Bible and Nature.* New York: AMS Press, 1970; Taylor, Archer. *The Literary History of Meistergesang.* New York: Modern Language Association of America, 1937.

Edward Green

MENSTRUATION. The age of consent for women in medieval **canon law** was twelve and this probably coincided with the onset of the menses. However, since menstruation, in part, is dependent upon body size and weight, it is quite possible that it occurred somewhat later in northern climes or during famine. Medieval people in general had a fear of menstrual blood, which was considered unclean. It was the curse of Eve, and menstruation revealed that a woman's body was not the closed, smooth, and autonomous body of the male. Some writers such as Isidore of Seville in the seventh century claimed that after coming into contact with menstrual blood, fruits would not blossom, flowers would fade, and grasses would wither, and dogs that tasted it would turn rabid.

While this was an extreme view, the idea of menstruating women receiving holy communion was frowned upon, although this was more a self-imposed abstinence in the West than an ordered one. Women were not usually asked, although they were in the Byzantine church. One way a woman could demonstrate her holiness was to cease having her menses, something possible through heroic fasting, which many nuns did. By suppressing their menstruation, they rid themselves of the inherently "polluting nature" and allowed themselves to transcend their alleged sexual disability and become forgetful of their sex, and in essence become like a male. Apparently, young girls who wanted to avoid a forced or unwanted **marriage** delayed their menses through fasting, perhaps with the hope that they later might be allowed to have some choice.

It was not only blood from menstruation that was unclean but also the blood associated with **childbirth**. Women were required to purify themselves after delivery before they could be admitted to church services, while women who died in childbirth and were therefore not purified were often denied burial in the cemetery. Even a funeral procession was often denied them because of the possible pollution of others through their blood. Sexual intercourse during menstruation was said to result in the conception of lepers, epileptics, or even demons, or otherwise impaired children. **Albertus Magnus, Thomas Aquinas**, and Duns Scotus all prohibited intercourse with women during their menses. Some of the church writers said that one reason deaconesses (who existed in the early Christian church and continued to exist in the Byzantine church) were abolished in the West was that a menstruating woman was not allowed to approach the altar.

There were, however, special saints to whom menstruating women could turn, and most notable among them was St. Radegund of Thuringia, who died in 587.

Though menstruating women were not isolated from society in the medieval period, their activities were certainly confined if others knew of their condition. *See also* Medicine; Misogyny in Latin Christendom.

Further Reading: Bynum, Carolyn. *Holy Feast and Holy Fast*. Berkeley: University of California Press, 1987; Ranke-Heinemann, Uta. *Eunuchs for the Kingdom of Heaven: Women, Sexuality and the Catholic Church*. New York: Doubleday, 1990; Schulburg, Jane Tibetts. *Forgetful of Their Sex*. Chicago: University of Chicago Press, 1998.

Vern L. Bullough

MESOAMERICA. Because of the extensive trade routes; the large, cosmopolitan urban populations; and the powerful empires that rose and fell in Mesoamerica from 250 BCE till the arrival of the Europeans in 1519 CE, Mesoamerican elites shared similar cultural and social practices. Most direct information on pre-Hispanic Mesoamerica comes from archaeological records, along with the very few remaining precontact manuscripts. While these do not specifically address sex and love, some inferences can be made from the information they offer. In the Mixteca-Puebla bark-paper manuscript, known as the *Codex Zouche-Nuttall*, an account of the **marriage** between Lady 3 Flint from the polity of "Hill of the Wasp" and Lord 12 Wind from "Hill of Flints" in 957 shows the couple being ritually cleansed by two women before they appear in their marital bed. While certainly this image is meant to describe a military alliance between the two cities, it portrays the actual consummation of the marriage and thus offers some interesting commentary about the importance of sex in the establishment of that alliance.

Marital alliances in Mesoamerica had less to do with love and sex than with military power; nevertheless, links between sex and power permeate Mesoamerican narratives. A complete picture is difficult to reconstruct, however, since most of the ethnographic information about pre-Hispanic Mesoamerica comes from the vast encyclopedias of information gathered and reinterpreted by missionary priests as they attempted to catechize the inhabitants of New Spain. These materials, compiled nearly entirely by males under the supervision of males who were supposed to be celibate, do not present the voices of at least one-half of the participants in sex in Mesoamerica—indigenous women.

In the narratives and images that discuss love and sex, images of birth and the cycle of life abound. While themes of fertility, earth, and female reproduction were common among agrarian people, nomadic hunters and gatherers celebrated prowess in warfare and hunting. Conflicts between agrarian and nomadic groups were reflected in complex stories about the creation of the universe as a duality of earth and sky. The nomadic Mexica, who were attempting to integrate into established agrarian communities in central Mexico, combined their own narratives with those of local groups. For them, the earth was the realm of the feminine while the sky/sun was the realm of the masculine. The earth "monster" was represented as a female saurian figure from whose body the sun (the warrior Nanahuatzin) emerged every day and into whose body the sun entered at night to make its trip through the underworld.

It is especially telling that Cipactli (crocodile/saurian creature) is the name of the very first day in the Mesoamerican solar calendar in many Mesoamerican languages. The cosmological construction of the day as the male sun emerging from the female earth's body on a daily basis illustrates the power of "birth" (and its consequence, "death") as an important Mesoamerican frame. This frame extends to the military principles that helped organize empires dedicated to conquest, as illustrated by the narrative of the birth of the pan-Mesoamerican divinity Quetzalcoatl. While hunting

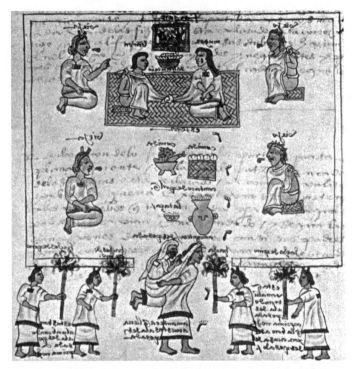

An Aztec wedding. From the Codex Mendoza, ca. Codex Mendoza. © The Granger Collection, New York.

in the desert, the Chichimec warrior Mixcoatl meets the female warrior and virgin Chimalman. After a fierce battle, Mixcoatl and Chimalman have sexual relations. In Mesoamerica, women were believed to have more power than men in the sexual realm since they controlled all aspects of reproduction from **menstruation** to giving birth, while men only participated in copulation. Although Mixcoatl defeats the female warrior in battle, Chimalman wields the power in the sexual act since she captures his "essence." She becomes pregnant with the divine Quetzalcoatl, and, after four days, Quetzalcoatl rips his way out of his mother's womb and emerges fully formed as a warrior himself. In the birth process, Chimalman perishes. This is significant because women who died in **childbirth** went to the same paradise as warriors who were killed in battle: Tamoanchan. Chimalman takes her rightful place in Tamoanchan as a warrior and as a woman who died in childbirth.

Certainly, both the battlefields and the birth rooms in Mexica society would have been bloody, and for the Mesoamericans, blood was the most precious fluid. Women's power in the sexual realm is reiterated by their monthly blood sacrifice, the menstrual flow. In many rituals, men and male divinities appear to imitate these natural female processes. The male rain (agrarian) divinity Tlaloc offers his blood as rain so that the crops will be successful. While Tlaloc's sacrifices often came from his hands, men would also draw blood for auto-sacrifice from their earlobes, tongues, and penises. In some areas of Mesoamerica, very elaborate penis perforators have been recovered in sacrificial caches. Many rulers are depicted in the process of performing auto-sacrificial rituals to assert their right to rule. Blood and water were linked by their power to cleanse and to give life, and cleanliness was an important aspect of Mesoamerican life.

Cleanliness was so important, in fact, that the Mesoamericans had a female divinity who governed the area of cleanliness, both physically and spiritually. This divinity, Tlazoteotl (Divine Eater of Filth), was responsible for the ritual cleansing of those who were out of balance. Interestingly, Tlazoteotl was also the patron of **midwives**, whose role was to assure the cleanliness of the entire birthing process. The women shown bathing the couple in the Mixteca wedding are probably midwives. This role was very important because midwives ultimately presided over the most powerful and dangerous moments in the sexual process: birth. Cleanliness was certainly important in preventing death by infection, but the midwife would also wash away any evidence of imbalance that the newborn child might bear. For example, the vernix, a milky coating often present on newborn babies, was seen as a sign that the parents had overindulged in sexual intercourse during the pregnancy. It was the midwife's role to "clean up" this indiscretion, as it was Tlazoteotl's role to perform the same type of cleansing on a cosmological level.

Tlazoteotl offers another frame linking sex and female power to military prowess. In the celebration of "Ochpaniztli" or "Sweeping," Tlazoteotl gives birth to the warrior/corn divinity Centeotl, while the midwives play the part of warriors. In this celebration, the midwives would sing and dance and would dress as warriors and engage in mock battles as they prepared for the birth of the new war season. They bless the weapons and help the personification of Tlazoteotl give birth to Centeotl as the season for the ritualized battles to collect warriors to offer as sacrifice to the Mexica sun, Nanahuatzin, is also born. While cross-dressing by males and females appears to have been common in rituals and for entertainment, and although the second most powerful figure in the political hiercharcy was a male called Woman Snake, issues of homosexuality are not addressed in great detail in the sources. It is also difficult to separate the pre-Hispanic information from the missionary process that considered the practice of sex for any nonreproductive purposes as inappropriate.

In a colonial collection of songs called the *Cantares mexicanos*, a series of "cradle songs" describe the birthing of warrior kings. While bringing warriors safely into the world was an important role for females, caring for the infant warriors and nurturing them were equally important tasks. Several cradle songs celebrate the pleasure of the suckling baby. Several of the same songs also present the pleasure of the female body and the pleasure afforded the adult male warrior by female songs. Catholic missionaries documented a group of women know as Joy Women, whose duty was to give pleasure to military classes. These women lived in a place called Joy House. The vagina itself was called Joy Place. The women are treated in a derogatory manner in the missionary narratives. They are called prostitutes and concubines, and their residence a brothel, reiterating the missionary attitude toward sex for nonreporductive purposes. Nevertheless, these women appear to have been well educated and trained in the arts of singing, dancing, composing songs, and possibly writing and painting as well as the arts of physical pleasure.

In Mesoamerican society, there were no such concepts as good and evil or sin. Problems could occur, however, when things went out of balance. As Louise Burkhart explains, the world was a slippery place where one could fall down and become "dirty" (28–33). Excesses were often the cause of being out of balance. When the ruler Quetzalcoatl becomes drunk on pulque and has sexual relations with his sister, his shame is so great that he abandons his kingdom, Tollan. Overindulgence in sex and alcohol caused the loss of a great empire. Sexual pleasure in moderation was seen as a divine gift, and Inga Clendinnen explains that female pleasure was an important consideration in sexual relations. Elders warned young, unmarried men not to "use up all their honey," that is, not to overindulge in sex before they are married, because they would "dry up" and not be able to please their wives (165–66). Precious body fluids like water, blood, and semen continue the metaphors of birth as important organizing principles for Mesoamericans. For the Mexica, the physical pleasure of sex, as well as the pleasures of the arts, were gifts from the divinities. Those pleasures, like everything else, must be enjoyed in moderation.

Further Reading: Bierhorst, John, trans. *Cantares Mexicanos: Songs of the Aztecs*. Stanford, CA: Stanford University Press, 1985; Bierhorst, John, ed. *A Nahuatl-English Dictionary and Concordance to the Cantares Mexicanos*. Stanford, CA: Stanford University Press, 1985; Burkhart, Louise. *The Slippery Earth: Nahua and Christian Moral Dialogue in Sixteenth-Century Mexico*. Tucson: University of Arizona Press, 1989; Byland, Bruce E., and John M. D. Pohl. *In the Realm of 8 Deer*. Norman: University of Oklahoma Press, 1994; Clendinnen, Inga. *Aztecs*. Cambridge: Cambridge University Press, 1991; Gillespie, Jeanne. *Saints and Warriors: Tlaxcalan Perspectives on the Fall of Tenochtitlan*. New Orleans: University Press of the South, 2004; Lopez Austin, Alfredo. *Tamoanchan, Tlalocan: Places of Mist*. Translated by Bernard Ortiz de Montellano and Thelma Ortiz de Montellano. Niwot, CO: University Press of Colorado, 1997; Nuttall, Zelia, ed. *Codex Zouche-Nuttall: A Picture Manuscript from Ancient Mexico*. New York: Dover, 1975; Sahagun, Bernardino de. *Florentine Codex: General History of the Things of New Spain*. 13 vols. Edited by Arthur J. O. Anderson and Charles Dibble. Santa Fe, NM: School of American Research and University of Utah Press, 1950–1982; Velsquez, Primo F., ed. "Leyenda de los soles." *Anales de Cuauhtitln. Cûdice Chimalpopoca*. Mexico: Imprenta Universitaria, 1945.

Jeanne L. Gillespie

MIDWIVES. To understand the history of women who helped deliver children during the European Middle Ages, one must realize that their fate was connected to wider socioeconomic trends. Considered members of a profession in antiquity, by the early Middle Ages (c. 500–1000) midwives had probably lost their professional standing. As cities in western Europe dwindled during the decline of the Western Roman empire and the continent became more rural, Western European midwives appear to have lost their status as specialized professionals. The term midwife soon came to mean any woman who assisted in **childbirth**.

Around 1300 midwives gradually regained professional status in growing urban centers. Contributing to this trend was a general concern that midwifery be made available cheaply, or even at no cost, to the poor. Formal licensing, though, came later—probably during the fifteenth century. It was also during the late Middle Ages (c. 1300–1500) that midwives encountered stiff competition from male doctors as **medicine** became increasingly professionalized.

Another reason midwives became professionalized in the later Middle Ages was the Roman church's growing emphasis on baptism. Maintaining that the souls of children who died without having been baptized would not be saved, by the thirteenth century the church began to require that those involved in delivering children know how to perform the sacrament in extreme circumstances. For this reason the church paid close attention to those women routinely assisting in births, and by the early fourteenth century it pressured individual towns to make available trained midwives who could help deliver babies and, if necessary, baptize them.

Little is known about how medieval midwives were trained. Most of them, it seems, were not of high social status, though under the right conditions they could earn prestige and standing. Many learned their trade through the oral transmission of knowledge that occurred during an apprenticeship. Surviving guidebooks provide glimpses into the support midwives and their assistants offered to laboring women. Midwives were responsible for monitoring the labors from beginning to end. In communities where birth stools were used they were also supposed to know when it was time to transfer the laboring woman from a standing or lying-down position to the chair. They kept the parturient lubricated and monitored the presentation of the baby, working to ensure a head-first presentation; if a fetus presented with a body part other than its head, the midwife would most often gently push the baby back into the uterus and attempt to rotate the child so that the head would descend first. Throughout the birth the midwife and her assistants offered words of support to the woman. The midwife would also do her best to keep the woman calm and help her manage her pain. Strategies to do so might include touching relics, saying prayers, reciting charms, and holding amulets. Yet another responsibility of the midwife was to keep the room warm so that the mother would be comfortable. Once the birth was successful (including delivery of the afterbirth), the midwife would lead the mother to a clean bed in which she could rest, and the newborn would be placed in a cradle. It is clear from surviving Jewish, Christian, and Muslim sources that midwives played extraordinary supportive roles as they helped countless numbers of medieval women bring into the world the generations that would succeed them.

Further Reading: Greilsammer, Myriam. "The Midwife, the Priest, and the Physician: The Subjugation of Midwives in the Low Countries at the End of the Middle Ages." *Journal of Medieval and Renaissance Studies* 21 (1991): 285–329; Hellwarth, Jennifer Wynne. "'I wyl wright of women prevy sekenes': Imagining Female Literacy and Textual Communities in Medieval and Early Modern Midwifery Manuals." *Critical Survey* 14 (2002): 44–63; Taglia, Kathryn. "Delivering a Christian Identity: Midwives in Northern French Synodal Legislation, c. 1200–1500." In *Religion and Medicine in the Middle Ages*, edited by Peter Biller and Joseph Ziegler, 77–90. Rochester, NY: York Medieval Press, 2001.

Dawn Marie Hayes

MINNESINGER (*Minnesänger*). The lyric poetry of the French **troubadours** and *trouvères* set the stage for the appearance of the vernacular song in German-speaking lands: the songs of the *Minnesinger*. The term was coined in 1189, though the style was present as early as 1150. These poet-composers, who wrote for an aristocratic audience and performed in their courts, had their golden age during the glory days of the Hohenstaufen emperors—roughly from 1180 to 1230. Exactly when the Minnesinger epoch ended is hard to determine, for it gradually melded into that of the **Meistersinger**—songwriters who sang to, and themselves arose from, an urban audience of artisans. Perhaps the last of the Minnesinger was Oswald von Wolkenstein, a South Tyrolean knight.

Reflecting feudal culture, wherein every man was pledged to his superior, the love songs of these poets are actuated by the concept of *Minnedienst*—servitude to love. The lyrics characteristically express a yearning to obtain the grace of a lady nobler than oneself. In these songs, often there is a tension between a spiritual interpretation of that yearning and a corporeal one. The Minnesinger, however, did not restrict themselves to themes of love. At times their poetry was even didactic. There were songs of ethical and religious instruction as well as those with clear political content.

Minnesinger came from very diverse social backgrounds—ranging from the emperor Henry VI to children of the humblest classes. Most came from the lesser nobility. Among the greatest were Reinmar von Hagenau, Walther von der Vogelweide, Neidhart von Reuental, Hugo von Montfort, Ulrich von Lichtenstein, and Heinrich von Meissen—who was known as "Frauenlob," meaning the Praise of Women. Another Minnesinger, famed in the modern world for a Wagnerian opera named after him, is Tannhäuser—who, according to legend, visited the mountain of Venus, lingered with the Goddess of Love, and then asked the pope to absolve him for that sin.

Musically, Minnesinger song was, at first, closely modeled on the songs of the troubadours and trouvères, but one can also see, in the genre of the *Leich*, a reflection of the medieval Latin *sequence*, and in their hands the French *ballade* evolved into the *Barform*—a tripartite, AAB structure, that had a powerful influence on all later German music.

Further Reading: Richey, M. F. *Essays on the Mediaeval German Love Lyric*. Oxford: Oxford University Press, 1942; Sayce, Olive. *The Medieval German Lyric, 1150–1300*. Oxford: Oxford University Press, 1982.

Edward Green

MISOGYNY IN LATIN CHRISTENDOM. Although the Christian Middle Ages has the reputation as a time when women were exclusively depicted in negative terms, the issue of misogyny in Latin Christendom is actually complex. While the vocabulary of misogyny remained static, textual uses of woman-hating language shifted throughout the period. In the early Middle Ages misogynistic texts were often written by monks and clerics to sexually regulate monastic communities dedicated to **celibacy**. With the growth of vernacular literature in the twelfth century, the discourse of misogyny was adapted to shape the depictions of duplicitous women found in later medieval secular stories of **courtly love** and **marriage**.

Medieval authors inherited and continually recycled misogynistic language and attitudes from the writings of the early church fathers, particularly **Jerome** (c. 340–420), **Augustine** of Hippo (354–430), and Tertullian (c. 160–c. 230), and from classical philosophy and medical texts, as well as the stories of the Hebrew Bible and Christian Gospels. Due to women's biological reproductive role, many classical and late antique texts held that women were ruled by nature, their senses, and the physical world. Men, whose role in reproduction appeared less polluting, and therefore less problematic, were thought to be governed by the mind and the spirit. Following *Genesis*, Christians believed that God had first created the male, and the female was subsequently formed from Adam's rib. Christian writers attributed the downfall of humanity to the initial deception of Eve, and this suggested that women also had a greater responsibility for Jesus's suffering and death on the cross. Thus, in most early Christian and medieval texts, women were depicted as mentally and spiritually inferior to men, and women's redemption required additional and often exaggerated penitential suffering. For the early church fathers, and the medieval writers who continued to use their words, women's only means of expunging the stain of Eve was adherence to a regime of strictly enforced **virginity**, often achieved through total seclusion from society, and consecration to Christ.

Christianity's association of celibacy with purity and holiness contributed to the expansion of misogynistic writings and attitudes. The female form symbolized the possibility of ultimate sin and the mysterious nature of feminine sexual pleasure, and female reproductive organs gave religious and secular authors additional scope to suspect women. Medieval medical theories, also based on earlier classical models, associated women with humors and conditions that were cold and moist. As the secretion of sexual fluids was also considered to dry out the body, women with their cold and moist composition were believed to desire, and capable of sustaining, unlimited sexual intercourse.

Throughout the Middle Ages, philosophical, theological, and secular texts tended to view women through a lens that was hostile to female sexuality and the possibility that feminine temptation could lead good men astray. During the Gregorian reform in the late eleventh century, however, certain writings exhibited a distinctive vehemence in connecting the impurity of women's sexuality with calls for a celibate clergy. When urging clerics to renounce their wives, monastic authors like **Peter Damian** (1007–1072) claimed that the priest's hands, which touched the body of Christ through contact with the Eucharist, should not be allowed to touch the genitals of women whose bodies he likened to vipers and wallowing hogs. Eleventh-century legislation ordering that the former wives and children of priests be enslaved to the church echoed the tone of this misogynistic language. However, while the writings of the eleventh-century reform movement had serious repercussions for the former wives of the clergy, the most extreme misogynistic texts were usually intended as exemplar for the celibate brethren of the author. Additionally, some religious texts also used maternal or feminine imagery to describe abbots and even Jesus. This metaphor was particularly popular during the twelfth and thirteenth centuries when the attributes of motherhood were becoming more closely associated with the growing cult of the Virgin Mary.

With increased veneration of the Virgin, tensions arising from the impossible dichotomy of Mary and Eve were reinterpreted in vernacular literature dealing with courtly love and marriage. During the later Middle Ages, secular literature often represented women as either the objects of unattainable love or adulterous hussies, or both simultaneously. Using literary structures based on classical authors, and ancient associations between women and animals such as pigs and snakes, texts like Jean de Meun's (c. 1240–c. 1305) **Romance of the Rose** and **Giovanni Boccaccio's** (1313–1375) *The Corbaccio* argued that women's inherently wicked and deceptive nature made marital happiness impossible for men. While the authors of these late medieval texts may have adapted the historical rhetoric of misogyny partially for intellectual amusement, as the fifteenth-century feminist author **Christine de Pisan** (c. 1364–c. 1431) noted in her *Book of the City of Ladies*, the result perpetuated the indictment of all women indiscriminately. Thus, during the later Middle Ages, textual representations of women in both secular and clerical literature remained conflicted. *See also Fifteen Joys of Marriage*; Menstruation.

Further Reading: Blamires, Alcuin, ed. *Woman Defamed and Woman Defended: An Anthology of Medieval Texts*. Oxford: Oxford University Press, 1992; Bloch, R. Howard. *Medieval Misogyny and the Invention of Western Romantic Love*. Chicago: University of Chicago Press, 1991; Dalarun, Jacques. "The Clerical Gaze." Translated by Arthur Goldhammer, chapter 1. In *A History of Women in the West: Silences of the Middle Ages*, edited by Christiane Klapisch-Zuber. Cambridge, MA: Belknap Press of Harvard University, 1992.

Susan W. Wade

MONASTICISM, FEMALE. Monasticism is a religious practice of renouncing worldly desires to focus upon spiritual life. During Christianity's early days, monasticism arose as a way to prove one's faith once persecution ceased and martyrdom was no longer possible. The primary function of the medieval Christian female monastic was to work toward the salvation of humanity. Like their male counterparts, monastic nuns were generally required to adhere to the *Rule of Saint Benedict*, which stipulated that they take vows of chastity, poverty, and obedience. (Composed by the eponymous saint in the sixth century, the *Rule* draws on both Eastern and Western traditions of asceticism to create guidelines for a balanced cenobitic life of work and prayer.) Nuns also celebrated the same liturgy and learned the same psalms as monks.

However, nuns and monks participated in quite different consecration ceremonies. While the ceremony for nuns emphasized their symbolic role as a spouse of Christ who surrenders her personal belongings and productive assets to Jesus, the ceremony for monks emphasized their independence as a symbol of Jesus himself. To this end, monks were able to be ordained as priests and celebrate mass. This both increased their status over nuns and spared male monasteries the cost of paying for a priest to administer sacerdotal functions. As "brides of Christ," female monastics had to rely on *cura monaliam*, the monks' responsibility to care for the nuns. The issue of *cura monaliam* became particularly problematic during the middle and the late Middle Ages when claustration (separation of nunneries from the outside world) increased and many nunneries were in financial distress.

One of the first important female monasteries was founded in Kildare, Ireland, in the fifth century by Saint Brigid, who is, along with Saint Patrick, the patron saint of Ireland. According to Cogitosus's (620–680) *Life*, Brigid made a childhood vow to God that she would remain a virgin and was reputed for her great charitable works and hospitality. Saint Brigid created a double monastery, that is, one consisting of both men and women monastics. Brigid selected Saint Conleth to perform episcopal and sacerdotal functions that she, as a woman, was unable to carry out. Nonetheless, as abbess, she was still ultimately able to maintain power and authority over the monastery, which prospered greatly under her rule. Saint Brigid also founded a school of art within the monastery, which produced the Book of Kildare, a famous illuminated manuscript.

Another influential Christian double monastery was founded by the Saxon King Oswy in 657 at Whitby, Northumbria. Oswy appointed Saint Hilda (614–680) as Whitby's first abbess. Under Hilda's reign, Whitby became a major center of learning in both Latin and Old English. In fact, five of the men whom Saint Hilda trained went on to become bishops, and Caedmon composed his famous religious verses in Old English at Whitby.

One of the earliest and most influential abbeys in continental Europe was the Monastery of the Holy Cross near Poitiers (originally named St. Marie Abbey), founded in 560 by Saint Radegunde (520–587). Radegunde was a Frankish queen who had been captured and forced to become King Clothar's fifth wife. It is said that Radegunde paid more attention to her charity work than to her husband: she used to abandon her marital bed in favor of spending hours prostrated on the cold church floor. Radegunde finally left her husband and the royal court after the king had her brother murdered. Radegunde renounced her possessions, fled to Poitiers, and adopted a daughter, Agnes, whom she named abbess of the new monastery that she founded. Saint Radegunde's monastery grew quickly and boasted 200 nuns at her death.

Of course, not all influential female monastics were as committed to their role as a bride of Christ during their early life as Saint Radegunde was. Heloise (1100–1163), the first abbess of the famous Paraclete monastery near Nogent-sur-Seine, quite brazenly wrote that her love for Peter Abelard (1079–1142) exceeded her love for the Lord. After Heloise had accidentally gotten pregnant as a result of her affair with Abelard (before her taking of the veil), the young lovers gave the child to Heloise's sister and joined separate monasteries. Heloise was a good abbess from a managerial standpoint, although the letters she exchanged with Abelard later in life clearly demonstrate that she never forgot her earthly love for him. In his last letter to Heloise, Abelard asks her to pray for his salvation, thereby granting her the status of intercessor. Seen in this light, Abelard asks Heloise to see through her carnal love for him and to turn that love toward God, an idea akin to St. Bernard's description of love in his famous treatise *On Loving God*. *See also* Abelard, Peter, and Heloise; Bernard of Clairvaux; Catholic Europe; Hildegard of Bingen; Monasticism, Male.

Further Reading: Eckenstein, Lina. *Woman under Monasticism*. Cambridge: Cambridge University Press, 1896; Johnson, Penelope Delafield. *Equal in Monastic Profession: Religious Women in Medieval France*. Chicago: University of Chicago Press, 1991; Warren, Nancy Bradley. *Spiritual Economies: Female Monasticism in Later Medieval England*. Philadelphia: University of Pennsylvania Press, 2001.

Kathryn O'Keeffe and K. Sarah-Jane Murray

MONASTICISM, MALE. Monasticism is a religious practice of renouncing worldly desires to focus upon spiritual life. During Christianity's early days, monasticism arose as a way to prove one's faith once persecution ceased and martyrdom was no longer possible. Hence monasticism came to be called "white" martyrdom as opposed to "red." Men subjected themselves to tribulation practicing chaste lives rather than being tried by state-inflicted torture. People who chose this existence were known by the Greek word *monachos*—"solitary individual." Significant to monastic ideology is abstention from sinful practices, most notably, sexual relations.

Two main forms of monasticism exist—eremitic and cenobitic. Saint Anthony of Egypt (c. 251–356) helped establish eremitic monasticism by withdrawing from society into the Egyptian desert to become a hermit. He longed to escape distractions, which would afford the solitude necessary for prayer. Anthony suffered a series of temptations recorded in the *Life of St. Anthony* by St. Athanasius (c. 296–273), in the third of which the devil came to him in female form. Anthony had to conquer his carnal yearnings in order to center all his energy upon God. Saint Pachomius (c. 292–346), also an Egyptian ascetic, is credited with developing the cenobitic system. This method allowed monastics, unable to endure the rigors of isolation, to live communally in groups of single gender to avoid enticement.

Saint Basil of Caesarea (c. 330–379) affirmed the cenobitic technique and sought to bring monasticism under church authority. The *Rule of St. Basil* functioned as the first handbook to create order within monasteries by structuring the day into periods for work, dinner, and devotion, and it made all monks responsible to an abbot. This provided more time for God, which is important because monks believe they engage the world through prayer. This is why monasticism stresses **celibacy**; the sacrifice helps free a person's mind so that they can better focus upon God. Saint Paul addresses this concern when he urges Christians to remain unmarried if they are able (1 Corinthians 7:32–35). Rather than caring for a spouse and children, a person will be at liberty to serve God. Saint Basil's *Rule* is the foundation of Orthodox monasticism, which centers on Mt. Athos (in northern Greece). After the gradual split between the two branches of Christianity, Eastern monasticism matured separately from the West.

Saint **Augustine** of Hippo (354–430) had great influence on the development of monastic thought in Western Christendom. His writings especially convey that sexual intercourse resulted from the Fall of man. Augustine bases his understating of human weakness on his own predilection toward "concupiscence" (fleshly desires), recounted in *The Confessions*. In his work *On Holy Virginity*, Augustine rates **virginity** above **marriage**, but his *On the Good of Marriage* confirms some of the benefits of wedlock, one of which is to contain inordinate longings. However, marriage must not interfere with an individual's dedication to God. This is similar to Paul's apprehension concerning marital commitment. According to Augustine, intercourse within marriage for the purpose of children is a venial sin: it does not keep a person from heaven. Copulation for the sake of pleasure, though, is a mortal offence: it consigns a person to hell, unless confessed. Augustine, like Paul, taught that the best way to honor God and to insure one's salvation was to refrain from sexual interaction.

Saint Benedict of Nursia (c. 480–547) is considered the founder of Western monasticism. The *Rule of St. Benedict* defines the virtues by which monks must live—poverty, obedience, and chastity. Monks should not burden themselves with possessions because this also will not allow them to concentrate solely upon God. Furthermore, monks have to be humble and submit to their superiors, whose job it is to shepherd their flock. Most important, monks must remain chaste. Benedict's work does not explain the need for celibacy in detail like Augustine's. He simply states that a monastic ought to love chastity in reverence of God. To become a monk, a man partakes of the sacrament of holy orders. It is analogous to the sacrament of marriage, except that one is swearing one's life to God. A monk becomes the bride of Christ; however, this motif works better with female monastics. Male monastics often dedicate themselves to the service of St. Mary the Mother of God to create a representative relationship.

Significant for the preservation and growth of Roman Catholic monasticism was the influence of Celtic Christianity. After St. Patrick (c. 387–461) converted the Irish, the foundations that formed were governed not by bishops but by abbots. Indeed, monasteries served as churches. Peculiar to the Celtic Rite is that women and men often lived in the same establishments. Saint Brigid's monastery of Kildare is a famous example. Dual monasteries were favored because nuns could be better protected from marauding invaders and more easily attended by priests who could perform the sacraments. But this method presented a greater chance for abuses, and it quickly began to decline with pressure from the church.

When Irish monks traveled to the Continent after the Germanic migrations that devastated Europe, beginning in the fourth century, they reinvigorated the ecclesiastical systems that were falling into moral ruin. In particular, St. Columbanus's (543–615) monastery at Bobbio (northern Italy) became a hub of pious civilization. The Irish monks emphasized a need to return to the path of righteousness, which included rules on celibacy. Individuals who broke regulations were not punished; rather, they were expected to live up to the standards of the monastic reforms. If they did not, a secular life was always available. Through their work, the monasteries of Western Christianity became seats of intellectual dissemination—manuscripts of classical scholarship were copied—and were united through their ethical organization. *See also* Catholicism; Monaticism, Female; Monophysite Churches; Orthodox Christianity.

Further Reading: Cahill, Thomas. *How the Irish Saved Civilization*. New York: Anchor Books, 1995; French, R. M., trans. *The Way of a Pilgrim and the Pilgrim Continues His Way*. San Francisco: HarperCollins, 1965; Laboa, Juan Maria, ed. *The Historical Atlas of Eastern and Western Christian Monasticism*. Collegeville, MN: Liturgical Press, 2003.

Hannah Zdansky

MONOPHYSITE CHURCHES. The Monophysite religious movement arose in the fifth century in the Byzantine empire as a result of a long-term debate on the nature of Christ. According to Monophysites, there is one and only one divine reality. Therefore, the person of Jesus could have only a single (mono) divine nature (physis). In 451, the Fourth Ecumenical Council held at Chalcedon condemned Monophysitism and formulated a creed that said that Christ had two natures, human and divine, inseparably united. The Byzantine emperor Zeno (474–491) attempted to settle the dispute, but his efforts led to a schism within Eastern Christianity. During the later decades, the Monophysites successfully disseminated their doctrine in the empire's periphery.

In the sixth century, the Monophysite church was established in Syria. It was named Jacobite after the charismatic bishop Jacob Baradaeus, who was supported by the Byzantine empress **Theodora**. He traveled throughout Asia and Egypt and consecrated several hierarchs. Most of the Armenian and northern Egyptian (Coptic) churches also rejected the Chalcedonian creed and declared their independence from Constantinople. Some years later, Monophysitism was accepted in the Nubian kingdom and in Ethiopia. In the seventh century, Arab invaders conquered Egypt and Syria. However, the Coptic and Jacobite churches survived under Muslim dominion through the Middle Ages. Armenia was also included in the sphere of Arab influence, but had certain administrative autonomy.

Monophysite Christians recognized the New Testament and the writings of the first church fathers including St. Athanasius (298–373), the famous bishop of Alexandria, who formulated regulations for clergy and laymen regarding **marriage** and sexual behavior. Most of Athanasius's writings are preserved in Coptic, Syrian, and Armenian. Saint Basil the Great (330–379), bishop of Caesarea in Cappadocia, was another popular author in Monophysite Christology. His canons include duties of widows, virgins, and clergy.

The Monophysite churches considered sexual relations within marriage as legitimate. Marriage belonged to the nature of humanity, and was regulated by **canon law**. The church required married couples to limit sexual contacts by abstention from intimacy during numerous religious holidays. Athanasius condemned marital sex undertaken only for pleasure, claiming that the purpose of marriage is procreation. He also prohibited sexual intimacy during women's menstrual period and pregnancy. Married couples were encouraged to practice continence in order to exercise their will to control the body. Voluntary renunciation from sexual relations was regarded as a form of **celibacy**. To a certain extent, temporary abstinence from sex allowed married Christians to approach the ideal ascetic life of monks and virgins.

As in other Eastern churches, Monophysite clergy was divided into two categories. The lower ranks of priests and vicars were allowed to be married, but they could not be promoted to higher ranks of the church hierarchy. Bishops were appointed only from the celibate monks who lived in monasteries. Monks represented the first rank of Christians together with virgins, who were considered brides of Christ. Saint Athanasius devoted a number of his writings to **virginity**, describing it as a higher form of marital unity. On the whole, the Monophysite churches were hostile to human sexuality. They exalted asceticism, monastic life, and virginity.

Further Reading: Atiya, Aziz S. *A History of Eastern Christianity*. Notre Dame, IN: University of Notre Dame Press, 1968; Brakke, David. *Athanasius and the Politics of Asceticism*. New York: Oxford University Press, 1995; Frend, W.H.C. *The Rise of the Monophysite Movement;*

Chapters in the History of the Church in the Fifth and Sixth Centuries. Cambridge: Cambridge University Press, 1972.

Sergey Lobachev

MURASAKI SHIKIBU (c. 970–c. 1031). Born in the 970s, probably in the Japanese capital city, Kyo, Lady Murasaki Shikibu was the daughter of Tametoki, a scholar and official in the ministry of ceremony. Her family was a minor branch of the Fujiwara dynasty, which had secured power over the Japanese emperors through **marriage** and regencies. Murasaki studied classical Chinese and Japanese alongside her brother, Nobunori (d. 1013), which gave her a far more thorough education than her female peers. Married around 999 to a much older relative, Murasaki had a daughter, but in 1001 her husband died in an epidemic. She remained in seclusion in the family home until both her father and brother became provincial officials and Murasaki acquired a court post in 1004 as lady-in-waiting to Empress Fujiwara no Akiko, the consort of Emperor Ichijo.

Although she had kept a diary since adulthood, Murasaki only began writing her masterpiece, *The Tale of Genji*, in 1008. Its fifty-four chapters detail the life and adventures of an illegitimate son of an emperor and his experience in Heian Japanese society. Rich with details about clothing, social customs, and manners of court life, the chapters circulated amongst the elite and gained popularity for their evocation of the imperial court and the elaborate rituals of love, courtship, and seduction. Murasaki wrote the work in *kana*, the phonetic Japanese of women, allowing her both a greater audience and the ability to mimic different classes of speech. Genji is an admirable hero, who was particularly popular amongst female readers for his loyalty and affection for all the women he had connections to, even long after their relationships ended. In a polygamous society like Heian **Japan**, jealousy between wives and concubines, legitimate and illegitimate children, and former and present lovers was a crucial threat to good manners and social harmony, which Murasaki uses as a theme in her work.

Murasaki, a literary rival and a contemporary of *Pillow Book* author **Sei Shonagon**, shows a synthesis of **Buddhism**, Shinto, and classical Chinese Confucianism in her intricate and epic work, which contains many original poems written by the characters. She disappears from court records after 1025, and probably retired to a convent, dying around 1031. *The Tale of Genji* and her diary continued to circulate as admired court literature.

Further Reading: Bowring, Richard, ed. *The Diary of Lady Murasaki.* New York: Penguin, 1996; Morris, Ivan. *The World of the Shining Prince: Court Life in Ancient Japan.* New York: Alfred A. Knopf, 1964; Puette, William. *The Tale of Genji: A Readers' Guide.* Rutland, VT: Charles Tuttle, 1992.

Margaret Sankey

MUT'A MARRIAGE. *Mut'a* means pleasure, enjoyment, or delight. This term is used to refer to a temporary **marriage** contracted for a fixed time period and for an agreed amount of compensation. *Mut'a* marriage is only permitted in Shia **Islam**. Shia jurisprudence refers to it as "discontinued marriage" or "temporary marriage." The Qur'anic basis for this type of marriage is found in the verse "So those of them [women] whom you enjoy, give them their appointed wages" (4:24).

A *mut'a* marriage could only be legitimately contracted between a man and a free woman, or with a female slave who has the permission of her master. Typically, it was a temporary marriage of pleasure, arranged by men who traveled or were away from their families for extended periods of time.

The fixed period of time for the *mut'a* marriage could be of any length, only an hour or even years. The woman was often referred to in juristic texts as a "rented woman." The conditions of the marriage contract stipulated the amount of financial compensation in cash or kind due to the woman for the fixed time period. *Mut'a* marriages established legitimate sexual partnerships, which were extremely flexible. They provided a legal and socially acceptable alternative to **prostitution**.

Mut'a marriages could only be contracted between a Muslim man and a believer (i.e., a Muslim, a Christian, or a Jew). Muslims were admonished to abjure women of bad reputation and to only marry women who are honest and who have followed the religious laws regarding marriage. It was unlawful to marry a woman of ill repute. If a man doubted the virtue of a woman, he was urged to make inquiries about her and her marital status before a marriage contract was concluded. It was also considered extremely objectionable to marry a virgin in this type of marriage. However, this was possible with the permission of the woman's father.

If a marriage contract was concluded and the start of the contract was postponed, it was possible for the woman to enter into a second *mut'a* marriage. However, the first marriage must be concluded before the commencement of the second and in time for the woman to observe her waiting period to ascertain that she was not pregnant.

The marriage contract required both a declaration and an acceptance. The complete dowry or financial compensation was payable once the contract was concluded. Contracts could stipulate a specific number of sexual acts. If so, when the specified number had been preformed, no further sexual relations were allowed even though the marriage period had not elapsed.

Under this arrangement the man was under no legal obligation to provide his wife with food or shelter as under regular Islamic law in a permanent marriage. Additionally, this type of marriage excluded any possibility of inheritance. However, while *mut'a* marriage was extremely flexible and set for a fixed time, it was theoretically possible to write the contract for an extended length of time and to include provisions for inheritance. Conditions for **divorce** in Islamic law are very easy; however, in this kind of marriage divorce was impossible. The *mut'a* marriage was purely for pleasure and not for progeny. However, in the case of offspring, children in all cases reverted to the man. **Contraception** was practiced in these types of marriages.

Further Reading: Heffening, W. "Mut'a." In *The Encyclopaedia of Islam*. Second ed. Leiden: Brill, 1960, 2005 Vol. VII, p. 359; Murata, S. *Temporary Marriage (mut'a) in Islamic Law*. London: Muhammadi Trust, 1987.

Mark David Luce

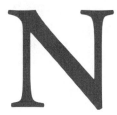

NESTORIAN CHURCHES. The Nestorian church, or the church of the East, was established in Persia in the fifth century, when the local bishop's council at Seleucia declared independence from the Roman empire. The church was named after Nestorius, the former bishop of Constantinople (428–431), who became famous for his involvement in the dispute about the nature of Christ. Nestorius claimed that the Virgin Mary gave birth only to the man Jesus, not to God; therefore, she could not be described as Theotokos (bearer of God), but rather as Christotokos (bearer of Christ). In 431, the opponents of Nestorius, Cyril of Alexandria and Celestine, bishop of Rome, gathered the ecumenical council at Ephesus for the final dispute. Nestorius, however, considered the assembly unrepresentative and refused to participate in its debates. He was removed from the patriarchal see and sent into exile in Asia Minor. He spent the rest of his life in Egypt, dying soon after the Council of Chalcedon in 451.

During the Middle Ages, Nestorian Christianity penetrated into **central Asia**, reaching **India** and **China**. However, it survived in cultural isolation from **Orthodox Christianity**. The Nestorians preserved original rituals and practices and established their own theological doctrine at the school of Nisibis. They had specific opinions on everyday life and social behavior, including **marriage** and sexuality. Although Nestorian Christians recognized marriage as one of the seven sacraments, their matrimonial law was not strictly regulated. **Divorce**, for example, was allowed on numerous grounds, which was unusual for a Christian church.

The church of the East did not require **celibacy** among clergy. During the first centuries of Nestorian history, even monks and nuns were permitted to live together and raise children. Thomas of Marga, a historian of the ninth century, described a monastic settlement as a village where **concubinage** was a normal practice. At a later time, monastic life was radically reformed with the introduction of celibacy. The Nestorian tradition, however, did not require staying in the monastery for one's entire life. Anyone who took monastic vows could easily obtain a dispensation to leave the cloister without disgrace.

Priests were allowed to marry at any time, both before and after ordination. Remarriage upon the death of their wives was permitted only for lower clergy. The higher clergy, on the contrary, might live in celibacy. Nevertheless, some sources point out the existence of married bishops. Another Nestorian custom was that the offices of patriarchs and bishops were hereditary within certain families, usually passing from uncle to nephew.

Nestorian Christianity was challenged by other cultures and religions. In the seventh century, Persia was conquered by Muslims. Islamic rulers tolerated Christians, and Nestorians played a significant role in translating Greek philosophical writings into Syrian and Arabian languages. The church of the East also survived under the Mongols, who spread their authority throughout Asia in the thirteenth century, when the caliphate had declined. However, at the end of the fourteenth century, the Nestorian church was almost destroyed as a result of persecutions of Timur, the Muslim ruler of central Asia, who had subjugated Iran and other lands formerly part of the Mongol empire.

Further Reading: Atiya, Aziz Suryal. *A History of Eastern Christianity*. London: Methuen, 1968; Moffett, Samuel. *A History of Christianity in Asia*. Vol. 1, *Beginnings to 1500*. San Francisco: Harper San Francisco, 1992; Vine, Aubrey Russell. *The Nestorian Churches*. New York: AMS Press, 1980.

Sergey Lobachev

NEW SONGS FROM A JADE TERRACE. *New Songs from a Jade Terrace*, the earliest Chinese collection entirely devoted to love poems, was compiled by the poet Xu Ling (507–583) in 545. The project was commissioned by Xiao Gang (503–551), also known as Emperor Jianwen (r. 550–551), himself a brilliant poet. The Chinese title of the book was *Yutai xinyong*. *Yutai* means "jade terrace," and generally indicates terraces of imperial palaces; *xin* means "new," and *yong* means "song," "sing," or "recite." The collection contains 656 poems in ten volumes arranged in chronological order from second century BCE to the mid-sixth century CE. *New Songs from a Jade Terrace* is considered a Chinese literary treasure because it best represents the "palace style poetry," which fully developed during the period of Southern dynasties (420–589) of **China**. During this era, twenty-seven non-Chinese kingdoms controlled northern China while six Chinese dynasties successively ruled southern China. Largely shielded from wars and chaos, literary aristocrats, under the patronage of the Southern courts, devoted their talent to poetic expressions of their life and emotions. The poems in this collection carried on the tradition of *The Book of Songs* of the Zhou dynasties (1050–221 BCE) and paved the way for the literary efflorescence of the Tang dynasty (618–907), the golden age of Chinese poetry.

The most recurring theme among the poems in this collection is the everlasting longing and sorrow of a love-stricken beauty. She is profoundly despondent but waits submissively for her lover. She appears emotionally vulnerable to the doomed love, yet is quite determined to fulfill her passion and desire. The women portrayed in these love poemsare all divinely feminine and remote. While continuing the earlier Chinese poetic tradition of depicting facial characteristics and style of dress, such as silkworm eyebrows, red lips, jade-like fingers, artful smiles, and light skirts, poems in *New Songs from a Jade Terrace* added new sensuous and erotic elements by stressing the beauty's fragrant dress and her delicate body. Such emphasis on sexual appeal was typified by Shen Yue's (441–512) "For a Young Bridegroom" in the collection: "She is lovely and pretty in face and figure, courteous and clever the way she talks. Her waist and limbs are graceful, her clothes so sweet and fresh. Her round red cape reflects the early chill, her painted fan welcomes the first spell of heat. On brocade slippers is a pattern of like flowers, on embroidered sash twin heart lettuce design. Gold leaf brooches fasten her bodice edge, flower jewel pins hold up her cloudy hair" (Birrell 137).

In Confucian tradition, palace style poetry was often criticized for its lack of masculinity and its avoidance of broader social issues. Thus *New Songs from a Jade*

Terrace never gained the same status as *The Book of Songs* and *The Complete Tang Poetry* in Chinese literary history. *See also* Chinese Paintings of Elite Women.

Further Reading: Birrell, Ann. *New Songs from a Jade Terrace: An Anthology of Early Chinese Love Poetry*. London: Allen and Unwin, 1982.

Ping Yao

NIZAMI (1141–1203). Abu Muhammad ibn Yusif Nizami Ganjavi, one of the great Persian poets, is best remembered for the emotional and immortal love story between Laila and Majnu. Details of his life had remained obscure. An author of **ghazals**, rhymed couplets, and long narrative poems, Nizami was born in Ganja, Azerbaijan, to Yousef-ibn-Zaki and Raiseh, an affluent couple. He had a sound education in arts and science, which was applied in his poetry. All his life was spent in the Ganja, a flourishing trade center remaining independent. Nizami married thrice. Each of his wives died when Nizami began to author a new work, and he remarked that he sacrificed a lot with every book!

Nizami's works included the five *masnavis* (poems in rhymed couplets), having 30,000 couplets and a *divan* (collection of lyrics). The *masnavis* dealt with romantic themes. One could glean philosophy, history, humanism, fatalism, deep love, and a little bit of eroticism. Each *masnavi* had a separate subject and was composed in a different meter. Nizami's language was not vulgar and obscene even when dealing with passionate love. Nizami portrayed his women characters as learned, tender, subtle, beautiful, and intelligent. In 1175 Nizami authored the *Khusrau u Shirin* (the story of Khusrau and Shirin), a tragic and semihistorical love story having 6,500 *distichs*, involving the Sassanian king Khusrau Parviz, his Armenian queen Shirin, and the stonecutter Farhad.

One of the classic love stories, Nizami's *Laila u Majnun* (Laila and Majnu), containing 4,700 *distichs*, was written in 1188. Translated into many languages of Asia and Europe, enacted in operas, filmed in different countries, and memorialized by Eric Clapton in his album *Layla and Other Assorted Love Songs*, the romantic tragedy was set in the exotic Arabic nomadic-aristocratic life in the period of *jahiliyah* (ignorance) predating the coming of **Islam** by about a 100 years. Nizami deals with the love between Laila and her lover Majnu, their meeting, and the ultimate death out of insanity of their love. Nizami wrote that although time had passed, true love remained, which was real without beginning or end. In another verse, the lover cried in agony saying that the grief of his partner was also his and that he belonged to her and her alone.

Nizami's 1191 epic, *Eskandar Nama* (*The Book of Alexander*), is devoted to Alexander the Great of Macedonia. It contained 10,500 stanzas in two parts and narrated Alexander's story from an Islamic viewpoint. The *Haft Paykar* (The Seven Beauties), written in 1198, was about Bahram V, the ideal Sassanian king. The king fell in love with seven princesses from **India** to **China** up to Kharazm after seeing their portraits, and married them. In the same year, Nizami also compiled his collection of lyrics.

Nizami died in 1203 and was buried in Ganja, where a beautiful mausoleum was constructed in 1991 along with a metal statue commemorating his poems. One of the craters of planet Mercury had been named after him.

Further Reading: Arberry, A. J., ed. *Persian Poems: An Anthology of Verse Translations*. New York: Dutton, 1964; Nizami. *The Story of Layla and Majnu*. Translated by R. Gelpke. New Lebanon, NY: Omega Publications, 1978; Yarshater, Ehsan, ed. *Persian Literature*. Albany, NY: Bibliotheca Press, 1988.

Patit Paban Mishra

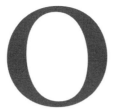

ORGASM, FEMALE. Women's pleasure in sexual intercourse was taken seriously in medieval European cultures. While it is not often possible to draw a distinction between sexual pleasure and orgasm in particular, women's ability and right to satisfaction in intercourse were widely assumed.

The "two-seed" theory of generation, inherited from Hippocratic treatises and Galenic works of antiquity, was dominant until the thirteenth century. Its premise was that both the male and female partners needed to emit "seed" (semen or sperm) for conception. Thus, it was argued in university textbooks from the twelfth century that prostitutes did not become pregnant because they had sex for money, not for pleasure. Conversely, according to the same scholarly dialogues, a woman who was raped and bore a child as a consequence had not been truly raped because she must have felt some pleasure for conception to occur. A woman's pleasure in climax was twofold: emitting her own seed and receiving the man's. **Albertus Magnus** (d. 1280) added a third source—the motion of the uterus—while others referred to the sensation of the penis against the cervix. Some authors queried whether women, being "wet" and "cold" creatures, experienced more sexual pleasure than "hot and dry" men. A stock answer was that a man should be likened to kindling, while a woman was like a damp branch—slow to catch fire but burning longer. **Hildegard of Bingen** (d. 1179) was unusual in arguing that men's pleasure in sex was greater. Foreplay (usually stimulation of breasts, perineum, or navel) was sometimes counseled as a way to ensure a woman's arousal and orgasm and aid conception. From the thirteenth century onward, the translation of Aristotle's works on animals saw the partial displacement of the two-seed by the one-seed theory, where the man alone contributed active seed to conception and women's orgasm was not necessary. The one-seed theory remained important among philosophers, but medical authors mostly held to the two-seed model.

Orgasm was seen as healthy for women: virgins, nuns, and widows ran the risk of a buildup of seed that could cause "suffocation of the uterus." **Midwives** could massage a woman's vulva to release the seed. Women's right to pleasure was acknowledged in **canon law**, as witnessed in late medieval church court cases where impotent men were condemned by women because they had failed to give their wives satisfaction. One London prostitute advised prospective brides about the sexual prowess of their husbands-to-be. Medieval Jewish custom saw a wife's orgasm as important in lessening the chance of her seeking satisfaction outside the **marriage**.

Women's sexuality was thought to be penis-focused. The clitoris, although mentioned in Arab sources and occasionally described in Latin texts, was not understood by Christian writers as a site of pleasure until the sixteenth century. Due to this phallocentrism, medieval authors rarely mentioned "lesbian" sex. French fabliaux included tales of women with phallic fantasies: one wife wished her husband's body were entirely covered with penises. Medical writers, however, occasionally mentioned manual stimulation, and a seduced maiden of an English lyric tells of a cleric who "groped so nicely in my lap, I had no power to say him nay." We lack women's real-life testimony about experiences or regularity of orgasm, but some women mystics wrote of divine union in quasi-orgasmic terms. Mechthild of Magdeburg (d. c. 1282) wrote of receiving God's word as a womb receives seed and thus conceiving her book of revelations. *See also* Orgasm, Male.

Further Reading: Cadden, Joan. *Meanings of Sex Difference in the Middle Ages: Medicine, Science, and Culture*. Cambridge: Cambridge University Press, 1993; Karras, Ruth Mazo. *Sexuality in Medieval Europe: Doing Unto Others*. New York: Routledge, 2005.

Kim M. Phillips

ORGASM, MALE. While no explicit discourse on male orgasms existed within medieval culture, many writers discussed orgasm while considering other matters. Commentators debated the purpose and function of orgasm in relation to procreation and overall bodily health in a teleological context, while moral and psychological health was a focus of philosophical discussion. In the early Middle Ages, male sexual pleasure was associated with the generative act and maintenance of the bodily humors. By the late medieval period, male orgasm was directly connected with ejaculation, but its influence on procreation was debated. It is evident within the medical and philosophical texts of the fifth through fourteenth centuries that sexual pleasure was viewed skeptically in European culture, less so within Judaic tradition, and as an important part of Islamic sexual relations.

When discussing the relationship of orgasm and generation, medieval writers followed two traditions. Galenic theory held that orgasm was required for conception, while Aristotelian thought did not, and related pleasure only to the force of ejaculation. Constantine the African wrote that males experienced orgasm only through seminal issue and connected coital pleasure psychologically with procreation. **Albertus Magnus** believed that conception could occur without orgasm, and Bernard of Gordon made a distinction between sex for production of offspring and for pleasure. Arabic writers such as **Ibn Sina** and **al-Razi** echoed the ideas of Galen. Thomas Sanchez concludes philosophically that a man who withdrew from intercourse with a prostitute before ejaculation would be repenting his act since illicit pleasure would not have a result. While a connection between ejaculation and sexual pleasure is broadly evident in the sources, male orgasm and conception were not inextricably tied.

Health and morality's relationship to orgasm drew upon the connection between sexual pleasure and ejaculation. The physical side of the issue relied upon the theory of bodily humors, while the psychological aspect considered the emotional and spiritual condition. Since seminal fluid was related to the balance of heat and moisture within the male body, many writers concluded that ejaculation was an important excretory activity of the body. Galenic theory argued that moderate intercourse was therefore good for optimal health, allowing Ambrose to proclaim its value to participants of the Third Crusade and Albertus Magnus to conclude that this type of sexual activity accelerated growth in adolescents. Epicurean and Stoic philosophy idealized constancy, leading Christian thinkers **Augustine** and Gratian to view sexual pleasure as diverting attention from religious salvation. Peter Lombard supports these ideas with his sinful assessment of passionate love. The importance of orgasm to physiological health is evident in Talmudic stories stressing that widowers remarry and childless **marriages** remain intact. While morality influenced the ongoing philosophical debate, Galenic medical thought enjoyed broad acceptance after the eleventh century. *See also* Medicine; Orgasm, Female; Theories of Sexual Difference.

Further Reading: Bullough, Vern L., and James A. Brundage, eds. *Handbook of Medieval Sexuality.* New York: Garland Publishing, 1996; Cadden, Joan. *Meanings of Sex Difference in the Middle Ages: Medicine, Science, and Culture.* New York: Cambridge University Press, 1993.

T. Brice Pearce

ORTHODOX CHRISTIANITY. Orthodox Christianity, or the Eastern Orthodox Church, was the product of hundreds of years of evolution during the Middle Ages. In the fifth century, five patriarchates existed within the Catholic Church: Rome, Constantinople, Alexandria, Antioch, and Jerusalem. Each ruled its own region and tried to follow the teachings of Christianity. Because Western Romans were proving slow to convert to Christianity, the first Christian Roman Emperor, Constantine I the Great (c. 280–337), made **Byzantium** capital of the Eastern Roman empire and renamed it Constantinople in 330 CE. Constantine took the opportunity to create a spiritual center for Christians of the Roman empire. Eventually, most Romans did embrace Christianity, and Constantine's "second Rome" theoretically came under the jurisdiction of the pope, while retaining de facto independence until a schism over doctrine in 867. The church settled its differences briefly, but a second schism in 1054 forever split the Catholic Church into the Roman and Eastern Orthodox branches.

The growth of Christianity in the two branches must be viewed within the context of their political and social cultures. Roman **Catholicism** actively spread throughout western Europe by means of traveling priests backed by an increasingly wealthy and powerful Roman pontiff. Christianity in the East evolved into a largely monastic culture with great emphasis on solitary prayer and worship. There were many attempts to conquer Constantinople in the seventh and eighth centuries, but they failed. The troops of the Fourth Crusade successfully invaded in 1204. When they left, the city never regained its former glory, and the invasion cemented the enmity between the East and the West.

Because of its origins and location, the seat of the Eastern Church had to deal with cultural influences from Europe, Asia, Egypt, and the nations of **Islam**. The area itself is predominantly Greek. In addition, the secular and religious were never completely separate. The area was governed as much by the church patriarch as by the emperor. This overall culture contributed to Orthodox treatment of various sexual issues.

HOMOSEXUALITY. The Eastern Church struggled with male homosexuality and, indeed, all kinds of sexuality. (A dearth of documentation leaves us with little knowledge of female homosexuality in medieval Orthodoxy.) The enjoyment of non-procreative sexual relations was the main objection the church had to homosexuality. Because Constantinople was a Hellenistic society, male homosexuality in itself was not vilified within the culture for most of the medieval period. The Christianization of the area imposed its sexual mores on the society but could not suppress its nature completely. In the twelfth century, however, there was a very sudden reversal of the issue, and most of the public became very intolerant of the practice.

There is a uniquely Orthodox service called the Adelphopoiia Rite that has come under some scrutiny. The rite was originally used to consecrate fraternization, a relationship that bound together people who were not blood relatives. It is similar to blood-brother practices in ancient Greece, Rome, and other areas of western Europe. The rite is used today to provide consecration of same-sex unions, and there are some who believe it was used this way in the Middle Ages also. There is some controversial evidence of cases of this, but it has not been proven conclusively.

PROSTITUTION. The most famous group of Orthodox monasteries is on Mount Athos, located on the peninsula of *Athos* or *Halkidiki*. To this day, no women are allowed within 500 meters of the mount. This edict has been in effect since the eleventh century, when some women, probably prostitutes, disguised themselves as shepherds in order to lure younger monks away from their religious duties. The church purports that the ban is because the Virgin Mary appeared at the mount and fell in love with it, declaring it her special garden. She will be the only woman ever allowed to set foot on the Holy Mount.

Prostitution was a thriving business in the Byzantine empire long before it became the seat of Orthodox Christianity. The church only wished to make male homosexual and child prostitution illegal. Many theologians did not have a problem with prostitution per se. Women prostitutes were considered necessary even by St. **Augustine** (354–430), who promoted not only procreative sex between husband and wife, but also recognized a man's need for nonprocreative sex. He advocated the use of prostitutes for this function. The only issue the medieval church seemed to have with adult female prostitution was the possibility that prostitutes may actually enjoy themselves. Courtesans were even known to climb the social ladders in the empire. **Theodora**, wife of the first Byzantine emperor Justinian (483–565), was a former actress, which almost certainly meant that she worked as a prostitute.

The church's opposition to male prostitutes was based on the idea that the body of a man was superior to that of a woman. The church could not abide that the body of a grown man would be used in the same way a woman's was. The traditional sexual relationship between males in Greek tradition was of an active adult male with a passive pubescent male. Although the culture of the area supported a rather large homosexual community, grown men were not normally passive partners in relationships. Much of the prostitution trade was fed by the sale of children and procurement of abandoned babies. The church entered into a debate about this practice that eventually cut child prostitution significantly. The clergy feared that since babies were abandoned or sold at such an early age, they would be unrecognizable to their families in the future, when working as prostitutes. This could lead to **incest**, albeit unknowingly.

EUNUCHISM. While homosexuality and prostitution were issues not unknown to the Roman church, eunuchism was uniquely an Eastern entity. Although many attempts were made to outlaw the practice, it continued to thrive in the Byzantine empire, despite the public's hatred of the **eunuchs** themselves, simply because of the wealth and power associated with the condition. The emperor's palace was always full of eunuchs, where they served in many trusted positions. There are letters to emperors even in the ninth and tenth centuries about the numbers of eunuchs sent as gifts.

Slaves were often made eunuchs, which was difficult to prevent because of ownership laws. Parents authorized the surgery for sons, which was impossible to stop because of their absolute rights over their children. Some men even chose to undergo the surgery themselves. Eunuchs were found in every class of the society. Two different kinds of eunuchs were recognized. The *ektomoi* or *ektomiai* had undergone surgery to remove all means of procreation. The *spadones* or *thladiai* were impotent men, although still intact physically.

The Orthodox church did not reject eunuchs, and they were even allowed into high offices within the church. The only stipulation was that they could not have undergone the surgery electively. If they had been forcibly castrated or it was necessary because of illness, there were no impediments to promotion within the church, even to bishop or patrician. There were several monasteries built specially for eunuchs, and eunuchs alone were given positions of steward and vice-steward in women's convents. *See also* Chrysostom, John; Orthodox Europe; Theophylactus of Ochrid.

Further Reading: Boswell, John. *Same Sex Unions in Pre-Modern Europe*. New York: Villard, 1994; Clark, Victoria. *Why Angels Fall: A Journey through Orthodox Europe from Byzantium to Kosovo*. New York: St. Martin's Press, 2000; Dauphin, Claudine. "Brothels, Baths and Babes: Prostitution in the Byzantine Holy Land." *Classics Ireland* 3 (1996), University College Dublin, Ireland. See www.ucd.ie/classics/96/Dauphin96.html; Guilland, Rodolphe. Les Eunuques dans l'Empire Byzantin (English). From *Études Byzantines*. Vol. 1 (1943). See www.well.com/user/guilland-eunuques.htm; Mantzouneas, Evangelos K. "Fraternization from a Canonical Perspective." Athens, 1982. See www.qrd.org/qur/religion/judeochristian/eastern_orthodox/church.of.greece.on.adelphopoiia.

Jennifer Della'Zanna

ORTHODOX EUROPE

HISTORICAL BACKGROUND. **Orthodox Christianity** came into existence in the Byzantine empire. In the early Middle Ages, the differences between Eastern and Western Christian traditions concerning religious practices, theological matters, liturgical language, and relations between church and state grew rapidly. The final schism emerged in 1054 when Pope Leo XI excommunicated the patriarch of Constantinople, Michael Cerularius. The primary issues were debates about the authority of the bishop of Rome and the so-called *Filioque* clause. The Eastern Church recognized the supreme jurisdiction of ecumenical councils, but the western Roman tradition granted the pope authority to make changes in councils' statements. In addition, Leo XI added to the creed established at the Council of Nicaea the *Filioque* clause asserting that the Holy Spirit proceeds from the Father "and the Son" (*filioque*), an innovation vigorously rejected in Constantinople.

Byzantine culture influenced neighboring countries inhabited by Slavic tribes. In the seventh century, Orthodox Christianity penetrated into Serbia, in 865 it was adopted in Bulgaria, and in 988 in Russia. In the Middle Ages, the Orthodox religion preserved cultural unity on the vast territory from the Balkans to the Baltic rim. Slavic states became a part of Orthodox Christendom with the center in Constantinople. In the fifteenth century, however, **Byzantium** faced the threat of Ottoman invasion. The emperor asked for help from the West in a change of compromise in religious matters. In 1439, the highest clergy of Roman Catholic and Orthodox churches gathered at the Council of Florence and declared the union of the East and the West. Byzantine patriarchs accepted the *Filioque* clause and papal authority, as well as other rituals established in Catholic Christianity but did not save the empire from Turkish conquest in 1453. The downfall of Byzantium made local Orthodox churches autonomous, although the ecclesiastical influence of Constantinople remained considerable.

LOVE AND MARRIAGE. The cultural unity of Orthodox Europe did not exclude local peculiarities. Byzantine traditions, in many respects, differed from the customs of medieval Slavs. For centuries, ecclesiastical law officially adopted in Slavic countries existed side by side with pagan practices. **Marriage**, for example, was primarily regulated by the common law, especially in rural areas. Pagan **wedding rituals** were prevalent, and the Orthodox clergy had to make considerable efforts to encourage couples to attend a religious ceremony. The purpose of marriage was political and economic, rather than moral and emotional. Personal desire and physical attraction were totally neglected. The idea of romantic love, popular in western Europe, was unknown in the Orthodox East. Sometimes the bride and groom did not see each other before the wedding. The first **marriage** was usually arranged by the parents of a young couple, who became husband and wife at early ages. Although the **canon law** recognized children's right to refuse to marry against their will, in reality, objection to a parent's choice might lead to dishonor and shame.

Legal marriage in Orthodox Europe was possible when both partners were Orthodox Christians. Nonbelievers needed to be baptized in the Orthodox faith. Such restrictions allowed multiethnic societies to preserve their identity. The only alternative to marriage was monastic life, which required chastity and asceticism. While monks and bishops might observe **celibacy**, the parish clergy, on the contrary, had to be married in order to avoid temptations of the secular world.

The church did not forbid second and third marriages, but certain penances and a waiting period were required. The termination of legal marriage was possible under some circumstances. The most common reason for **divorce** was **adultery**. Other motives included political and criminal matters. For example, a wife could leave her husband if he committed treason against the monarch, or ruined her reputation by raping her or forcing her into **prostitution**. The ecclesiastical law also allowed divorce if one spouse took a monastic vow.

SEXUAL RELATIONS. The church authorities exercised complete control over moral standards of the society in Orthodox Europe. Clergymen demanded that lay people obey regulations of the canon law, which contained numerous limitations of sexual behavior even within legitimate marriage. Ecclesiastical rules, for example, required spouses to abstain from intimacy during religious holidays and **Lent**, on Wednesdays and Fridays throughout the year, and when the wife was menstruating. Many types of sexual intercourse were regarded as sinful. Married couples were allowed to practice only vaginal penetration and missionary position. The church approved of marital sex only for reproduction. All forms of birth prevention were considered evil. From the religious point of view, **contraception** and **abortion** were nothing other than infanticide. Violation of canon rules related to sexual behavior entailed certain penalties, which might include praying, fasting, and prohibition from church services. More serious offences, which disturbed the social order, required stricter punishment and involvement from secular authorities. **Rape**, for example, fell under lay jurisdiction. Both church and state were interested in the maintenance of social peace and stability in a well-structured medieval society. They granted certain privileges to high-ranking aristocracy and imposed different punishment for the same crime depending on the social status of victim and violator. For example, sexual relations with a married woman, which could destroy a family as an important social institution, were considered a more dangerous crime than premarital sex. The churchmen were also concerned about the anti-Christian behavior of the population. For clergy, male homosexuality represented a minor threat in comparison with lesbianism, which was associated with pagan rituals.

Many examples suggest that attitudes to sexual behavior in Orthodox medieval Europe were highly pragmatic. Church and state regarded intimacy as a public matter that might challenge social order, but they never took into account human desire and emotion.

Further Reading: Brundage, James A. *Law, Sex and Christian Society in Medieval Europe.* Chicago: University of Chicago Press, 1987; Bullough, Vern L. *Sexual Variance in Society* *and History*. New York: Wiley, 1976, 317–41; Levin, Eve. *Sex and Society in the World of the Orthodox Slavs, 900–1700*. Ithaca, NY: Cornell University Press, 1989.

Sergey Lobachev

OSCULUM INFAME. See Kiss of Infamy

OVIDIANISM. The poetical works of Ovid (Publius Ovidius Naso, 43 BCE–17 CE) provided the Middle Ages with a treasury of amorous literature, including ancient tales of love and lust, and witty, first-person commentary on the game of love. During the early medieval period, Ovid's erotic lyrics from the *Amores* (Loves), *Ars amatoria* (Art of Love), and *Remedia amoris* (Remedy for Love) were the stuff for student grammar lessons, but the content eventually came into its own in later medieval works. The famous twelfth-century *De arte honeste amandi* of **Andreas Capellanus**, often called "The Art of Courtly Love," hands down Ovid's ideas (perhaps not to be taken seriously in either age) that love can only exist outside **marriage**; that it involves deceit, suffering, and jealousy; and that it ends inevitably in boredom once the prize has been won.

Ovid's *Metamorphoses*, a compendium of mythological tales, rose to popularity in the twelfth century, spawning numerous commentaries, redactions, and borrowings on into the early modern period and beyond. Its wealth of ancient stories covers the gamut of desire and gender conflict, from **rape**, **incest**, same-sex desire, and sex change, to devoted spousal love and matrimonial disasters, both tragic and comic. Often, medieval writers who make use of the *Metamorphoses* also use other Ovidian sources, particularly the *Heroides*, a collection of melancholy letters from the perspective of various women (Dido, Ariadne, and Medea, for example) who have been separated from their men. These complex portraits of female emotion, along with the female self-assertion so common in the *Metamorphoses* (be it positive or negative), have prompted modern debates regarding Ovid's attitude toward women and love. It is equally difficult to be certain as to how medieval writers understood Ovid. The medieval French texts surveyed by Norman Shapiro in *The Comedy of Eros* give evidence that while some twelfth- and thirteenth-century writers took up Ovid's erotic material to denounce it and others to promote it, few preserved any of Ovid's literary flair, and most captured little, if anything, of his ambiguously ironic tone. Far from addressing the varied issues of sex and gender that Ovid raises, the commentaries of the later Middle Ages are notorious for reducing Ovid's *Metamorphoses*, in particular, to a series of unrelated allegories, fodder for sermon-ready morals or an excuse to rehearse traditional Platonic cosmology.

A more thorough and authentic Ovidianism appears in some of these commentaries, particularly the fourteenth-century *Ovide Moralisé* (Moralized Ovid), wherein Ovid's text survives in fairly accurate translation, and the commentary includes subtle sexual puns and bawdy tales imported from non-Ovidian sources. Many scholars would concur that the thirteenth-century **Romance of the Rose** provides one of the most fascinating examples of Ovid's influence on medieval poetry. Although the work is not a response to or a rewriting of any particular Ovidian text, it addresses the trials of love in a strange allegorical epic that clearly draws on Ovid's erotic poems and the *Metamorphoses*, all the while preserving a certain ambiguity as to how cynical one should be about love. This ambiguity is achieved in suitably Ovidian fashion by ascribing much of the poem to various character-narrators, including the first-person protagonists, who offer dubious criticism, advice, and ostensibly instructive stories while relating their own experiences with desire. Geoffrey **Chaucer**'s unfinished fourteenth-century "Legend of Good Women," which might be called a parody of the *Heroides*, is more overtly based on Ovid, but similarly noteworthy for capturing Ovid's habit of letting a text cause its own interpretive problems. **John Gower**'s contemporary *Confessio Amantis* (The Lover's Confession) fits into a similar category, as it puts Ovidian tales into the mouth of a moralizing priest of Venus whose interpretations are too myopic to be trusted, and whose authority is therefore similarly suspect where love is concerned. The messages are mixed as to whether women, love, and sex are good, bad, both, or neither, and readers continue to be fittingly intrigued.

Further Reading: Allen, Peter L. *The Art of Love: Amatory Fiction from Ovid to "The Romance of the Rose."* Philadelphia: University of Pennsylvania Press, 1992; McKinley, Kathryn L. *Reading the Ovidian Heroine: "Metamorphoses" Commentaries, 1100–1618.* Leiden: Brill, 2001; Shapiro, Norman. *The Comedy of Eros.* Urbana: University of Illinois Press, 1971.

Elizabeth Maxey

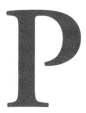

PAGAN EUROPE. The word "pagan" is derived from the Latin *pagus*, meaning "rural." When Christianity was adopted in Roman cities, most country people remained heathen, and townsmen used to call them *pagans* to distinguish themselves from non-Christians. In the early medieval period, when urban culture declined, a great part of Europe was populated by pagan tribes. The Celts settled mainly in Gaul, Britain, and Ireland. Germanic people lived on the Rhine and the Baltic shores. Some of them confederated in the third century as Francs and Saxons; others were known as Scandinavians, or Vikings, the famous sea-raiders of the epoch. Slavic tribes inhabited the vast territory from the Balkans in the south to the Baltic sea in the north, where they adjoined with Finns and Lithuanians. Most of these tribes observed heathen traditions through the Middle Ages, even after conversion to Christianity. Marital and sexual practices in pagan Europe varied in different cultures, but all of them obeyed certain regulations.

Medieval clerics complained about immoral marital and sexual customs in pre-Christian Europe, emphasizing **polygamy** and promiscuity. However, there is much evidence that pagan societies observed certain rules applying to relations between the sexes. The institute of **marriage** was established on the basis of the common law. Although polygamy was not prohibited, it was practiced only among the upper classes. The majority of population respected monogamy and penalized women for **adultery**.

Early German Law, the *Lex Salica*, and the Russian Legal Code of Prince Yaroslav legitimatized some traditional methods of marriage. A groom could purchase his bride by arrangement with her family and the payment of compensation. If a man was poor, he was able to marry by consent of his spouse without permission of her relatives, but he was to live in her family. Pagan law also recognized marriage by forcible abduction. Although the abductor might pay heavy fines, he was allowed to keep his bride.

Pagan tradition made no distinction between marriage and **concubinage**. No formal ceremony was required for young couples who wished to create a family, only an intention to live together and raise children. Sexual intercourse was indispensable for marital unions as the primary purpose of marriage was procreation. If the wife failed to become pregnant within a year, the husband might terminate their relations. There were only a few restrictions on marriage to prevent unions between close relatives. Both husband and wife had a right to initiate **divorce**, although pagan tradition granted men more freedom to do it. The most common motives for dissolution of marriage were adultery and **magic**.

Sexual relations in pagan Europe were closely connected with religious rites and celebrations. Pagan people used to live in accordance with natural rhythms. Their customs were based on the idea that human behavior has an impact on nature. The famous celebration of the summer solstice included ritual sex symbolizing the resurrection of fertility. Another popular tradition in pagan Europe related to the cult of the Earth. During sowing season couples had ritual sex to promote the growth of the crops. This ritual reflected the idea that sexual intercourse might influence vegetation. Adultery or fornication was considered a serious sin, because it could damage the harvest.

Some celebrations were devoted to the god of fertility. In pagan mythology, he was represented as an idol with distinctive sexual attributes. Images of the Slavic god Rod, or Scandinavian god Freyr, for example, had a prominent phallus. There was a belief that female virgins had magic power and special relationships with the gods. In Slavic mythology women who died as virgins reappeared as evil spirits of forests and rivers. During the wedding night a husband had to release his spouse from those charms and present evidence that she lost her maidenhood. Extramarital sex in pagan societies was treated as an offence and punished by fines or even death depending on the social status of the fornicators. Rapists, as a rule, merited a death penalty; however, they might survive by marrying their victims, if the woman's parents consented. Most pagan laws required different penalties for the same crime by taking into consideration the status of the violators. For example, a male slave who had sexual intercourse with a free woman faced harsher punishment. *See also* Freya/Frigg; Medb; Phallic Worship.

Further Reading: Brown, Peter. *The Rise of Western Christendom: Triumph and Diversity*. Oxford: Blackwell, 1996; Brundage, James A. *Law, Sex and Christian Society in Medieval Europe*. Chicago: University of Chicago Press, 1987; Fraser, James. *The Golden Bough: A Study in Magic and Religion*. 3rd ed. Parts 1–2. London: Macmillan, 1963; Jones, Prudence, and Nigel Pennick. *A History of Pagan Europe*. London: Routledge, 1995.

Sergey Lobachev

PEDERASTY. Since the age of consent was twelve for girls and thirteen for boys throughout the medieval period, pedophilia would not normally have been regarded as any different from homosexuality itself. While historians have debated whether Greek pedophilia was carried over into Roman times, there is now general agreement that it did exist among certain levels of Roman society. Sources for the medieval period are difficult to find, but recent studies of twelfth-century French literature emphasize intergenerational relationships that might better be called pederasty than pedophilia. It was also during this period that the close relationships of males with each other began to be seriously questioned, but still, if the literature is to be trusted, they existed. A good example is **Peter Abelard**'s poetic version of the lament of the biblical king David for Jonathan. In it, David regrets not rescuing Jonathan, which would have allowed death to join them more closely together.

Male friendships are at the heart of the twelfth-century *Roman d'Éneas* based on Virgil's *Aeneid*. Eneas is closely involved with the youth Pallas, who was killed in the conquest of Italy. Eneas calls him a "flower of youth" as he holds the dead Pallas in his arms and laments his death. Later in the text, where Eneas has fallen in love with Lavine, who is betrothed to his political rival, her mother attempts to dissuade Lavine by saying that Eneas would rather take a boy than be near her. She goes on to say how Eneas would use her to attract a boy whom he could mount. In fact, the anonymous redactor of the story seems to imply pederasty might be a part of the military culture.

Many writers of the twelfth century describe the erotic charms of youthful males with manly stature and girlish faces. The adolescent male, the bachelor with his first beard, appears in virtually all twelfth-century discussions of sexual intimacy. Some historians have described the sexual adventurousness of bands of adolescent males but assume it to have taken place entirely within a heterosexual framework. Others, mostly more recent scholars, see the relationships as more homoerotic. Hildebert of Lavardin, archbishop of Tours in the middle of the twelfth century, railed against what he called the Ganymede sin. He emphasized that a boy is not at all a safe thing and urged soldiers not to devote themselves to them. Bernard of Cluny writing about the same time complained of the Ganymedes of his day. **Marie de France** in the *Lai de Lanval* had Guinevere retort to a man who rejected her sexual advances that she had been told that he had no inclination toward women but loved well-built young men.

Obviously, writers were conscious of the attractiveness of adolescent boys to some older men, but how often such relationships led to sexual acts is unknown. Undoubtedly, it did in some cases, but when, where, why, and how is not yet clear. The more research there is on the topic, the more incidents are discovered. *See also* Homosexuality, Male.

Further Reading: Kuefler, Mathew. "Male Friendships and the Suspicion of Sodomy in Twelfth Century France." In *The Boswell Thesis; Essays on Christianity, Social Tolerance and Homosexuality*, edited by Mathew Kuefler, 179–214. Chicago: University of Chicago Press, 2006.

Vern L. Bullough

PENITENTIALS. Penitentials were guidelines used by confessors, which detailed appropriate penances for different sins. They were used from the sixth to the eleventh centuries, when they were criticized for their excessive legalism. In private penitence, sinners confessed their sins in private to the priest as many times as they wanted. The system of penitence for their guilt took the name of tariffed penitence. Every type of sin corresponded to subsequent obligations that the sinner must accomplish. The price was not a tax to pay in fiscal terms, but a punishment to expiate the committed guilt. These consisted of harder mortifications, alms, punishments by exile, and, above all, fasts of various kinds.

The dimensions of the penitentials varied considerably, and for the greater part they are anonymous or attributed to a great character. The categories of sins on which the penitentials were more stringent were sexual offences, theft of church property, murder, physical violence, false oaths, and alimentary and hygienic prescriptions. There were many and very remarkable divergences in the evaluation of sins and in the choice of punishment. In particular, the Breton penitentials differ from the others for their laxity toward sexual and matrimonial matters. All the penitentials have at least a canon that censors homosexuality and many of them dedicate ample space to the problem. There are two factors that influence the penitential treatment of homosexuality: the specific type of offence and the people involved. In the case of the people involved in this sin, we can gather the canons used; there were canons addressed to people not identified, and canons addressed to bishops, priests, deacons, and monks. It is interesting to observe that female homosexuality is rarely considered. Only in the penitential of Theodore and in the penitential of Beda are there references to lesbian relationships.

Burchard of Worms in his *Decretum* includes an additional enquiry for women, about which strange contraceptive and abortive practices were imputed. There are, in addition, references to unions between women and animals; this is a sin that is punished more severely than lesbianism, with forty days of bread and water for seven consecutive years, and with the obligation to make penitence one's whole life. Other sexual sins mentioned in the penitentials and punished more severely were **incest**, **adultery**, repudiation by the wife, sex with an indisposed wife, sex after having given birth, sex with a pregnant wife, sex on a Sunday, sex in **Lent** or in Advent, sex when drunk, sex in unusual positions, sex with animals, fornication in general, **masturbation**, masturbation in company, having an orgasm in the church, **abortion**, use of contraceptives or sexual prostheses, **magic** practices to attract a man, and magic practices to make a man impotent. *See also* confession.

Further Reading: McNeill, John T., and Helena M. Gamer. *Medieval Handbooks of Penance: A Translation of the Principal* Libri Poenitentiales *and Selections from Related Documents.* New York: Columbia University Press, 1990; Payer, Pierre J. *Sex and the Penitentials. The Development of a Sexual Code, 550–1150.* Toronto, ON: University of Toronto Press, 1984.

Elvio Ciferri

PETER DAMIAN (1007–1072). Peter Damian was a Camaldolese monk at Fonte-Avellana who followed the rule of Benedict. He worked for monastic and church reforms. Peter was born at Ravenna in 1007, the last child of an impoverished noble family. He was orphaned as a child. His older brother, a priest named Damian, arranged for his education. In gratitude Peter added Damian to his own name.

Peter Damian completed his studies at Ravenna, at Faenza, and finally at the University of Parma. Around 1035, repulsed by the worldliness of university life, he joined two hermits of Fonte-Avellana to become a hermit. Around 1042 Damian wrote about the life of Saint Romuald for the monks of Pietrapertosa. In 1043 he became prior of the monastery of Fonte-Avellana, a post he held until his death. Damian promoted monastic life with the founding of monasteries at San Severino, Gamugno, Acerata, Murciana, San Salvatore, Sitria, and Ocri. He oversaw the building of a cloister and the purchase of silver chalices, a processional cross, and many books for the library.

Even though Peter Damian remained secluded from worldly life, he was aware of events affecting the church. He worked with Hildebrand (later Pope Gregory VII) and others for reform. As a reformer Damian wrote *Liber Gomorrhianus* (1049) and *Liber Gratissimus* (1053) to denounce common clerical sins. The latter work denounced simony, but argued that the purchase of a church office did not invalidate ordination.

In *Liber Gomorrhianus* (*Book of Gomorrah*) Damian addressed four kinds of sexual practices, all of which he held criminally wicked. The first was **masturbation**, an activity done alone. The second was mutual masturbation. The third wicked sexual practice was interfemoral intercourse, which involves rubbing between the thighs of another. The most severe condemnation was left for anal intercourse. Damian taught that each of these sexual practices required a greater penance to rescue the soul from hell. *Liber Gomorrhianus* caused a sensational controversy. Hostility roused against Damian eventually affected the pope, who had at first looked on the book with favor.

Damian also wrote a minor philosophical book, *De divina omnipotentia*. During a dinner conversation about **virginity** at Monte Cassino, the question, can God restore the virginity of a woman who has lost it? had arisen. Another question was can God change the past? To answer that God cannot restore virginity denies God's omnipotence. However, to affirm that God can seems to deny the law of noncontradiction. Damian chose the latter answer.

Damian was frequently sent on papal missions as a legate. In 1057 Stephen IX made him a cardinal against his will. Damian died at Faenza of a fever on February 21, 1072.
See also Homosexuality, Male; Sodomy.

Further Reading: Gonsette, J. *Pierre Damien et la culture profane*. Louvain: Publications Universitaires, 1956; Payer, Pierre J. *Book of Gomorrah: An Eleventh-Century Treatise against Clerical Homosexual Practices*. Waterloo, ON: Wilfrid Laurier University Press, 1982.

Andrew J. Waskey

PETER OF ABANO (fl. late thirteenth/early fourteenth centuries).   Peter of Abano was a professor at the universities of Paris and Padua in the late thirteenth and early fourteenth centuries. He wrote extensively on philosophy and **medicine**. His two major works are the *Conciliator*, an attempt at reconciling seemingly contradictory statements from different sources, and a commentary on the Pseudo-Aristotelian *Problems*.

Peter's writings on sexual matters emphasized naturalism over supernatural explanations. His naturalism, however, included a large role for the influence of the stars. He took a Galenic approach to sex, emphasizing its positive aspects such as its contribution to good health. Peter's treatment of sexual pleasure describes male pleasure as more concentrated and intense, female pleasure as more diffuse and long-lasting. He was one of the few medieval European authors to identify the region of the clitoris as the seat of female sexual pleasure, although he did not identify the organ itself. Peter also provided one of the fullest discussions of sex between men in the medieval Latin medical literature, discussing various techniques such as mutual masturbation, intercrural sex (which he claimed to be the most popular in his own time), and anal sex. He distinguished between men whose "seminal vessels" leading to the penis were constricted or blocked, thus diverting the area that could be pleasurably stimulated to the anus, and depraved sodomites who voluntarily chose unnatural sex. *See also* Homosexuality, Male.

Further Reading: Cadden, Joan. *The Meanings of Sex Difference in the Middle Ages: Medicine, Science and Culture*. New York: Cambridge University Press, 1993.

William E. Burns

PETRARCH (or Petrarca), **FRANCESCO** (1304–1374).   A noted humanist, scholar, and poet, Petrarch was one of the most important figures of the Italian Renaissance. His work in recovering the literary legacy of ancient Greece and Rome provided much of the foundations for a flowering of new learning across Europe in the postmedieval period, and his romantic poetry in the Italian vernacular was widely read and imitated.

Petrarch was born in 1304 in the Italian city of Arezzo, near Florence, and grew up in the nearby town of Incisa. When he was eight, his family moved to the French city of Avignon, which at that time was the headquarters of the papal court. Petrarch's father wanted him to be a lawyer, and while he did spend time at the law schools of Montpelier and Bologna, he devoted much of his time in both places to studying literature. After his father's death, Petrarch returned to Avignon, took minor orders in the Roman Catholic Church, and began to write in earnest. His first major work, an epic poem in Latin about the Roman general Scipio Africanus, was widely praised. During this period, Petrarch traveled widely, mainly in Italy and also through northern France and Germany. He also began a voluminous correspondence with authors and scholars across Europe, including his compatriot **Giovanni Boccaccio**. Petrarch's scholarly and creative work attracted the attention, and eventually the patronage, of the powerful Colonna family, which culminated in him being crowned Poet Laureate in Rome in 1341, the first poet to be so honored since the fall of the western Roman empire. In 1352, Petrarch moved back to Italy permanently, although he spent most of the subsequent years moving from place to place in search of forgotten classical manuscripts. He is responsible for the recovery of several of Cicero's letters and fragments of a work by Quintilian, and during this period he also commissioned a translation of Homer's works. In 1367, he settled in Padua, and a few years later he had a villa constructed in the nearby town of Arquà, where he died in 1374.

Although Petrarch's Latin works and scholarship were the base of his fame among his contemporaries, they are not much read today. Among his more notable works in Latin are the bulk of his letters; *De Viris illustribus* (*On Famous Men*), which is a series of biographies of figures from classical history and myth; the epic poem *Africa* mentioned above; and a number of moral treatises. In the centuries after his death, Petrarch's fame rested mainly on his *Canzoniere*, a collection of Italian poems also known under the title *Rerum vulgarium fragmenta* (*Fragments of Vulgar Things*—"vulgar" here being used in the sense of "vernacular," not "crude"). Much of the *Canzoniere* consists of love poems to "Laura," a young woman who has traditionally been identified as Laura de Noves, the wife of a French nobleman. By Petrarch's account, the young poet first saw Laura in a church in Avignon in 1327 and immediately fell in love with her. Although they did not become romantically linked, primarily due to Laura's refusal to commit **adultery**, Petrarch considered her his romantic ideal for the remainder of his life. Although she died in 1348 and Petrarch later fathered children by at least one other woman, Laura remained his muse. His poems to her are considered among the best romantic verse written in the European tradition, and also helped fix the poetic form known as the "Petrarchan sonnet."

Further Reading: Foster, Kenelm. *Petrarch: Poet and Humanist*. Edinburgh: University of Edinburgh Press, 1984; Petrarca, Francesco. *Petrarch: The Canzoniere, or Rerum vulgarium fragmenta*. Translated by Mark Musa. Bloomington: Indiana University Press, 1996.

Stephen A. Allen

PHALLIC WORSHIP. In many areas outside Europe, particularly in **India**, phallic worship has been an established and popular practice since early times. Phallic worship was less central and visible in medieval Europe. Christianity adopted mainly ascetic values from ancient Greek and Roman philosophy and religion, but the less ascetic values of these cultures, as well as those of other pre-Christian societies, lingered on.

In the early Middle Ages, northern European societies still valued male sexual prowess in a manner that had become somewhat alien to the Christianized south. For example, a Norse tale recorded around 1390, but reflecting an earlier period, is focused on the *Völsi*, the phallus of the horse. The images of some of the Germanic gods, like Frey, the god of sexuality and fertility, included large phalluses. Some of the Scandinavian Romanesque churches contained various phallic symbols. Many of the fertility and phallus-worshipping ceremonies of the early Celts survived, openly at first, occasionally in defiance of the new religion of Christianity, and secretly later. Such were the May games, which took place around a maypole and were therefore eventually abolished by the Puritans in the seventeenth century; and the Christmas mumming, derived from the Roman Saturnalia. To this practice belongs the "great shaft of Cornhill" mentioned by **Geoffrey Chaucer** and from which the church of St. Andrew Undershaft, built in the twelfth century, took its name.

Besides the persistent manifestations of phallic worship there were also attempts to reconcile phallicism with the Christian doctrine. For example, Redwald, the king of East Anglia from 599 until his death, in c. 627, is said to have had two altars, one for Jesus and one for the devil. There are references to the persistence of phallic worship in the early **penitentials** and the edicts of the church councils. An eighth-century ordinance prescribed a penance of bread and water for three **Lent**s for addressing prayer to a *fascinum* (the Latin word for phallus, actually meaning shaft of light, and the etymological origin of the word "fascination"). Such prayers were forbidden in the ninth century by an edict issued by the council of the Church at Chelmsford, in England. In the eleventh century, Canute the Great (994/995–1035), king of England, Denmark, and Norway and governor of Schleswig and Pomerania, banned all heathen worship. The twelfth-century penitentials included many penances for the magical use of sex.

By the late Middle Ages the practice of phallic worship became so popular that it even had an effect on the clergy, who were occasionally influenced by it, as shown by the numerous church edicts addressing the matter. In the thirteenth century, a Scottish minister was called before his bishop for leading a fertility dance round a phallic figure in the churchyard at Easter. In the fourteenth century, the bishop of Coventry was accused before the pope of homage to the "devil."

Eventually, the Inquisition stepped in to ascribe phallic worship to witchcraft and heresy. However, the practices continued, even if in more obscure ways. The group flagellation that was practiced in Europe from the thirteenth to the sixteenth centuries is considered phallic in substance. And so is the intense eroticism that took over the mysticism of the Renaissance, the almost universal license of nuns and monks, such as illustrated by **Giovanni Boccaccio** in the *Decameron*, and the fantastic "ecstasies" of nuns like St. Catherine of Siena and St. Teresa of Avila.

Medieval society was patriarchal, that is, phallocentric. Some literary texts could also be regarded as manifestations of phallic worship in that they focus on male desire, of which the phallus is the symbol. However, as psychoanalysis would come to articulate later, phallic domination is mainly reinforced through the phallus's absence, through the presence of its referents. Such is *Le Livre de Manières*, written by Etienne de Fouguères between 1173 and 1178, while he was in England, at the court of King Henry II. It is a poem in favor of **marriage** and consequently phallocentric sexuality, and thus against "vile" homosexuality. But, surprisingly, it also manages to represent lesbianism as mutually satisfying, although it does so through phallic symbolism using objects like the fire poker, lance, pointer, handle, fishing rod, pestle, and fulcrum.

Phallic insignia were also used during the Middle Ages. In France phallic amulets were discovered, which are known to have been popular with the medieval Christian pilgrims. They show a phallus or a vulva on one side and a cross motif on the other. *See also* Kailasanath Temple at Ellora; Pagan Europe.

Further Reading: Bullough, Vern L., and James A. Brundage, eds. *Handbook of Medieval Sexuality*. New York: Garland Publishing, 1996; Scott, George Ryley. *Phallic Worship: A History of Sex and Sex Rites in Relation to the Religions of All Races from Antiquity to the Present Day*. Twickenham, UK: Senate, 1996.

Georgia Tres

PHILIP II AUGUSTUS, KING OF FRANCE (1165–1223). Son of Louis VII of France and his third wife, Adela of Champagne, Philip was born in 1165 and inherited the French crown in September 1180. Politically and militarily, he was an exceptional

French monarch, reclaiming lands lost to the English, subduing his fractious nobles, and establishing a strong central bureaucracy. His three **marriage**s, however, were the scandal of medieval elite and church circles, endangering his otherwise sterling relationship with the Vatican as a crusader, church patron, and suppressor of the Albigensian heresy.

Shortly before his father's death in 1180, Philip married Isabelle of Hainault, a descendant of Charlemagne, in an attempt to bind the powerful Hainault-Lorraine-Flanders family to the crown and enhance royal prestige. In 1184, the political winds shifted, making the childless match disadvantageous enough that Philip demanded a **divorce**. Resourcefully, fourteen-year-old Isabelle, dressed as a penitent, won over the church and the people of Paris, who successfully demanded Philip take her back. Isabelle gave birth to Philip's only legitimate son, Louis, in 1184, but died miscarrying twins in 1190.

On August 15, 1193, Philip married Ingeborg of Denmark, daughter of King Waldemar I, but hours after the wedding demanded an annulment on the grounds of **consanguinity**. The personal reasons for this, from Philip finding her unattractive or some *faux pas* to political calculations, are completely unknown. Ingeborg refused to cooperate, insisting that the marriage had been consummated. To pressure her, Philip kept Ingeborg confined for nearly twenty years in a series of isolated castles while she petitioned her family and the pope. Meanwhile, the French Gallican clergy granted Philip his annulment in 1196, allowing him to marry Agnes of Meran, daughter of Berthold IV, by whom he had two children, Philip "Hurpel" and Marie. Furious, Pope Innocent III, after several warnings, laid France under interdict in 1200 for this bigamous marriage. Under this serious threat, Philip stalled, producing Ingeborg and promising to restore her as queen. Only Agnes's death in 1201 allowed Philip to reconcile completely with the church, a deal that included legitimizing his children by Agnes while establishing the pope's ultimate authority over marital matters.

Ingeborg remained imprisoned until 1213, when Philip's foreign policy against John of England, in the campaign leading to the Battle of Bouvines (1214), required the assistance of the Danish fleet. She was received at court as queen, although the marriage was probably never consummated. Philip skillfully used all his children and sisters to make advantageous marital alliances with French nobles and European rivals. Philip died at Mantes on July 14, 1223, leaving the throne to his son, Louis VIII. Ingeborg lived on until 1236 at the convent Corbeil, treated as a dowager queen.

Further Reading: Baldwin, John. *The Government of Philip Augustus: Foundations of French Royal Power in the Middle Ages.* Berkeley: University of California Press, 1986; Bradbury, Jim. *Philip Augustus.* London: Longman, 1998; Duby, Georges. *The Legend of Bouvines: War, Religion, and Culture in the Middle Ages.* Berkeley: University of California Press, 1990.

Margaret Sankey

PHYLLIS LEGEND. See Aristotle and the Phyllis Legend

PHYSIOGNOMICS. Physiognomics is a technique that permits the user to know the psychological features of human beings from their physical traits. Arabic dictionaries and treatises of physiognomics refer to it as "the inference of the interior nature from the visible one." Physiognomics is an inductive process based on thorough observation of a person's appearance: indications of the character are drawn from the shape and color of hair, limbs, and face, and from movements and behavior. The theoretical foundations of this branch of knowledge and its methodological principles were fixed in the Greek world. Greek physiognomics strongly influenced the Arab tradition through the translations of Pseudo-Aristotle and Polemon of Laodicea, considered the most important authorities in this field. Arab scholars numbered physiognomics among the natural sciences and saw it as a branch of physics; being a divinatory technique it was also put side by side with other divinatory sciences as palmistry, examination of footprints, and examination of genealogical lines. Physiognomics in medieval Europe owes much to the Arabs, both for transmitting Greek works (for instance, Polemon's treatise is only extant in Arabic translation) and for original contributions. Arabic physiognomics treatises, like those on **medicine** and astrology, were translated into Latin and studied in European universities. Important Arab scholars, like **Ibn Sina** and **al-Razi**, are numbered among the authorities in this field.

Physiognomics was credited with many practical applications: it was considered useful in social and political contexts to make a careful choice of friends, wives, or courtiers and counselors of the king, or, in the Arab world, to purchase slaves suitable to the functions they had to perform. There is a peculiar branch of physiognomics commonly called "physiognomics of women" strongly connected to the purchase of slaves, particularly those destined to be concubines. It deals almost exclusively with the sexual behavior of women, their sensuality, and their suitability to procreate. For example, a treatise wrongly attributed to Ibn Arabi states that "protruding eyes point to a large vulva; a red mouth points to a great pleasure in having sexual intercourse; laughing frequently points to an intense desire." Along with these elements, sometimes there are observations about feminine anatomy and psychology, in the perspective of **marriage**. Even if mentioned under the label of physiognomics, all this pertains rather to erotology, from which it is drawn. A similar application of physiognomics is also attested in the European tradition, where some chapters in treatises dwell on signs of sensuality of women, as in the *Phisionomia* addressed by Michael Scot to the Emperor Frederick II.

Further Reading: Agrimi, Jole. *Ingeniosa scientia nature. Studi sulla fisiognomica medievale*. Florence: Sismel-Edizioni del Galluzzo, 2002; Förster, Richard, ed. *Scriptores physiognomonici graeci et latini*. 2 vols. Lipsiae: Teubner, 1893; Mourad, Yousef. *La physiognomonie arabe et le Kitab al-firasa de Fakhr al-Din al-Razi*. Paris: Librarie Orientaliste Paul Geuthner, 1939.

Antonella Ghersetti

POLYGAMY.   Polygamy means simultaneous **marriage** to more than one spouse. Of the two variants of polygamy, polygyny and polyandry (several wives/husbands at a time), polygyny was undoubtedly the more frequent. In medieval times, polyandry was practiced in certain regions in **India** and **Tibet**. Strictly speaking, polygyny involved contracting formal marriage with multiple wives, while institutionalized polycoity enabled men to licitly keep concubines, handmaidens, or slave girls as additional sexual partners.

The paramount function of polygamy was providing men with many potential heirs. Multiple wives could do chores and bring wealth to the household. Sexual gratification was another motive. Normally, only the wealthy could afford polygamy; it was a status symbol signaling prosperity and prestige. Generally, medieval potentates kept **harem**s of many wives, concubines, or both, while a large part of the population was monogamous even in cultures allowing polygamy. Occasionally, however, polygamy caused jealousy, rivalry, and conspiracies between the wives and their offspring. Polygamy also permitted rulers to ratify major political alliances by marriage.

The American Inca and Maya rulers were polygamous. In order to ensure the legitimacy of their reign, later Inca rulers took their own sisters as queens (*coya*) and half sisters as secondary wives in addition to concubines.

The Islamic world followed the Qur'anic norm (4. sura, 3. verse) authorizing men to have four wives in addition to concubines; for example, King Mansa Suleyman of Mali had four wives and 100 concubines. The wives had to be treated equally, though: prophet Muhammed gave his wives separate houses, each in turn being able to spend a day and night with him. The Qur'an presents polygamy as a charitable provision for orphans, and several of Muhammed's wives were widows and divorcees. Some men remained monogamous out of respect for their wives or in-laws, especially if their status was higher.

Mongol men had as many wives and concubines as they could support. The number of wives of the Îl-Khân rulers of Persia varied from five (Hülegü) to twelve (Öljeitü). One of these was the chief wife, but normally wives had separate households visited in turn by the husband. In India, polygamy was licit and practiced particularly by kings, members of upper castes, and the wealthy: for example, some medieval kings of the Hindu kingdom of Vijayanagar in southern India had over ten lawful wives in their harem consisting of thousands of women.

Polygamy was permitted in Jewish law and practiced, especially if the wife was childless or the husband's dead brother had left a childless widow (levirate). Medieval **Jews** under Muslim rule tended to be more polygamous, whilst monogamy became obligatory in some European communities. Wives' parents could insist on clauses in marriage contracts forbidding husbands to take other wives or concubines without spousal consent. Breach of contract could entail **divorce**, payment of the wife's marriage portion, or a penalty fee. This interpretation of marriage law was accepted even by some Islamic law schools.

In medieval **China**, polygamy was illegal but emperors formed an exception. Albeit only one wife at a time held the title of empress, the secondary high-status consorts were infrequently called concubines. Some emperors of the northern Song dynasty (960–1127) had over ten simultaneous consorts in addition to over a 100 hierarchically organized concubines. Eighth-century Japanese legislation officially forbade polygamy. Yet it was practiced, albeit the fact that the majority of unions were probably monogamous. The first of the multiple wives was usually considered the principal wife: she was called by a special title, her husband normally resided with her, and her sons had higher official standing.

Monogamy being a major tenet of Christian marriage dogma, polygamy was rejected. The Orthodox church even labeled serial monogamy and **remarriage** at widowhood as polygamy. Yet, when politics demanded, Orthodox princesses were given as additional wives to cement alliances with fourteenth- and fifteenth-century Ottoman rulers and Mongol khans. In western Europe, Merovingian and Carolingian kings, largely unconcerned about ecclesiastical canons, lived in confusing domestic circumstances with many wives and concubines, freely repudiating and divorcing them. The church castigated such practices: marital indissolubility made remarriage during one's spouse's lifetime into polygamy. The church was engaged in an increasingly successful battle to enforce monogamy and indissolubility in royal and aristocratic circles.

All converts to Christianity also had to embrace monogamy. In America, the rigid marriage system of the Spanish conquerors, forced upon Indian communities, caused havoc on traditional marriage and inheritance systems. When the native elites finally abandoned all wives but one, most Indian aristocratic children were bastardized and their mothers repulsed. *See also* Bigamy.

Further Reading: Ebrey, Patricia Buckley. *Women and the Family in Chinese History.* London: Routledge, 2003; Falk, Ze'ev W. *Jewish Matrimonial Law in the Middle Ages.* Scripta Judaica 6. London: Oxford University Press, 1966; McCullough, William H. "Japanese Marriage Institutions in the Heian Period." *Harvard Journal of Asiatic Studies* 27 (1967): 103–67.

Mia Korpiola

POPE JOAN. Pope Joan was a legendary female leader of the Catholic Church, who according to tradition filled the Pontifical See for two years, seven months, and four days during the ninth century. Her occupation of the papal throne is said to have occurred between the reigns of Leo IV (847–855) and Benedict III (855–858). This most famous version of her story comes from the *Chronicon Pontificum et Imperatum* of Martin Polonus, a Dominican monk. However, Martin's record first appeared in 1265—400 years after the reputed reign of Pope Joan.

Some earlier accounts exist, such as Anastasius Bibliothecarius's (d. 886) *Liber Pontificalis*, the Benedictine Marianus Scotus's (1028–1082) *Historiographi*, and the Dominican Jean de Mailly's (d. 1250) *Chronica Universalis Mettensis*. However, only one surviving manuscript copy of Anastasius's work, dating from 1602, contains a reference to Joan. It exists in a footnote with penmanship different from the rest of the text. Marianus is the first to attribute the name "Joanna" to the she-pope, but not all manuscript copies contain his brief report. Jean de Mailly's chronicle achieved little renown and places Pope Joan's reign in 1099 rather than the more conventional time of c. 855.

The most widely circulated story of Joan was the work of Martin Polonus. It states that she was of English stock though born in Mainz, and while a young woman was taken to Athens dressed in men's clothes by her lover. She excelled in all areas of learning and later came to Rome, where she taught the liberal arts still in the guise of a man. Because of her unparalleled intellectual capabilities, she was unanimously elected Pope John VIII. During her reign, however, Joan became pregnant by her unnamed lover, and while in procession from St. Peter's to the Lateran Church, delivered in a side street between St. Clement's Church and the Coliseum. This being discovered, she was punished severely, and both she and the child were killed and buried near the road. This is the reason why subsequent popes refuse to take the lane as a shortcut and turn aside in condemnation of the foul event. Her name was thence removed from pontifical listings. *See also* Transgenderism and Cross-Dressing.

Further Reading: Pardoe, Rosemary, and Darroll Pardoe. *The Female Pope: The Mystery of Pope Joan.* Guildford, Surrey: Thorsons Publishing Group, 1988; Stanford, Peter. *The Legend of Pope Joan: In Search of the Truth.* New York: Henry Holt, 1998.

Hannah Zdansky

PORNOGRAPHY. Pornography originally meant "writing about prostitutes," from the classical Greek roots πορνη and γραφειν. It derived from a Greek term for men who chronicled the well-known "pornai," or skilled prostitutes of ancient Greece. Pornography's content and status have varied substantially throughout history.

Outside Europe during the Middle Ages, pornography was more easily accessible and culturally embedded, almost legitimate, as it was in Greco-Roman antiquity. The advent of Christianity, with its asceticism, affected public perception and reception of pornography and increased its titillation through prohibition. It has even been claimed, from Pietro Aretino's sixteenth-century *I Modi* (The Ways) and Boyer d'Argens'

Thérèse philosophe (1748) on, that very ascetic yet arousing religious practices of the Middle Ages, like flagellation, gave birth to modern pornography.

Under the church's influence, the base sexuality that pornography depicted was generally associated with Satanism, witchcraft, and heresy. From early Christian times secular women (as opposed to nuns and saints) had been depicted as loose, malevolent, or ridiculous. In the heavily patriarchal culture of the Middle Ages, they were also depicted as the devil's easiest victims and most willing allies. However, there was also a middle-of-the-way genre of sex literature, specifically the French fabliaux (the diminutive for "fables"), which have been regarded as an expression of authentic medieval life. They are collections of short tales, usually in verse, about sexual activities. Among the related genres are the *dits*, obscene fables about beasts. They differ from the courtly epic, **romance**, and lyric in that they are less idealized versions of actual practice. The characters are depicted realistically, their language is generally vulgar, and **lust** is displayed with unfettered delight. It takes things in a different direction than the medieval romance like *Tristan and Iseult* does, where desire dissolves in affection. In the fabliaux, desire is consummated not routinely, but in an amusingly bizarre or acrobatic way, which some critics have regarded as a parody of **courtly love**. The humor arises many times from the humiliation of a character. In "Beranger Longbottom" ("Béranger au Lonc Cul") by Garin, a cowardly knight is humiliated by being forced to kiss his wife's crotch. In "The Knight Who Conjured Voices" ("Le Chevalier Qui Fist Parler les Cons") a woman is embarrassed when a knight forces her anus to tell him why her vagina would not answer his question and the anus responds that the vagina had been stuffed with cotton so it could not speak.

There is another possible interpretation of the fabliaux, one which reads their obsessive focus on sexual organs as the opposite of naturalism, as a fragmentation and distortion of identity in agreement with the guilt-centered ideology of Christianity, particularly because these sexual organs (either the penis or the vagina) are frequently detached, **castration** being a recurrent motif. Pornographic elements appear also in *The Canterbury Tales* by **Geoffrey Chaucer** (c. 1340–1400), particularly in *The Reeve's Tale* and *The Merchant's Tale*, which have been ascribed to the fabliau genre.

Further Reading: Berger, Sidney E. "Sex in the Literature of the Middle Ages." In *Sexual Practices and the Medieval Church*, edited by Vern L. Bullough and James A. Brundage. Buffalo, NY: Prometheus Books, 1982; Bullough, Vern L., and James A. Brundage, eds. *Handbook of Medieval Sexuality*. New York: Garland Publishing, 1996.

Georgia Tres

PRITHVIRAJ III (r. 1178–1192). Prithviraj III of the Hindu Rajput Chauhan dynasty, who ruled over the Delhi-Ajmer region of **India**, was immortalized in literature and folk tales for his chivalry, fair dealings, and the romantic legend of his affair with the princess of Kannauj, Sanjukta. Two contemporary rulers became his bitter enemies: the Gaharwar ruler of Kannauj, Jaichandra (r. 1170–1193) and Muhammad of Ghur (r. 1192–1206), the Afghan Muslim ruler over an area between Ghazni and Herat. One of the important sources for Prithviraja III was the epic poem *Prithvirajaraso* written by his court poet Chand Bardai. But the poet mixed facts and fiction. According to the legend recounted by Bardai, Prithviraj and Sanjukta had a love affair much to the dislike of her father Jaichandra. By the custom then prevailing in the royal families, the princess could choose her husband among the persons invited to the court. Jaichandra did not invite Prithviraj to this function known as *Svayamvara* and to humiliate Prithviraj erected a statue of him as a *dwarapala* (gatekeeper) near the gate. Sanjukta garlanded the statue and eloped with Prithviraj, who was hiding nearby. The traditional year for Prithviraj and Sanjukta's elopement is 1175. The scene of the garlanding has been frequently recounted in the ballads and folklore of Rajasthan as well as represented in art. The affair has made Prithviraj a romantic hero in India. But Jaichandra did not forgive him and sided with the Afghan Muhammed of Ghur.

Muhammed of Ghur met the army of Prithviraj in 1191 at the battle of Tarai. After a crushing defeat, Muhammed was captured and brought before Prithviraj, who magnanimously released him. Muhammed defeated Prithviraj in the second battle of Tarai the next year. This marked the end of Rajput control over North India and the beginning of rule from the northwest, which culminated in the Delhi sultanate. If Chand Bardai is to be believed, Prithviraj, an expert archer, killed his enemy in the latter's capital. Many historians doubt this story and believe that Prithviraj remained a vassal to Muhammed.

In addition to the romantic legend of Prithviraj, his legacy also haunts communalists in India and Pakistan. For some Indians, his defeat marks the end of Hindu rule in India. Muslims have depicted Muhammed of Ghur as one of the greatest Muslim warriors, and Pakistan has named its ballistic missile after him.

Further Reading: Chandra, Satish. *Medieval India: From Sultanat to the Mughals*. Delhi: Har Anand, 1998; Hasan, Masudul. *History of Islam*. Vol. 1. Delhi: Adam Publishers, 2002; Mithal, Akhilesh. "The Power of Myth." *Deccan Chronicle* (Visakhapatnam), May 1, 2005.

Patit Paban Mishra

PROSTITUTION. In the twenty-first century, the term "prostitution" means "commercial sex." In the medieval era this term encompassed the sexual activities of all promiscuous women. In the culture of Christian Europe, where **virginity** and chastity were highly esteemed and a woman was defined by her sexual behavior, prostitutes were considered notorious sinners.

The hagiographic tradition reveals through the lives of repentant prostitutes, who became saints, some of the reasons medieval people believed that a woman became a prostitute—pride in her beauty, greed, **lust**, and a love of pleasure. Contemporaries also realized that many women sold sex because of poverty (though this did not excuse their behavior). The scholar Jacques Rossiaud has revealed that in Dijon many women ended up working in the local brothels because as victims of gang **rape** they had lost all hopes of **marriage** or honorable employment. European brothels often had a large number of foreign women working in them, partly because no one else would hire them and partly to protect the wives and daughters of citizens. Other women were forced into prostitution by parents or husbands or masters in order to increase their income.

There were basically two types of prostitutes in medieval Europe—those who worked in brothels and those who did not. The former

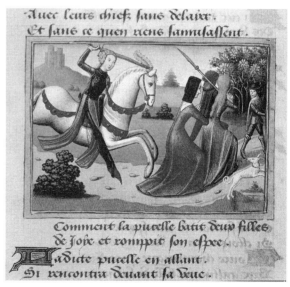

Iluminated page from a 15th century French manuscript of Joan of Arc driving the prostitutes out of the French army. © Bildarchiv Preussischer Kulturbesitz/Art Resource, NY.

could be further subdivided into those who did so regularly and those who did so only occasionally. Jeremy Goldberg has posited that brothels were a southern European phenomenon suited to the honor-and-shame culture of the region. This linked male honor with the sexual purity of female kin while demanding sexual proof of male virility from young men who had no hope of marriage until late in life. Brothels provided these men with a sexual outlet while maintaining the chastity of female relatives. Goldberg further argues that streetwalkers and women who sold sex occasionally to supplement their income were more common in northern Europe, where women had more independence and often married relatively late.

Prostitution was seen as a "necessary evil," sinful while preventing even greater sins, such as **adultery** and **sodomy**. Communities alternated between outlawing it, containing and regulating it, or profiting from it. In the fourteenth and fifteenth centuries, many European cities established municipal brothels (most of which were subsequently closed in the mid-sixteenth century). Brothels, whether municipal or not, were heavily regulated. Often they were confined to a certain area of the town or were built outside the city's walls. Some municipal brothels checked the women periodically for signs of venereal disease or pregnancy. Relations between prostitutes and clients were controlled; price scales were set and only certain men were supposed to use the services of these women. Married men and clergymen were to be turned away. (This rarely occurred, though. The surviving records indicate that clergymen formed a large portion of the clientele.) Byzantine law permitted a wife to **divorce** her husband if he consorted publicly with a prostitute. The relations between the prostitute and the brothel keeper or bawd were also regulated, though often not successfully. They were only to charge the women a set price for meals and for the use of the premises. Where the brothel keeper was not the owner of the establishment, relations between these two were also laid out. In England, women were not to be prevented from leaving the profession.

In many areas of Europe, laws were instituted periodically in an attempt to control prostitutes' attire. This made it easier to distinguish them from the respectable wives and daughters of the community and to prevent the latter from being accosted. The form of regulation varied considerably. Sometimes prostitutes were required to wear an identifying marker when in public (e.g., Parisian prostitutes sported a red knot on their shoulder). Sometimes they were restricted to certain types of clothing. In other cases, it was other women who were only allowed to wear certain clothing.

Streetwalkers conducted their business almost anywhere. Alehouses, churchyards, and bathhouses appear to have been popular places. Street names often revealed the areas where prostitutes were commonly found. Gropecuntelane and Maiden Lane in London are obvious ones. Rose Alley in London refers to the slang phrase for sex with a prostitute, "to pluck a rose."

Prostitutes probably practiced birth control. Contemporaries remarked on the low level of fertility amongst these women. The contraceptive and abortifacient properties of various plants appear to have been common knowledge. As well, vaginal sex was probably avoided, with anal, interfemoral, manual, or oral methods being used.

A prostitute's life was not an easy one. Referred to as "common women," they were treated as the joint property of the men of the community. As a common woman, a prostitute could deny her body to no man (with the exception of **Jews**), and as a result most places did not recognize the rape of a prostitute. A Sicilian law code of 1231 was exceptional in condemning the rape of prostitutes. It was difficult for a woman to leave the profession. While the church encouraged women to give up a life of prostitution, these women often had few other choices. In the later Middle Ages, religious houses for repentant prostitutes were established in some communities. In 1227, Pope Gregory IX established the Order of St. **Mary Magdalene** for former prostitutes.

Some prostitutes left to marry. The feasibility of this option varied. In the early Middle Ages, marriage to a former prostitute was strongly discouraged by the church. However, as time passed, the church became more accepting of such marriages as long as the woman was no longer a practicing prostitute and had performed penance. In medieval Serbia, marriage between an aristocrat and a prostitute was forbidden.

Prostitutes, though considered morally repugnant, played an integral part in medieval communities. They protected the "good" women by bearing the brunt of what was believed to be the uncontrollable male sexual drive. They helped to police community boundaries. David Nirenberg has shown how in Spain they played a key role in maintaining the bounds between Jews, Christians, and Muslims. R. I. Moore has argued that prostitutes were one of several groups whose labeling as "outsiders" allowed the state to establish, exercise, and define itself and its powers. Finally, the possibility of their repentance and salvation as exemplified in the stories of Mary Magdalene provided hope and reassurance for the common Christian.

Further Reading: Goldberg, P.J.P. "Pigs and Prostitutes: Streetwalking in Comparative Perspective." In *Young Medieval Women*, edited by Katherine J. Lewis, Noel James Menuge, and Kim M. Phillips, 172–93. Thrupp, Stroud, UK: Sutton Publishing, 1999; Karras, Ruth Mazo. "Prostitution in Medieval Europe." In *Handbook of Medieval Sexuality*, edited by Vern L. Bullough and James A. Brundage, 243–60. New York: Garland Publishing, 1996; Moore, R. I. *The Formation of a Persecuting Society: Power and Deviance in Western Europe, 950–1250.* Oxford: Basil Blackwell, 1987; Nirenberg, David. *Communities of Violence: The Persecution of Minorities in the Middle Ages.* Princeton, NJ: Princeton University Press, 1996; Otis, Leah Lydia. *Prostitution in Medieval Society: The History of an Urban Institution in Languedoc.* Chicago: University of Chicago Press, 1985; Rossiaud, Jacques. *Medieval Prostitution.* Translated by Lydia G. Cochrane. Oxford: Blackwell, 1988.

Tonya Marie Lambert

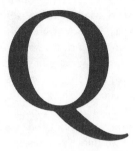

QIYAN.   *See* Singing Girls

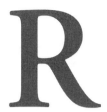

RAPE. The definition of rape in the premodern era was much more restrictive than it is in some countries today. In late medieval England, vaginal penetration by the penis, physical force (as evidenced by cuts and bruises), lack of consent, and cries for help were all necessary components of the crime of rape under secular law. Furthermore, the man and woman could not be married to each other because **marriage** vows were seen as granting consent to all future sexual acts. Finally, if a woman became pregnant, the act was no longer considered to have been rape. According to the ancient physician Galen, both men and women produced "seed." This seed was released through orgasm, which occurred only if the experience had been enjoyable and hence consensual. (Some church **penitentials**, however, followed the Aristotelian notion of conception and recognized that pregnancy could result from rape.) This definition of rape was common to secular law codes throughout much of Europe.

Under **canon law**, physical force, lack of consent, and vaginal penetration were also considered necessary components for an action to be defined as rape. Canon law further required a woman to have been abducted, thereby conflating rape and ravishment, crimes that were governed separately under secular law. In England, however, from the late thirteenth to the late sixteenth century, these two crimes were conflated in secular law, as well.

The law codes of medieval Europe, both ecclesiastical and secular, were based upon two main legal traditions—Roman and Germanic. Most of western Europe had been part of the Roman empire before its collapse in the fifth century, and many of these areas retained numerous Roman legal customs. The earliest known Roman rape law, the *lex Julia de vi publica*, dates from the late first century BCE. This law applied the death penalty to rapists (unless the victim was a slave, in which case monetary compensation was due to her owner). Monetary compensation was the preferred method of dealing with many crimes in the Germanic legal tradition. According to this tradition, each person was assigned a *wergild* or value based upon their social rank. In sixth-century Burgundy, some provision was made for the status of the rapist—a slave, unable to pay the wergild, would be subjected to physical punishment instead, whipping or death.

The crime of rape was variously classified as a property crime, a violent crime, or a sexual crime. Classification was important because it determined both what actions were considered criminal and what penalties were merited. It also identified the legal victim of the crime. As a property crime, it was the father, husband, or nearest male relative of the woman who was wronged. This was the man who brought forward the

RAPE

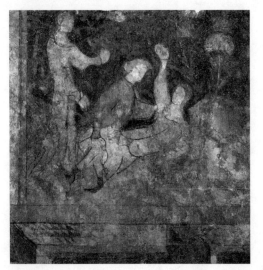

Rape of the mirror, a story from the summer and winter songs of Neidhard von Reuenthal (1200–1250). From a house in downtown Vienna, around 1397. © Erich Lessing/Art Resource, NY.

charge, and he was also the person to whom compensation was paid. As a violent or sexual crime, the person wronged was the woman herself. In fourteenth-century Venice, the rape of a noblewoman (especially if by a lower-class man) was considered a crime against the state and was punished accordingly.

The penalty given to rapists throughout this period varied according to the age, rank, and marital status of the woman (and sometimes of the rapist, as well). The rape of a child was most likely to be punished severely. However, this was not always the case, as children were seen as sexual beings. Numerous men accused of raping a girl claimed (often successfully) to have been seduced by her.

Unsurprisingly, the higher the social status of the woman, the more grievous the crime was considered. Canon law and many secular law codes deemed it impossible to rape a prostitute because, as common women, their bodies were available to all men. The German *Sachsenspiegel* was one of the few law codes that stated it was possible to rape a prostitute and, furthermore, that the penalty for doing so was the same as for the rape of any other woman—death.

The manner in which a woman's marital status affected the perceived heinousness of this crime varied. In fourteenth-century Venice, it was more difficult for a young single woman to prove she had been raped than it was for a married woman, since the former was assumed to be seeking to attract a husband through any means possible. Married women, on the other hand, were not covered by Anglo Saxon rape laws. Rape was considered a property crime, and since the **virginity** of a married woman had already been lost, it could not be stolen from her. In fact, a married woman caught in an act of sexual intercourse with another man, consensual or not, could be charged with **adultery**. Scandinavian law made no distinction between the rape of a virgin and that of a sexually experienced woman.

Most medieval law codes listed death as the penalty for rape. This penalty was seldom applied in practice, though. Nonetheless, the Scandinavian Konungsbok and the sixth-century law code of the Salian Franks granted immunity to anyone who killed a rapist. In thirteenth-century Normandy and England, as well as in Carolingian France, **castration** (rather than death) was the penalty for rape.

The rapist's life was spared if the woman agreed to marry him. In the Middle Ages, this was often the only way a woman could restore her honor and secure her future. However, such a practice was easily abused. Couples would stage an abduction and "rape" to force unwilling parents or guardians to let them marry. These false rapes led to actual assaults being viewed with more skepticism. Such rapes became so numerous in England that in 1382 a law was implemented barring women involved in these deceptions from inheriting. In Sicily, in 1231, marriage between a woman and her rapist was prohibited, while the *Sachsenspiegel* bastardized the children of such a union. It was not always possible for a woman to marry her rapist. If the rapist was already married, he might be required to provide the woman with a dowry as in thirteenth-century Ceneda and Mantua. *See also* Domestic Violence.

Further Reading: Brundage, James A. "Rape and Seduction in the Medieval Canon Law." In *Sexual Practices & the Medieval Church*, edited by Vern L. Bullough and James A. Brundage, 141–48. Buffalo, NY: Prometheus Books, 1982; Orr, Patricia. "Men's Theory and Women's Reality: Rape Prosecutions in the English Royal Courts of Justice, 1194–1222." In *The Rusted Hauberk: Feudal Ideals of Order and Their Decline*, edited by Liam O. Purdon and Cindy L. Vitto, 121–59. Gainesville: University Press of Florida, 1994; Ruggiero, Guido. "Sexual Criminality in the Early Renaissance: Venice, 1338–1358." *Journal of Social History* 8 (1975): 18–37; Winer, Rebecca Lynn. "Defining Rape in Medieval Perpignan: Women Plaintiffs before the Law." *Viator: Medieval and Renaissance Studies* 31 (2000): 165–83.

Tonya Marie Lambert

RAZI, ABU BAKR MUHAMMAD IBN ZAKARIYA AL- (Rhazes) (865–925).

Abu Bakr Muhammad ibn Zakariya al-Razi, known in the Latin West as Rhazes or Rasis, was an early Islamic philosopher-physician. Al-Razi was a Persian born in Rayy near Teheran. His studies included ancient Greek philosophy and **medicine**, with which he had several disagreements, as well as many other subjects. Al-Razi traveled widely throughout the eastern part of the Islamic empire, where his medical knowledge gave him easy entry into the courts of many rulers. His medical success attracted many students to him. Some of his writings sought to address his students' instructional needs.

Al-Razi often conducted empirical research. He experimented on animals to test medical ideas. He was the first to use alcohol (*al-kuhl*) for medical purposes. He used opium as an anesthetic, plaster of Paris for casts, and animal guts for sutures. He promoted sound diet as an aid to healing and used psychological techniques to promote health. For a time al-Razi served as the chief physician at the hospital in Rayy. Later he served as chief physician at a hospital in Baghdad. He published the first known description of smallpox as distinguished from measles in a work known as *Liber de pestilentia* (*A Treatise on Smallpox and Measles*).

Al-Razi wrote over 200 books. His major contribution to medicine, which was produced from notes made throughout his professional life, was an encyclopedic twenty-volume work titled *Kitab al-Hawi fi al-tibb* (*Continens Rhazes, The Comprehensive Book on Medicine*).

Al-Razi's ten-volume *Kitab al-Mansoori* (*Liber Almansoris*) included a detailed discussion of human anatomy in volume nine, including the nervous system and the reproductive system. The disorders he discussed included diabetes and its harmful impact on the sexual organs, as well as other sexual disorders. In the *Khulasai-al Tajarib* (*Quintessence of Experience*) al-Razi also described male and female sexual organs in considerable detail, discussing the mechanism of conception and difficulties in conceiving. In *Aghrabadin* (*Therapeutics*) al-Razi described **impotence** and *glactorrhea*—lactation without pregnancy—as well as treatments for these conditions. In *About the Menstrual Cycle* he described menstrual irregularities, including symptoms presented as *amenorrhea* (absent periods), *dysmenorrhea* (menstrual cramps), or vaginal bleeding. Al-Razi discussed the sex drive (*libido*) and sexual dysfunctions in his book *Kitab al-Bah*. He developed a therapeutic outline that prescribed both male and female **aphrodisiacs**. His discussion of *ubnah* in his book *Hidden Illness* (*ad-da' of-khafi*) deals not only with passive male homosexuality but also with intersexual conditions. Al-Razi died at Rayy in 925.

Further Reading: Ranking, G.S.A. *The Life and Works of Rhazes. Proceedings of the Seventeenth International Congress of Medicine*, London, 1913, pp. 237–68; Taylor, Julius

Heyward. *Rhazes: The Greatest of the Arabians*. Charlotte, NC: Southern Medicine and Surgery, 1934.

Andrew J. Waskey

REMARRIAGE. Throughout the Middle Ages, remarriage was discouraged and held in disdain under most circumstances, although its practice was not at all rare. Upon the rise of Christianity, **marriage** came to be regarded as an indissoluble bond to be broken only upon the death of a spouse. Throughout the period, legislators and theologians debated the exceptional circumstances that permitted **divorce**, marriage annulment, or both; in these directives lay the framework for conditions guiding remarriage. In Byzantine and Eastern cultures, remarriage was similarly ill esteemed and generally discouraged.

In the West, partly due to the influence of Gnosticism and asceticism on Christian theology, a second marriage for widows and widowers was considered sinful and unfortunate, although forgiven based on the weakness of the flesh. Saint **Jerome** (c. 340–420) and St. **Augustine** (354–386) both commanded that even adulterous marriages were indissoluble; the partners could separate but neither could remarry.

A series of legislative and ecclesiastical rulings in the early Middle Ages marked a trend toward tighter restrictions on remarriage after divorce along with an observable double standard in favor of men. By the time the early Christian emperors legalized the practice of divorce in the fourth century, Catholic teaching on the indissolubility of marriage had already infiltrated civil legislation through all of **Catholic Europe**. Constantine allowed women to dismiss their husbands if they had committed homicide, sorcery, or tomb desecration, whereas he allowed husbands a divorce if their wives were guilty of **adultery**, had acted as procuresses, or were proved to be sorceresses. The Council of Elvira (c. 306) ruled that a divorced woman who had accused a husband guilty of adultery and had remarried be excommunicated until her first husband died. The Council of Arles (314) advised against the remarriage of a man who had repudiated his adulterous wife. The Council of Carthage of 407 forbade remarriage because of adultery by either mate. Honorius and Theodosius (c. 400) added that a woman who had succeeded in obtaining a divorce could remarry only after five years while she could not remarry at all for a less serious crime. The husband could remarry immediately if he had repudiated her for a serious crime; he was to wait for two years if he had divorced based on a defect in her character.

Eventually, the affluent found a way to get around these strict rulings through the costly and intricate process of marriage annulment by the pope. An annulment, in the Catholic Church, remains to this day a declaration by an ecclesiastical tribunal that the marriage in question is invalid in the true sense of the word. There are many different reasons for annulment, such as immaturity or lack of true marital commitment. Once a marriage was annulled, the individuals involved could marry freely. Second marriages were frowned upon while third marriages were forbidden by Pope Leo VI (c. 928).

With the rise of the feudal system in ninth-century Europe, particular circumstances fell into place that discouraged widowed women from remarrying. The unmarried widow (*femme sole*) often chose not to remarry in order to enjoy financial independence and social status that she could otherwise never obtain. In this context, for example, the widow might rise to a powerful position and become a guild member, running the family business. An ambitious businessman might seek out a landowning widow of the noble class for control of her assets. Under English Common Law, for example, the rights and duties of the female landowner were equal to the man's. During the later Middle Ages, however, because of concern over carrying on the family line, the widow's right to inherit family property was restricted in favor of male heirs. A widow was bound to relinquish her rights as legal guardian of her own children to her overlord, who would take charge of the children's property and marriage plans.

In the Arab world, marriage was considered virtuous. Although divorce did not require burdensome legal proceedings, it was very rare and operated according to double standards. Women could only obtain a divorce if their marriage contract said they had this right. Once divorced, either person could remarry freely. In the Byzantine tradition, a woman could divorce her husband only if he was impotent for three years after the wedding, if he tried to kill her, or if he were a leper. Neither the husband's adultery nor his madness was seen as sufficient cause for divorce. A woman, on the other hand, could be divorced for adultery, leprosy, or a plot against her husband's life. When the husband of a Byzantine family died, the wife acquired legal possession and control of all family property; she gained full responsibility for supporting her children and arranging their marriages. If the wife remarried, however, she retained control only of her dowry and marriage gift. *See also* Bigamy.

Further Reading: Herlihy, David. *Medieval Households.* Cambridge, MA: Harvard University Press, 1985; Murstein, Bernard I. *Love, Sex and Marriage through the Ages.* New York: Springer Publishing, 1974; Stuard, Susan Mosher, ed. *Women in Medieval Society.* Philadelphia: University of Pennsylvania Press, 1976.

Sinda K. Vanderpool

RHAZES. *See* al-Razi, Abu Bakr Muhammad ibn Zakariya

ROMAN LAW. Roman law, a complex set of rules and principles, was constituted by different sources, including laws, senatorial consults, imperial decrees, jurisprudence, and jurists' opinions. Although of ancient origin, Roman law was not collected and compiled until the times of Emperor Justinian, who between 530 and 535 unified all rules into a single collection, later known as the *Corpus Iuris Civilis*. This *Corpus* was composed of the *Codex* (a collection of *leges* or imperial constitutions, divided into twelve books), the *Digestum* or *Pandectas* (the compilation of the opinions of previous *iurisprudentes* in fifty books, which constitutes the largest part of the *Corpus*), the *Institutes* (an elementary handbook of law for teaching), and the *Novellae* (which included the new imperial constitutions from Justinian).

This codification was essential in the development of late Roman law, since it reconstructed legal aspects of classical Rome, as well as created the Byzantine context in which passages were gathered and new statutes were added to the laws. Besides, the *Corpus Iuris Civilis* was the source of teachings on Roman law in the eleventh century, when it was rediscovered, and set the grounds for the growth of both church or **canon law** and the civil law of most continental European countries. In medieval times, the development of Christendom and the identification of a cultural Roman heritage stood as the two pillars for the progressive acknowledgment of the existence of a common legal system, the *ius commune*. Roman law, in this form, survived for nine hundred years after Justinian, all over the continent. In **Byzantium**, by the end of the ninth century, Basilius the Macedonian had ordered the creation of a Greek abridged version of the *Corpus*, which was published as the *Basilics* by his son and which managed to replace Justinian's work in the coming centuries. In the West, where barbarians overthrew the Roman empire in 476, several Roman law principles already extended throughout the region. After Justinian regained power over Italy, in 554, he promulgated the constitution *pro petitione Virgilii*, where he imposed the *Corpus* as obligatory law in the whole territory.

By the end of the seventh century, different legal systems emerged in the kingdoms of Europe. Whereas Germanic law drew upon Roman law to a great extent, the northern Italian communes soon started to issue their own statutes, based on the *ius commune* and local customary principles. The remains of Roman law during this transitional period are scarce, limited to some isolated commentaries.

The rediscovery of a manuscript from the *Corpus* at the Library of Pisa in 1094 transformed the University of Bologna with a new interest in Romanist studies. Promoted by generations of jurists, Roman law was permanently reinterpreted and changed by the constant activity of interpreters and legal commentators. Legal teachers, the "glossators," wrote copious *glosses* to clarify the meaning of different passages in the *Corpus*. As a result of this exegetic method and some difficulties in the textual transmission of the *Digest*, a medieval *Corpus iuris civilis*, known as the *Littera Bononensis*, was shaped differently from Justinian's compilation. In this rearrangement, the *Digest* was divided into three parts (*Digestum vetus, Infortiatum*, and *Digestum Novum*), the *Codex* split into two sections, and the *Novellae* reordered.

Some sexual regulations coming from the Roman historical context were reshaped by the *ius commune*. **Marriage**, as regulated by classical Roman law, found its basis on *affectio maritalis*, conceived as a continuing consent required for the existence of the bond. This concept continued in the postclassical period, but the union required only initial, rather than continuing, consent. As for ways of ending the affiliation, **divorce** was allowed by Roman legislation. Women were not allowed to initiate the procedure, which was left to the husband. The Christian doctrine that strongly influenced the previous body of Roman law introduced several modifications in accordance to the new religious values. Sex was classified following three models: the natural function of sex and its reproductive aim; the idea that sex was a contaminating activity and, therefore, a cause of impurity and shame; and, finally, that sexual relations were a demonstration of marital affection. Consequently, in medieval times, both **prostitution** and homosexuality were repudiated as deviations from the normal and natural purposes of sex. See also *Collatio Legum Mosaicarum et Romanarum*.

Further Reading: Brundage, James A. *Law, Sex, and Christian Society in Medieval Europe.* Chicago: University of Chicago Press, 1987; Brynteson, William E. "Roman Law and Legislation in the Middle Ages." *Speculum* 41 (1996): 420–37; Müller, Wolfgang P. "The Recovery of Justinian's *Digest* in the Middle Ages." *Bulletin of Medieval Canon Law* 20 (1990): 1–29; Pennington, Kenneth. "Medieval Law." In *Medieval Studies: An Introduction*, edited by J. M. Powell, 333–52. Syracuse, NY: Syracuse University Press, 1992.

Emiliano J. Buis and Silvana A. Gaeta

ROMANCE. The medieval romance depicts two primary activities, adventure and the pursuit of love. Often the two threads are interconnected, as a lady's wishes or the lover's desire for her may lead the hero, typically a knight, to embark upon often dangerous enterprises. The heroine of the romance is usually highborn, cultured, and, of course, beautiful. Her love, actual or sought, ennobles the knight who aspires to it. The lover is typically courageous and skilled in battle, but other qualities—courtesy, good manners, accomplishments in the arts, and fidelity—are often as important.

Romances began to appear in the twelfth century in France, where the first great creator of romances, Chrétien de Troyes, flourished between 1155 and 1185. One of his contributions to the genre was wedding material from the **Arthurian legend** to **courtly**

love conventions. In *Lancelot*, the suitor is Lancelot himself, who pursues Queen Guinevere. In *Erec* and *Yvain*, Chrétien has his two heroes achieve **marriage** with the women they love, Enid and Laudine, respectively. However, the knights' inability to understand how to function in love leads to many difficulties before they reclaim their wives. One of the more modern-seeming aspects of Chrétien's romances is their sustained effort to explore the nature of love.

A number of French romances involve **Tristan**, perhaps the finest of which is an unfinished poem by a person about whom nothing is known except his name, Thomas of Britain, and the probable date of composition, around 1170–1180. After drinking a love potion, Tristan and Isolde are bound permanently in love. For a time, they live together in perfect happiness in a grotto far from court. Banished by a jealous king and wounded mortally in battle, Tristan waits for Isolde, who alone can cure him. Hearing a false report that she is not coming to him, he dies; Isolde arrives soon after and expires on her lover's body.

Stories of antiquity also supply the material for medieval romances. Benoót de Ste-Maure's *Roman de Troie*, written about 1165, transplants the Trojan War into a courtly love framework. Love affairs such as Achilles's relationships with Polyxena and Penthesilea receive considerable attention. Benoót also added the story of Troilus and Briseida, with the Trojan Troilus dying heartbroken when Briseida forsakes him for the Greek Diomedes. The tragic love story prompted many retellings, including **Giovanni Boccaccio**'s *Il Filostrato*, **Geoffrey Chaucer**'s *Troilus and Criseyde*, and Shakespeare's *Troilus and Cressida*. Other stories of antiquity, such as Virgil's *Aeneid* and the life of Alexander the Great, also yielded romances with the same fusion of love and martial conflicts.

Among the great German romances are Wolfram von Eschenbach's *Parzival* and Gottfried von Strassburg's *Tristan*, both from the early thirteenth century. In Wolfram's romance, the love between Parzival and Condwiramurs is marked by purity and fidelity. Gottfried's depiction of love is more complex. The relationship between Tristan and Isolde is both sensual and spiritual. The grotto in which the lovers find their sequestered happiness is described allegorically, each part conveying a particular dimension of love and a crystal bed in the center, the grotto as a whole representing the human heart in love.

The romance flowered later in England. Perhaps the single greatest English romance is the anonymous *Sir Gawain and the Green Knight*. The highly moral fourteenth-century poem features Sir Gawain in two relationships: with a seductress and the Virgin Mary. At Sir Bercilak's castle, the lord's wife seemingly attempts to seduce Gawain over three days while her husband is out hunting. Gawain, though, balances courtesy toward his host's wife and devotion to Mary. He resists the lady's advances but then yields to her offer of a green girdle that will protect him in battle against the Green Knight. In addition to hiding the gift from Bercilak, when an exchange-of-winnings agreement calls for them to give each other whatever they have received, Gawain fails to put his faith in Mary and God to protect him. Nonetheless, the failing is described as a small one, and Gawain returns home forgiven if also humbled by his temporary lack of faith.

In the fifteenth century, Sir Thomas Malory drew a wide range of Arthurian stories together in a lengthy prose account known as *Morte d'Arthur*. The work would forever formalize the fall of Camelot as caused by the adulterous relationship between Lancelot and Guinevere. After so many accounts of love in the medieval romances, the Middle Ages yielded to the modern age with this final lesson regarding love: how a world can truly be lost by loving badly.

Further Reading: Cooper, Helen. *The English Romance in Time.* New York: Oxford University Press, 2004; Jackson, W.T.H. *Medieval Literature: A History and a Guide.* New York: Collier Books, 1967; Krueger, Roberta, ed. *The Cambridge Companion to Medieval Romance.* New York: Cambridge University Press, 2000.

Edward J. Rielly

ROMANCE OF THE ROSE. The *Romance of the Rose* (*Roman de la rose*) is an allegorical poem about a man who falls asleep and dreams of falling in love with a woman and seeking, through various difficulties, to attain her. Composed by two authors (with an initial conclusion written by still another poet), the poem was highly influential throughout the Middle Ages.

Guillaume de Lorris began the *Romance of the Rose* around 1237 and composed 4058 lines before dying. An allegorical dream vision, Guillaume's incomplete portion depicts the Lover falling in love with a woman (the Rose) that he has seen in a garden. He is instructed by the God of Love but finds winning the Rose fraught with challenges, which are represented as personified abstractions. Resistance forces him away from the Rose, Dame Reason tries to dissuade him from his pursuit, and Warm Welcome leads him to the Rose but refuses to permit a kiss through fear of Chastity. Warm Welcome finally grants the kiss, but Bad Mouth informs Jealousy, who orders a new wall built around the Rose.

After Guillaume's death, possibly a friend of the poet wrote a brief conclusion in which Pity and her friends bring the Rose to the Lover, and the two spend the night in lovemaking. The next morning, they escort the Rose back into the garden, with Beauty assuring the Lover that so long as he serves Beauty well he will be master of the Rose.

Not long after Guillaume's death, Jean de Meun, who also translated **Peter Abelard**'s *Historia calamitatum* and the letters of Abelard and Heloise, continued *Romance of the Rose*, extending the poem to 21,780 lines. Less in the **courtly love** tradition than Guillaume and more grounded in scholastic learning, Jean adopts a comprehensive approach to examining the subject of love. He especially relates human love to the divine plan, which includes procreation.

Jean also introduces satire into the *Romance*. He presents **marriage** as a state filled with misfortune and depicts women as deceitful. Yet, through an account of the Jealous Husband, he argues for equality between husband and wife in order for love to endure. Nor are men exempt from criticism. Nature laments men's sexual sins, especially their rejection of procreative love. Forced abstinence is especially criticized.

A battle led by Venus against the opponents of love precedes the Lover's victory. The Lover finally reaches the rosebush and plucks the Rose. The act is described in terms of sexual union and the loss of **virginity**. The Lover breaks a small bit of skin to gain his goal. As he dislodges the rose, he spills some seed. The Rose afterward expands, suggesting pregnancy. After reflecting on his triumph, the Lover awakens, and the poem abruptly ends, to be widely read, copied,

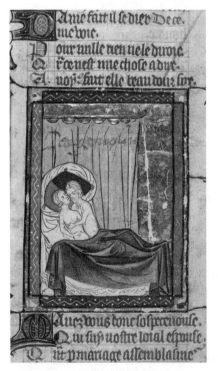

A couple in bed making love. From a French text discussing marriage, from *Le Roman de la Rose* (The Romance of the Rose), by Jean de Meun and Guillaume de Lorris, ca. 1300. © HIP/Art Resource, NY.

translated, attacked, and defended throughout the Middle Ages. *See also* Misogyny in Latin Christendom; Romance.

Further Reading: Arden, Heather M. *The Romance of the Rose.* Boston: Twayne, 1987; Lewis, C. S. *The Allegory of Love.* 1936. Reprint, New York: Oxford University Press, 1985.

Edward J. Rielly

RUIZ, JUAN. Written by a largely unknown author called Juan Ruiz, the *Libro de buen amor*, a fourteenth-century collection of verses in a broad spectrum of styles and with a variety of subjects, is regarded as one of the most important books in Spanish literature. It includes, among other things, religious and lyric poetry, popular fables and exempla, anticlerical poetry and religious parodies, pastoral verses and popular cantigas, all linked together by a pseudo-autobiographical frame in which a first-person narrator describes his amatory life. The book contains approximately 7,000 verses, most of them in *cuaderna via*, monorhymed quatrains of Alexandrine verses of fourteen syllables.

Little is known about the author. The only information is contained in the text, in which he introduces himself as Juan Ruiz, archpriest from Hita. The date of the book is also unclear. Three manuscripts have been found: Salamanca (S), Toledo (T), and Gayoso (G), and they indicate different dates for the book's composition. While in G and T, Ruiz writes that he finished the book in 1330; in S, he dates the year of its completion as 1343. Due to this discrepancy, some scholars have concluded that the *Libro de buen amor* was edited in two different versions.

There is also debate concerning the sources of the book. While some scholars believe the book is based on a Western tradition, and was specially influenced by Ovid, the anonymous comedy *Pamphilus*, and popular medieval and Greek fables and exempla, others believe that there are traces of Arabic and Hebraic influences in the book, such as *The Dove's Neck Ring* by **Ibn Hazm**, and the *Libro de las delicias* by Ibn Sabarra.

The *Libro de buen amor* is a series of fourteen love episodes of uneven length intertwined with poems, fables, and examples to illustrate them. The episodes in almost all cases follow the same pattern: the narrator unsuccessfully tries to conquer women with the help of a go-between. A partial listing of the women the go-between tries to furnish includes some widows, a Muslim woman, four peasants, and a nun. During these episodes, the moral position of the narrator shifts. He shows an ambivalent moral stand regarding sins of the flesh; he can be either a sybaritic sinner or a pious ascetic. It is also interesting to note the wide range of sins of the flesh exhibited throughout the collection: **concubinage**, acts of **rape**, sexual relations without **marriage**, and love between persons under religious vows.

The most controversial issues regarding this book are the intentions of the author. In the prologue, Juan Ruiz expresses the purpose of teaching, by example, the importance of refraining from committing a sin of the flesh. However, the *Libro de buen amor* cannot be considered just an example of the religious didactic literature of the time. The final lines of his prologue make it a more complex and ambiguous piece of art, presenting the book as a guide to the art of seduction. His ambivalent moral stand regarding carnal acts; the presentation of sexual and religious parodies and the different connotations of the term *buen amor* along the book, at some times related to God, at others to carnal love, add to the ambiguous character of the *Libro de buen amor*.

Further Reading: Gybbon-Monypenny, G. B., ed. *Libro de Buen Amor Studies.* London: Tamesis, 1970; Ruiz, Juan. *Libro de buen amor.* Madrid: Cátedra, 1992.

Claudia M. Mejía

RUMI, JALALUDDIN (1207–1273). Maualana Jalaluddin Rumi was a notable Sufi saint and Persian poet. Born in Wakhsh in the Balkh region on September 30, 1207, he migrated to Iconium (present-day Konya), Turkey, in the wake of a Mongol invasion, along with his father Bahaduddin Valad, a reputed theologian, and his mother Mumine Khatun. Rumi married Gohar Khatun when he was eighteen. In his forties, after Gohar's death, he married a widow named Kira Khatum of Christian background. At twenty-four, he succeeded his father in the *madrassa* (religious school) as a teacher and became an accomplished scholar. Rumi became a *murid* (disciple) of Sufi-mystic Shams ad-Din Tabrizi (d. 1247), the wandering *dervish* who greatly influenced him. Rumi founded the Mawlawiyya (Mevlevi) Sufi order, which emphasized union with God through dancing and *sama* (musical gatherings). By rhythmically reciting "Allah-Al-lah, Al-lah," accompanied by music from drums, cymbals, and flutes, dancers attained ecstasy.

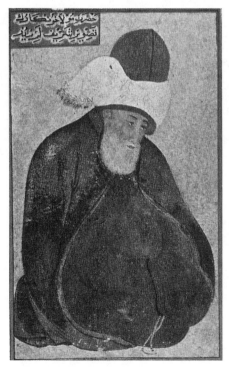

A Persian manuscript illumination of the Persian poet Jalaludin Rumi. © The Granger Collection, New York.

Rumi penned 33,135 lines of intense love poems in *The Diwan of Sams of Tabriz* in forms like **ghazal**s and rubaiyats. *The Diwan* was composed after Rumi's bereavement of his master, Shams ad-Din Tabrizi. Rumi had searched for his own identity and wrote the songs of love, desire, and loneliness. For him, love was infinite and identified with truth. The "wine of love" had created the poet himself. He wrote that one should die in love if he wanted to remain alive. Conforming to Sufi thinking, Rumi emphasized *wahdat al-wujud* (unity of being) and longing for union with God. Rumi used words like wine, dance, and gambling as metaphors.

Rumi's poetry is in the mystical tradition of Persian literature. *Masnavi-i-Ma'anavi* (the epic of spirituality), comprising 20,000 couplets in six volumes, is Rumi's *magnum opus*. Referred to as the "Quran in Pahlavi," it took about thirty years to complete. Throughout his life, Rumi recited these verses before his *murids*, preaching Sufi spiritual life and practice. The *Masnavi* was didactic. The anecdotes and lyrical poetry from various sources like the Qur'an and oral traditions had a moral purpose. The singing of *Masnavi* was an art in itself in the *sama*, which inculcated among the participants spiritual ecstasy and longing for merging with divinity. He also wrote a metaphysical discourse for his *murids*, the *Fibi ma fibi*.

Rumi died on December 17, 1273, in Konya, and his tomb became a pilgrimage center. Transcending national and religious borders, his influence has spread throughout the world. *See also* Sufism.

Further Reading: Helminski, E. Kabir, ed. *The Rumi Collection: An Anthology of Translations of Mevlana Jalaluddin Rumi*. Boston: Shambhala Publications, 2000; Schimmel, Annemarie. *I Am Wind, You Are Fire: The Life and Work of Rumi*. Boston: Shambhala Publications, 1992; Schimmel, Annemarie. *Look! This Is Love: Poems of Rumi*. Boston: Shambhala Publications, 1991; Wilson, Peter Lambon, and Nasrollah Pourjavady, eds. *Drunken Universe: An Anthology of Persian Sufi Poetry*. Grand Rapids, MI: Phanes Press, 1987; Wines, Leslie. *Rumi, a Spiritual Biography*. New York: Crossroad Publishing Company, 2000.

Patit Paban Mishra

S

SAGA LITERATURE. Related to the verb *segja*, meaning "to say," or "to tell," the Old Norse sagas are narrative accounts of events that occurred over a great stretch of time, from the imagined past of gods and legendary kings, through the so-called Viking Age (eighth to eleventh centuries), and into the times of the saga authors themselves (twelfth to fifteenth centuries). These writers were, with few exceptions, Icelanders working from oral traditions and older written material. Despite their literary mode of presentation, the sagas routinely feature historically attested persons, places (from North America to Constantinople), and events. Cited for their portrayal of violence within the contexts of large-scale political conflict as well as interfamilial, and even interpersonal, feuding, the sagas often treat matters of love, sex, and **marriage** as incidental but essential aspects of a society built upon kin relationships.

Several subgenres of saga literature are nevertheless noteworthy for their attention to, and expression of, love and sex as major themes, a characteristic perhaps traceable to royal prerogative. In Norway, King Hakon Hakonarson (r. 1217–1263) sought to replicate the great continental European cultural centers at his court. His initiatives resulted in the introduction of courtly literature, especially **romance**s on the French model, in Norway. Under King Hakon, for example, a Norse translation of the **Tristan** and Isolde story was completed by one "Brother Robert" as *Tristram's Saga* in 1226. *Tristram's Saga* and other translations like it became popular in Norway and then Iceland and also inspired the creation of original "sagas of chivalry" based on continental conventions.

The effects of these romances, indebted in turn to European conceptions of **courtly love**, were also felt elsewhere in saga literature. In the "legendary sagas" (Icelandic *fornaldarsögur*, literally "sagas of ancient times"), the deeds of figures like Sigurd the Dragon-Slayer or Arrow-Odd, respective heroes of *The Saga of the Volsungs* and *Arrow-Odd's Saga*, include passionate and fantastical sexual relationships. The influence of continental trends on the sagas can also be seen among the crowning achievements of Old Norse literature, the "sagas of Icelanders," also commonly known as "family sagas," which tend to focus on relations within or among families in Iceland from the period of the island's settlement in the late ninth century through the first several decades following Iceland's conversion to Christianity in 1000. In *The Saga of the People of Laxardal*, for example, the well-respected Olaf the Peacock and the inimitable Gudrun Osvifs's daughter, who divorces one of her four husbands, are praised in superlative terms for their physical beauty, much like the heroes and heroines of courtly romances. Likewise, the author of *Grettir's Saga* borrows material directly from the Tristan story.

Less dependent on foreign influences are a small number of sagas that form a subset of the sagas of Icelanders, the so-called skalds' sagas, named for the skalds or poets who are the protagonists of these stories. The texts in this group, such as *The Saga of Gunnlaug Serpent-Tongue*, share a number of common features, most notably the inability of their eponymous heroes to consummate relationships with their beloveds, and the consequent success of their rivals where they have failed.

In short, the presentation of love and sex within these narrative histories is as various as the sagas themselves, ranging from simple and heartfelt affection to the destructiveness of irrepressible passion.

Further Reading: Hreinsson, Víɛar, ed. *The Complete Sagas of Icelanders Including 49 Tales*. 5 vols. Reykjavík, Iceland: Leifur Eiríksson Publishing, 1997; Kristjánsson, Jónas. *Eddas and Sagas: Iceland's Medieval Literature*. Translated by Peter Foote. Reykjavík, Iceland: Hiɛ íslenska bókmenntafélag, 1997.

John T. Sebastian

SAKTHISM. *Sakthism* is a religion based on praxis, whose origin can be traced to the Tantric philosophy that developed in ancient **India**. The term *Sakthism* was derived from the word "Shakti," which literally translates as "power" in both its latent and manifest forms. The *Devi Shakti* is considered the "power" aspect of the omnipotent supreme spirit. The scriptures named *Tantra Shastra* constitute the various doctrinal aspects as well as ritual practices of Sakthism. It is believed that through following the specifications of this holy book, spiritual truth can be realized.

Sakthism is signified by the conception of the goddess Shakti. This goddess is believed to be the creative source behind the entire universe and the power that drives it further. In fact, all that is manifest in the world is determined to have Shakti as its essential source. The universe is supposed to have two aspects—rational and empirical. In other words, the world consists of mind and matter. In her most refined aspect, Goddess Shakti becomes pure spirit or pure consciousness, and is called Chit-Shakti. At the same time, we know her nature only through the world of sensation, that is, our senses.

The follower of Sakthism or the worshipper of Goddess Shakti is called Shakta. *Tantra Shastras* describe Shakta beliefs and ideas. Shakti is the ultimate reality, the only truth. The principal doctrine of Sakthism—about the nature and relevance of the all-powerful Goddess Shakti—is described in immaculate detail, along with the cosmogony and the practical tenets of this radical philosophy.

Every system of Indian philosophical thought has its own worldview on the genesis, functioning, and evolution of the universe. One can even say that the foundational tenets of each philosophy derive from these very conceptions about life and the universe. For Sakthism, the goddess Shakti is that source, out of which the universe as mind and matter has evolved. She is, in other words, the Great Mother of the Universe. A point called Bindu, which is mere Spirit, represents her in her most concentrated form.

Shakta, that is, the worshipper of Goddess Shakti, is also oblivious of the caste system and its varied distinctions that play determining roles in the social relations in India. The Brahma Shakta would worship this goddess of power standing in line with the Shudra outcast, or the Pariah. Such a panhuman attitude is quite uncommon to Indian structures of social and religious thought, and hence it is contemplated that Sakthism might have drawn on traditions outside India, probably **China** or **Tibet**. The unique features of this philosophy, which allows the Shakta to eat meat as well as drink wine, apparently non-Indian, is also thus explained. Active inclusion of women in the

Shakti worship is another striking feature of this system of thought since women have usually been kept away from all social ceremonies in India. The Shakta treats women as equal, if not more. The Panchatattva Ritual, the most important ritual of Sakthism, is still alive in some parts of Bengal. The name "Panchatattva" is derived from the words "Pancha" (five) and "Tattva" (elements). It goes on to explain the five constituents of this ritual, that is, wine, meat, fish, parched corn, and sexual union. As part of the ritual, men and women meet as equal partners and sit together in a circle called Chakra. For a Shakta, a woman sitting by one's side is the highest form of the Goddess Shakti. It is believed that this union, as per the Maithuna rites, is symbolic of the bliss of the great union of Shiva and Shakti. So, sexual union is not for physical satisfaction but is a ritual to realize the highest union of the individual with the Goddess, the Cosmic-Whole.

Further Reading: Cotterell, Arthur. *A Dictionary of World Mythology*. New York: G. P. Putman's Sons, 1980; Dev, Usha. *The Concept of Sakti in the Puranas*. New Delhi: Nag Publishers, 1987; Jordan, Michael. *Encyclopedia of Gods*. New York: Facts on File, 1993; Rice, Edward. *Eastern Definitions: A Short Encyclopedia of Religions of the Orient*. New York: Doubleday, 1978; Walker, Barbara G. *The Woman's Encyclopedia of Myths and Secrets*. New York: HarperCollins, 1983.

Jitendra Uttam

SCHOLASTIC PHILOSOPHY. Scholastic philosophy, which arose in medieval universities, deepened and continued the patristic thought on sexuality, bringing new results, especially with regard to **marriage**. It fully agreed with the fathers of the church—any sexual activity outside of marriage is wrong and sinful—but defined with greater precision the goals and restrictions of matrimonial sexuality.

The first scholastic discussions of the subject, developed in the eleventh and twelfth centuries, depended tightly on the patristic one, finding justification for marriage in the double finality of good of kind and as a remedy for **lust**. For Peter Lombard, matrimonial choice, after the arrival of Christ, did not anymore find a valid motive in procreation, but could be considered only as a remedy for the weakness of the flesh. Thus, marriage was not a duty but a concession, a gesture of indulgence from God, an excuse for lust that man is not able to overcome with continence.

However, most authors continued to view procreation as the essential and objective goal of marriage. Procreation is the legitimate aim of marriage. Saint **Augustine** developed this doctrine, and **Peter Abelard** and Peter Lombard held this to be true. Abelard thought that procreation excuses lust, and that, therefore, every sexual action between consorts has to have from the beginning the intention of procreation. Only then can it find a justification on the overall moral plan. Hugh of Pisa distanced himself from this vision, claiming that procreation never eliminates completely the actual sin of sexual union in marriage, because of the lust that accompanies it, even if it is a venial sin and not a serious sin. Rufino faces the same matter, claiming that marriage offers a remedy to people who are satisfying their lust and find it attenuates their sin making it venial and not serious.

Hugh of St. Victor distinguishes himself by claiming that the primary purpose of marriage is the constitution of the conjugal community in love, excluding procreation as the primary goal. He looks at the different parts of marriage—the spiritual aspect and the actual physical union permitted. The main point is union of hearts and souls. Marriage is a figure of the alliance between God and the soul, while procreation would be only good of the kind, not intrinsic to the relationship. Also, the remedy to lust offered by marriage is extraneous to the authentic spousal relationship, which Hugh sees as a purely spiritual reality. Such vision idealizes the virgin relationship between Mary and Joseph, putting above all perfect chastity and confining sex, also in marriage, to a smaller role. **Virginity**, also in marriage, remained the model of perfect chastity to which all should aspire.

With **Thomas Aquinas** the complex problem finds a new formulation. He is convinced that natural desires and tendencies are good, as pleasure is good in the practice of marital sex. However, like everything else for Thomas, sexuality is ordered to objective ends. Chastity serves to contain the passionate urge, to direct it to objective values; therefore, chastity becomes a means and not a goal, as it was for preceding thinkers, from the fathers of the church to St. Augustine and the first scholastics.

Matrimonial chastity is perfect when it succeeds in directing lust to attainment of the objective ends of marriage—procreation. Marriage is therefore the remedy to lust, as the sacrament gives the necessary grace to direct sexual appetites toward their permissible goals. Thomas sees in this the holiness of the marriage, recovering and giving back to it the place of honour of a "great sacrament" in the wake of St. Paul. Thomas classifies any instance of sex outside marriage as serious sin, because it is outside the objective ends to which sex is orderly. In the *Summa Theologiae*, he classifies sexual sins in a hierarchical way, reserving the worse place to homosexuality and **bestiality**, because such sin is against nature.

The Franciscan John Duns Scotus, approving the death penalty in one of his writings, argued it was permissible for the legislator to apply it for various crimes, among which was **adultery**. Bonaventure of Bagnoregio confirms this sentence for sexual sins. *See also* Giles of Rome.

Further Reading: da Crispiero, Massimo. *Teologia della sessualità, approfondimenti sui temi del matrimonio e della verginità*. Bologna: Edizioni Studio Domenicano, 1994.

Elvio Ciferri

SECLUSION OF WOMEN. Seclusion of women generally refers to the segregation of women from public appearances and from the opposite sex. It commonly designates the custom of *purdah* (from the Hindi *parda*, meaning "curtain"), or the veiling and seclusion of women, that occurred throughout the medieval Arab world. While "Arab" originally referred to natives of the Arabian peninsula, the Arabic language and the Islamic religion spread to the Middle East and **Africa** in the seventh century; thus, "Arab" here refers to this larger context in the later Middle Ages. The seclusion of women is commonly practiced today in many parts of the Arab and Muslim worlds. In the West, this can also refer to the cloistering of women in convents and, in the case of aristocratic women, at home.

Protecting women from contact with strangers outside the sphere of kinship was the impetus behind most forms of *purdah* in the larger Arab world from the tenth century onward. In its strictest form, *purdah* involved the complete isolation of women within the female quarters of the family compound, where only female servants and relatives were permitted. Thus, aristocratic women had no form of contact with men other than their immediate family. In actuality, complete veiling and seclusion were only possible for urban upper-class women, since most women of lower classes were required to work outside their homes.

While it is commonly believed that female seclusion is intrinsically Islamic, the *purdah* tradition is rooted in both Mediterranean (ancient Greek) and

Mesopotamian-Iranian practices. Veiling and seclusion laws first appeared in legal documents under Assyrian law more than 1,000 years before the advent of **Islam**. By the time the Assyrians dominated Mesopotamia and the Near East (c. 600 BCE), laws about families had become more restrictive regarding women than in pervious times, as under Mosaic Law (c. 1000 BCE) where veiling had already been legislated. Prior to the Arab conquests, and during the life of the Prophet Muhammad (570–632), Muslim women of Arabia did not wear **veils** and were not secluded. After Muhammad condoned the practice of *purdah*, women of privileged families tended to stay at home, deliberately keeping themselves out of the public eye. Outside the home, they covered their faces with veils (*hijâb*). Lower-class women who needed to go out to work dressed so that the rest of their bodies, except the hands and face, were concealed. This practice spread to various groups of Hindus, especially in India.

Upon the rise of Christianity in Russia, women gradually became secluded from male society. By the mid-thirteenth to fourteenth centuries, under the Tatar-Mongol reign, the "Domostoroi" became the moral ethical code governing upper-class women. Required by law to live in seclusion, such women were not permitted to go out except when necessary and with the permission of their husbands, fathers, or other male guardians. Such practices were not fully revoked until the reign of Peter the Great (1682–1721).

Married Europeans were generally not secluded in the same way as women of the Arab world. However, late medieval society recognized a clear hierarchy of status with stricter regulations on codes of behavior for each class. Aristocratic women possessed less freedom than women of craft backgrounds, who were free to attend church services and festivals and circulate through town without chaperones. As key members of a family business, they were required to pursue their trades in public.

The only respectable option available to women outside **marriage** was religious vocation. Monasticism (from the Greek monos, meaning "alone") included giving up the secular world and taking on a simple, chaste, and communal existence following a religious rule. In the early Middle Ages, women sometimes labored in fields and farms belonging to the monastery. However, such activities were eventually banned in the *Periculoso* bull by Pope Boniface VIII in 1298, which universally mandated that increased seclusion of religious women would allow the nuns to dedicate their lives more completely to prayer. Modern feminists trace the bull's origins to the teachings of St. Paul as well as to the general mistrust of women by medieval monks. Indeed, early Christian writings indicate an exaggerated fear of women who could lure religious men away from their chaste lives. As strict seclusion of religious women became the norm, the nuns were forced to hire men to provide sustenance for the daily monastery life. *See also* Harem; Monasticism, Female.

Further Reading: Ahmed, Leila. *Women and Gender in Islam: Historical Roots of a Modern Debate*. New Haven, CT: Yale University Press, 1993; Lerner, Gerda. *The Creation of Patriarchy*. Oxford: Oxford University Press, 1985; Mernissi, Fatima. *Beyond the Veil: Male-Female Dynamics in Modern Muslim Society*. London: Saqi Books, 2003; Venarde, Bruce L. *Women's Monasticism and Medieval Society: Nunneries in France and England, 890–1215*. Ithaca, NY: Cornell University Press, 1997.

Sinda K. Vanderpool

SECRETS OF WOMEN (*De Secretis Mulierum*). This short but influential Latin tract on women's sexual and reproductive capacities has been falsely ascribed to **Albertus Magnus**. It was probably written by a disciple of Albertus in the late thirteenth or early fourteenth century for a monastic audience. *Secrets of Women* is primarily a work of natural philosophy in the Aristotelian tradition, drawing on Aristotle himself and the Aristotelian writings of Albertus, **Ibn Rushd**, and **Ibn Sina**. It also draws from medical and astrological writings and reflects some popular beliefs. Although the author agrees with medical writers, against Aristotle, that conception proceeds through the mixture of the female menses and the male semen, his medical ignorance is revealed by his belief that women urinate through the vulva.

Secrets of Women was part of a movement toward a more biologically based Aristotelian misogyny in the High Middle Ages. Throughout it treats women as innately deceitful. A man should be able to tell if a woman is a virgin or is "corrupted" by the condition of her vagina, but since women are adept at deceit, the text gives an alternate method, examining the urine, presumably harder to fake. (A virgin's urine is clear and sparkling, that of corrupt women golden.) Women's evil is explained by their menstrual fluids, which are corrupt and poisonous. The text claims that the mere glance of a menstruating woman can poison a child in the cradle, since the menstrual poisons can be emitted through the eye. *Secrets of Women* was extensively copied and eventually printed. It inspired voluminous commentaries and was one of the most influential works of **Misogyny in Latin Christendom**.

Further Reading: Lemay, Helen Rodnite. *Women's Secrets: A Translation of Pseudo-Albertus Magnus's De Secretis Mulierum with Commentaries*. Albany, NY: State University of New York Press, 1992.

William E. Burns

SEX MANUALS. The most widely available and the most read sex manuals in Europe in the early Middle Ages seem to have been produced and circulated by the Christian church in the form of **penitentials**, records of theological pronouncements, and required atonements for all known aspects of sexual activity. They were not official publications bearing the church's imprimatur, but local compilations by clerics for the use of fellow priests. Nevertheless, the range of listed variations of sexual possibilities is quite impressive.

From the middle of the eleventh century on, the penitentials evolved to a more elaborate confessional-handbook format known as *summa confessorum*. Also, the range of instructional writings on sex became more varied, including such formats as poems, **romance**s, historical chronicles, philosophical dissertations, and medical treatises. One remarkable work is *De coitu*, by the eleventh-century monk Constantine the African, which deals with topics like sexual pleasure and conception without mentioning women at all. At the opposite side of the spectrum is *De secretis mulierum* (**Secrets of Women**), wrongly ascribed to the German philosopher of nature **Albertus Magnus** (1206–1280), which, among other things, reflects the common belief among natural philosophers, regarding female orgasm, that a woman experiences two *delectatio* (delights) in coitus (one at the emission of her own seed and the other at the reception of the man's) and therefore her enjoyment of sex is greater. There was even one astrologer, **Peter of Abano**, who, in *Conciliator*, written around 1303, attempted to analyze the stars' impact on sexual intercourse.

The best-known medieval romance to have served as a sex manual is ***Romance of the Rose***, written in two stages. The first part was written by Guillaume de Lorris, around 1230, as a text of allegorical fiction about a courtier's efforts to conquer a lady's love (the Rose in the title). The second part was added by Jean de Meun, around 1275, and represents a philosophical discussion of love. The book depicts coital acts in which the characters display somber expressions and lack of enjoyment meant to represent the sex act as a moral duty for the sake of procreation. Also, the female partner is always passive, with the male completely in charge.

Outside Europe, sex manuals express a higher appreciation of coitus and treat it as very important and serious. **India** produced the all-time archetype of sex manuals, *Vatsyayana* **Kama Sutra** (Vatsyayana's Aphorisms on Love), written by Vatsyayana, belived to have lived during the Gupta dynasty (320–550). It describes eight ways of making love, each with its respective eight positions, for a total of sixty-four, which are depicted as arts.

Medieval Arab literature overflows with treatises on the art of love, written by philosophers, historians, theologians, and physicians. For example, *Kitáb al-Izáh fi'ilm al-Nikáh* (*The Book of Exposition in the Science of Coition*) by Jalál al-Dín al-Siyuti, an actively religious man, contains very detailed and intimate directions for coital technique, presented with the utmost reverential spirit. Other well-known titles are *Kitáb al-Báh* (Book of **lust**) by Al-Nahli, *Kitág Jámi' al-Lizzat* (Compendium of Pleasure), and *Kitáb al-Munákahah wa al-Mufátahah fí Asnáf al-Jimá' wa Alátih* (Book of Carnal Copulation and the Initiation into the Modes of Coition and Its Instruments) by Aziz al-Dín al-Masíhí. One of the most important titles in this category is Shaykh al-Imám Abú 'Abd-Allah al-Nefzawi's *Al-Raudh al-'Atir fí Nouzhat al-Khawátir* (*The Perfumed Garden for the Delectation of Souls*), probably written between 1394 and 1433. It contains twenty-one chapters dealing with topics like "The Causes of Enjoyment in the Act of Generation" and "Everything Favorable to Coition." *See also Ananga Ranga.*

Further Reading: Bullough, Vern L., and James A. Brundage, eds. *Sexual Practices and the Medieval Church*. Buffalo, NY: Prometheus Books, 1982.

Georgia Tres

SEXUAL DIFFERENCES. *See* Theories of Sexual Difference

SEXUALLY TRANSMITTED DISEASES. The early history of sexually transmitted diseases is difficult to recover, since many medical writings describe symptoms that could be caused by many different diseases, and diseases themselves have changed in historical time.

The symptoms of venereal syphilis, caused by a spirochete, *treponema pallidum*, can be confused with many other diseases, particularly its fellow trepanomatosis, yaws. Although there is some evidence of the bone lesions caused by syphilis in both America and the Old World in the medieval period, the most virulent strain did not emerge until the end of the fifteenth century when it was perceived as a new disease. Gonorrhea, identified by discharges and painful urination—fourteenth-century French physicians called it "hot piss"—was described in its present form by Arab physicians of the tenth and eleventh centuries. (The term had appeared in the writings of the ancient Greek physician Galen, but he had used it to describe a different condition, in which the penis leaked semen.) Medieval European physicians prescribed injections into the genitals as a treatment—John of Arderne suggested a mixture of the milk of a woman, sugar, oil of violets, and barley water. Physicians were also aware of genital warts and ulcers. The Roman imperial physician

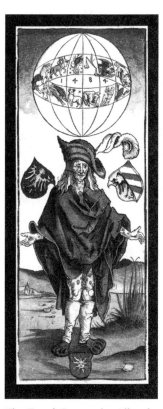

The *French Disease*, by Albrecht Dürer. Made in response to a syphilis epidemic in 1484. © Bildarchiv Preussischer Kulturbesitz/Art Resource, NY.

Oribasius (325–397) and the seventh-century Alexandrian Paul of Aegina compiled lists of conditions of the genitals, and soft chancre and vaginitis were discussed in Indian texts of ayurvedic **medicine**.

Leprosy, which medieval Catholics viewed as a punishment for sin, particularly the sin of **lust**, was also viewed as a sexually transmitted disease. Inmates in leprosaria were strictly required to be chaste, even if married.

Further Reading: Kiple, Kenneth F., ed. *The Cambridge World History of Human Disease*. Cambridge: Cambridge University Press, 1993; Oriel, J. D. *The Scars of Venus: A History of Venereology*. London: Springer-Verlag, 1994.

William E. Burns

SHAJARAT AD-DURR (fl. thirteenth century). Shajarat ad-Durr was one of the few women in Islamic history to rise from the **harem** to the position of sultan in her own right. The slave and later the favorite wife of the last ruler of the Ayyubid dynasty of Egypt and Syria, she took power on the death of her husband in 1249, concealing his death until his son and heir Turanshah arrived at the capital, Cairo. Following Turanshah's murder, Shajarat ad-Durr seized power in her own right. Although she ruled only for a few months, Shajarat ad-Durr exercised the prerogatives of a traditional Muslim ruler, being named in the Friday prayers at the mosques and having coins minted with her name. Her reign also saw the expulsion of a crusader army from the Egyptian port of Damietta.

Shajarat's ability to openly rule may be connected with her own Turkish origins as well as those of the Mamluk commanders of the Egyptian army, as the Turks accepted women's leadership roles more easily than the Arabs. Her connection with the Ayyubid dynasty was also an important symbol of continuity and legitimacy. After the leading Mamluk emirs, facing problems from Syria and condemnation from the Abbasid caliph for submitting to a woman ruler, forced her off the throne, she married her successor, Aybak, and continued to exert great power. Shajarat ad-Durr had Aybak murdered in 1257 shortly after she learned that he had planned to take a second wife, but soon was murdered herself. Beaten to death by the slaves of the new sultan's mother, Shajarat was finally reduced to the harem from which she had come.

Further Reading: Walther, Wiebke. *Women in Islam from Medieval to Modern Times*. Princeton, NJ: Markus Wiener Publishers, 1995.

William E. Burns

SHARIA. Sharia, Islamic religious law, is central to Islamic faith and practice. In Islamic theology ignorance is the human condition. **Islam** teaches that Allah gave Mohammed the Qur'an to guide believers to paradise. In addition to the Qur'an the life and sayings of Mohammed (*sunnah*), the prophet (*rasul*) of Allah, can also be used for guidance. The combination creates Sharia. Sharia originally meant a path for people to walk that was pleasing to Allah. Literally the word means a path to a place of water. It offers Muslims the means for being "rightly guided" in every aspect of life. Specific guidance is given as *fatwas* to the questions of the faithful by religious scholars and judges. Sharia is completely comprehensive, so there are no human actions outside its concern. All human behavior is included in one of the five categories of things that are obligatory (*fard*); things recommended (*mandub*); things permitted (*mubah*); things discouraged, but not prohibited (*makruh*); and things that are absolutely forbidden (*haram*). Most of Sharia was formulated in the Middle Ages. It was closed to changes by the 1200s.

Sharia was used to create a comprehensive order in which the whole society lives by the same law. The order is moral, sexual, social, economic, and political as well as religious. It includes religious and ritual rules such as the rules that govern fasting during Ramadan, the payment of alms, foods that may be eaten, sumptuary rules, and even the attitudes toward the choosing of a spouse, contracts, and worship. "Fiqh" is an Arabic word for law that is intimately connected with Sharia. It means the human action of translating the will of Allah into specific rules. The practice of *fiqh* is the science of jurisprudence. Rules are derived from the raw materials of the issues of life and the materials of Sharia.

The content of Sharia includes the "divine decrees" of Allah. The decrees are usually binding upon everyone. They are duties owed to Allah (*ibadat*). The word *ibadat* comes from the word for slave (*abd*) so that the Muslim believer is the slave (*abd*) of Allah in that his word is the believer's command. In contrast, duties that are owed to people are called *muamalat*.

In the early history of Islam many schools of law emerged. Four of them assembled a large following among Sunni Muslims. The four schools (*madhahib*) each took their name from one of their leading legal scholars. The Al-Shafi school emerged in Egypt and expanded into Syria, Indonesia, and East **Africa**. The Abu-Hanifa (d. 767) became the school with the greatest number of adherents in **India**, Pakistan, Bangladesh, Turkey, Afghanistan, and **central Asia**. Malik ibn Anas founded the third school, the "Maliki." He was a conservative-minded man from Medina. It was widely received in North and West Africa. The Ahmad ibn Hanbal or "Hanbali" School was the strictest of the four schools. It rejected innovation and adopted traditionalism. Through the influence of Ibn Taymiyah and Mohammad ibn Abl Al-Wahab, it became the foundation of the Wahhabi sect. Shii'ite Islam developed its own school of Islamic law. It differs only in details from the Sunni schools.

An extremely important scholar in the early history was Abdullah Mohamed Ibn Idris Al Shafi'i (d. 820). His work created a generally accepted jurisprudence by arguing that there are four sources of law (*usul al-fiqh*) which stand in a definite order of rank. The first is the Qur'an with its clear commandments of Allah. The second is the *sunnah* of the prophet if transmitted by a valid *hadith*, or tradition. The third is the legal scholar (*faqih*) who may look for consensus (*ijma*) of the community in the past. The use of consensus is derived from a saying of Mohammad that declared that the Islamic community should never agree in an error. This means that the consensus of the learned and pious of previous generations and the contemporary community can be trusted as a sure guide. Another tool of the science of Islamic law is analogical reasoning (*qiyas*). It was to be used when the other rules could not provide an answer to a question.

The criminal laws in Sharia recognize three types of offenses—crimes against Allah (*hudud*), crimes against the person (*quesas*), and crimes without penalties fixed by the Qur'an or Sunna (*ta'azir*). Islam accepts human sexuality as natural and normal. However, Sharia treats sexual offences (*zinah*) harshly, whether violent or deviant. Sexual crimes such as **adultery**, **rape**, and other sexual assaults can be punished with death. Homosexuality and **sodomy** are treated as adultery because they are sexual acts with an illicit partner. However, lesbianism is treated less harshly. It is condemned as sex outside **marriage**, but since penetration does not occur the punishment is reduced. Premarital sex and pregnancy are also punishable offences.

To prove rape under Sharia, four male witnesses to the same act are required. If the woman cannot prove her charge, she will be punished for illicit sex—death if married, but whipping if unmarried. Sharia makes marriage voluntary. Arranged marriages are permissible. A man may have up to four wives, but he must treat them all equally. In addition a man can have slaves and women taken in war as captives. **Divorce** is easy for a man, but virtually impossible for a woman. *See also* Genital Contact in Islamic Law.

Further Reading: Ali, Maulana Muhammad. *A Manual of Hadith.* 2nd ed. Lahore, Pakistan: Ahadiyyha Anjuman Ishaat Islam, 2001; Coulson, N. J. *A History of Islamic Law.* Edinburgh: University of Edinburgh Press, 1999; Schacht, Joseph. *An Introduction to Islamic Law.* Oxford: Clarendon Press, 1982; Swarup, Ram. *Understanding the Hadith: The Sacred Traditions of Islam.* Amherst, NY: Prometheus Books, 2002.

Andrew J. Waskey

SHEELA-NA-GIG. A *sheela-na-gig* is a stone carving of a naked woman with an exaggerated vulva. Other features vary widely, but they typically include an oversized, bald, triangular head; bulging eyes; protruding ears; a wedge nose; grimacing or gaping mouth with gritted teeth; depleted and misplaced breasts; striations on the face or chest; prominent ribs; exaggerated navel; short splayed legs; and short arms either framing or grasping the vulva. She may be standing, sitting, or squatting; the posture has reminded some of **childbirth**.

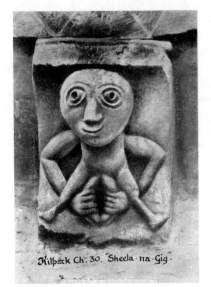

Sheela-na-Gig, from the church of St. Mary and St. David, Kilpeck, Herefordshire. © HIP/Art Resource, NY.

Over 110 sheelas have been found in Ireland, over forty in England, and a few as well in Wales, Scotland, France, Germany, and Denmark. The earliest dates to the eleventh or twelfth century, and the latest to the seventeenth. Most are from ecclesiastical milieux: the exterior of Norman churches, especially above doorways; but also from graveyards, baptismal fonts, and the underside of the lid on a bishop's tomb (Kildare). Most of the remainder are from castles. Some have suffered vandalism—of the genitals especially—and it seems that parish priests, at least in Ireland, were instructed from the 1600s onward to remove and hide them. A reference to burning sheelas does imply that some were wooden.

Where and how these figures originated, what they signify, and what the term *sheela-na-gig* actually means, all defy consensus. It has been suggested that they represent a pagan Celtic or Norse fertility goddess, a protective talisman, a folk deity assisting in childbirth, or on the other hand they were inspired by exhibitionist figures on Continental churches along pilgrimage routes, which were meant to vilify the sin of **lust**.

The term *sheela-na-gig* was first applied to the sculptures in the 1840s (*Proceedings of the Royal Irish Academy*, 1840–1844), having previously described a Royal Navy sloop of the 1780s (the *Shelanagig*), and a type of dance. In Irish, *Síle-na-gCíoch* was understood to mean "Sheela (old woman or hag) of the Breasts" and *Síle-ina-Giob*, "Sheela on Her Hunkers," both of which are problematic. St. Patrick's wife in Irish folklore, Shelagh, and *gig*—a slang term in some English sources for a vagina, a flighty girl, a prostitute, or anything that spins (a whirligig)—may be related.

Further Reading: Freitag, Barbara. *Sheila-na-Gigs. Unravelling an Enigma.* London: Routledge, 2004.

Matthieu Boyd

SHINÜ HUA. *See* Chinese Paintings of Elite Women

SHONAGON, SEI (fl. tenth–eleventh century). Sei Shonagon was a woman of the Japanese Imperial Court nobility. The title "Shonagon" meant minor counselor, and "Sei" refers to her father's family. In the late tenth century, Sei Shonagon served the Empress Sadako, to whom she was devoted, as a lady-in-waiting. Shonagon's beloved Sadako was eventually displaced by a young cousin, Empress Akiko, and shortly afterward died in **childbirth**. Shonagon left the court around this time. Her life was obscure, and after her departure from court became totally unknown.

Nearly all of what little we know of Shonagon's life comes from her sole surviving book, *Makura no Soshi*, or *Pillow Book*. The *Pillow Book* is a miscellany of lists, vignettes, descriptions, and thoughts, none of them longer than a few pages, and arranged in no obvious order. Sections recount events at the Heian court or vignettes of Shonagon's life and observations. There are over 300 sections in all, some only a few sentences long. Although not sexually explicit, the *Pillow Book* speaks forthrightly of Shonagon's—and others'—love affairs.

Sei Shonagon's approach to life was primarily aesthetic. Okashi—charming—is one of her favorite words. She evaluates things by the feelings they give her of beauty or ugliness, subtly analyzing both qualities as displayed both by things and by men and women. Her many lists include those of shameful things, such as a man who shows no regret when meeting a lady with whom he has broken off a love affair, and people who seem to suffer, such as a man whose two mistresses do not get along. Like her contemporary and acquaintance, Lady **Murasaki Shikibu**, Shonagon as a writer displayed keen awareness of the transitoriness of life and love. *See also* Japan.

Further Reading: Morris, Ivan. *The World of the Shining Prince: Court Life in Ancient Japan*. New York: Kodansha, 1994; Sei Shonagon. *The Pillow Book of Sei Shonagon*. Translated and edited by Ivan Morris. New York: Columbia University Press, 1991.

William E. Burns

SINGING GIRLS (*Qayna*, sing./*Qiyan*, pl.). Qiyan were musically and literarily trained Arab female slaves, sometimes members of a **harem**, who entertained the nobility and provided sexual services beginning in pre-Islamic times. Their role originated in the Arabian Peninsula. Trained by singers and poets, their qualifications were a clear and powerful voice, good singing technique, and the ability to recite poetry. Beauty, intelligence, and gentleness were also highly desirable qualities. Their position as sexual objects allowed a certain freedom of movement and access to male gatherings that were inconceivable for "free" women living secluded within the confines of their homes. Eventually, the *qiyan* became popular throughout the Arab world, as well as the Roman empire. Syrian musicians in particular settled very successfully in Rome, where they were called *ambubae*, after the instrument they played, the *embubu*, a kind of short-handled lute. They were generally admired, but not by everybody. The ancient Roman poets Horace and Juvenal mention them, decrying the corrupting effect their music had on the city's mores. Mohammad himself declared unlawful the teaching, selling, or buying of singing girls, but this was interpreted as a disapproval of all sensual dancing and singing, by either men or women, such as it was regularly performed in public taverns. In contrast, the prophet approved of masters listening to their singing girls reciting the Qur'an.

The *qiyan* are first mentioned in Arab literature only much later, in the ninth century, after the advent of **Islam**, by the Basra-born and Baghdad-educated essayist al-**Jahiz**. In *Kitab al-qiyan* (*The Book of Slave-Girl Singers*), he describes their art as venal and erotically stimulating for mercenary purposes. In Mecca and Medina the *qiyan* were used to entertain not only the pilgrims, but also political envoys and businessmen, by singing and dancing for them, and even providing sexual services. The local nobility had in fact a reputation for heavy drinking, gambling, and womanizing. Also in the ninth century, in Spain, at the other end of the Arab world, al-Hakam I, the emir of Cordoba, is said to have given a singer named Aziz 10,000 dirhams, a considerable sum. There is mention also of many noblemen making expensive gifts to the *qiyan*, especially jewelry and luxurious fabrics.

Rich and powerful men, including several caliphs, would frequently fall in love with the *qiyan* and marry them or make them concubines. The slave-girl singers actually constituted an artistic elite that catered to the political authorities and most rulers kept in their palaces a large number of *qiyan* to entertain them, their families, and their guests. They continued to do so through the first half of the twentieth century, when, for example, in Tunis, the bey still kept in his palace several such musical entertainers. However, after the birth of Islam, male musicians started joining the *qiyan* on stage and, consequently, the singing-girls' creative and performative authority decreased. By the twelfth century, they were commonly traded in the slave market, although many times for considerable prices. One of the most famous *qayna* markets at the time was in Seville, Spain (under Moorish occupation at the time), where the singers were displayed with a repertoire list pinned to their clothing. In fact, the first al-Andalus musician mentioned anywhere was a *qayna* named al-Ajfâ. Another famous *qayna* was Salâma al-Zarqâ, mentioned in the **Thousand and One Nights**.

Further Reading: Deguilhem, Randi, and Manuela Marin, eds. *Writing the Feminine: Women in Arab Sources (The Islamic Mediterranean)*. London: I.B. Tauris, 2002; Idrissi, Zebeida. *Qayna: Balades Arabo-Andalouses* [Qayna: Arabo-Andalusian Ballads]. CD. Night & Day, 2003.

Georgia Tres

SLAVERY. Chattel slavery, ownership of one person by another, was the form of slavery practiced most commonly during the Middle Ages. Slaves could be bought and sold, forced to work in any type of environment or fight in wars, and were used for sexual purposes. Although most slaves were kept destitute, some female slaves married their masters, and both male and female slaves were capable of gaining significant personal and political power.

During the Middle Ages, international trade routes became more established than they had been in the classical period, and the slave trade became big business. Many major cities of the time had significant slave markets, including Marseille, Dublin, and Prague. Caffa, in the Crimea, was considered the medieval capital of the slave trade, and Cordoba was a bustling center for slaves from West Africa and those sold by the Vikings.

Christianity, Judaism, and Islam all discouraged enslavement within their own faiths. The Vikings were major slave exporters because they had easy access to both Slavic Pagans and Anglo Saxon Christians and had no compunctions about enslaving them. So many Slavic people were exported for trade that the word "slave" came into universal use by the thirteenth century, derived from "Slav." They were one of the largest ethnic groups in Europe and did not practice Christianity until the middle of the period, after which concentration of the slave trade moved to Africa and India. The Far Eastern countries, such as Japan and China, tended to use debt or crime-slavery as a means of slave labor and did not dip into the pool of foreign slaves.

The **Islamic society** is the most well-known consumer of slaves during this period. It is also the most infamous for sex slavery, although all slave-owning societies have records of female, and sometimes male, slaves being intimately used by their captors. In fifteenth-century Florence, a foundling hospital estimated that up to a third of the babies abandoned there were children of slaves and, most likely, their masters. Documentation abounds with wives jealous of their husbands' relationships with slave women.

Slaves taken by the Muslim community were required to convert to Islam. Because they were slaves first and then converts, it was acceptable for them to remain slaves, and they could be bought and sold even though they were now Muslim. It was also acceptable, after conversion, to marry a slave. Once married, though, she was no longer considered a slave and could not again, even in case of divorce, be treated as such. Concubines retained their slave status. The child of a female slave and a male slave or other freeman was born a slave and remained the property of the mother's master. The child of a female slave fathered by her master was free and equal in status to any of his other children. The mother thereafter gained certain privileges, becoming *umm walad*, literally, "mother of a child." In cases of captured women who were already married, slavery annulled any existing marriage. Therefore, a captor could take as concubine, or even marry, a slave whose husband was still alive.

Islamic and many other societies of the time engaged in homosexual behavior. For this reason, young beardless males were in demand in the slave markets. These were known as *ghilman*, named after the mythical cupbearers of the Islamic heaven. These slaves, usually Turkish, were treated well and given important positions. In some societies, *ghilman* were tapped for special duty as *mamluk*, a class of slaves who were trained as soldiers.

There was a large market for **eunuchs** in the Muslim and Byzantine empires, with prices for these castrated males being as much as thrice that of an intact slave. Eunuchs were often given sensitive and powerful positions. The main job for a eunuch was to guard and care for the **harem**. Women could not be entrusted with this job, so "harmless" men were required. Many eunuchs were required for each harem, as concubines could number in the hundreds or even thousands.

It was considered a great act of charity for a Muslim to free a slave, and many masters manumitted slaves on their deaths. Because the slaves were then free and Muslim, it was unlikely that they would be enslaved again by a Muslim, even if they were obviously foreign. This gave a great boost to the Muslim population of the time.

In France, before the feudal system was fully developed, the rulers of the largely agrarian society found that moving slaves from the manor into individual huts on the property proved to be more efficient. With this arrangement, however, they lost some control over their slaves' lives. To correct this, slaves were required to report to the manor for one or more days a week, and were required to allow their masters admittance to their dwellings at any time. In this way, masters could continue any intimate relationships and limit relationships with other slaves. Human nature, however, dictated that slaves in this situation found ways to have more of a private life than before. Even though the master technically still owned their lives, privacy led to more autonomy.

Eventually, the feudal system came into use in most of western Europe, so serfs performed much of the work previously done by slaves. While serfdom can be seen as a form of slavery, there are critical differences that require separating the two conditions. Slavery is complete ownership of a person and his property, to the point of debasing a person to a thing. Although at times they were difficult to uphold, a serf had legal rights on which to rely. *See also* Concubinage; Singing Girls.

Further Reading: Ali, Kecia. "Muslim Sexual Ethics: Islam and Slavery." See The Feminist Sexual Ethics Project Web site: http://brandeis.edu/projects/fse/muslim/mus-essay/mus-ess-slav.html; Duby, Georges, ed. *A History of Private Life: Revelations of the Medieval World.* Cambridge, MA: Harvard University Press, 1988; Lal, K. S. *Muslim Slave System in Medieval India.* New Delhi: Aditya Prakashan, 1994.

Jennifer Della'Zanna

SODOMY. Sodomy is the sin that takes its name from the biblical city of Sodoma, where male homosexuality was widespread. This form of sexual behavior was opposed at first without much action in the early Middle Ages, but then bitterly repressed at the beginning of the eleventh century.

In 533 the emperor Justinian put homosexual relationships in the same category as **adultery** and submitted them for the first time to civil sanctions. In 538 and 544 the emperor decreed further laws, to push all those people that fell into similar sin to seek the pardon of penitence. Around 650 the government of Visigothic Spain approved legislation against homosexual acts as far as that it established the **castration** of those who committed them. The church did neither take part nor agree with this provision and it did not cooperate with the Visigothic government for over forty years after the promulgation of these harsh laws, but at the end, under direct order of the monarchy, the church was forced to promulgate ecclesiastical legislation based on these laws. A conciliare decree was released that established the degradation, excommunication, and exile for clerics who were guilty of homosexuality; for laymen, the punishment consisted of lashes and exile.

In civil circles, after the Visigothic legislation, no other law was passed on the subject up to the time of Charlemagne. An edict exhorted priests and bishops to look in every possible way to prevent and eradicate this "evil," but it did not prescribe any punishment and was intended only as an ecclesiastical admonition. Subsequent decrees of the French monarchy against homosexual practices were almost uniformly based on the relatively mild provisions of this edict.

At the onset of the Middle Ages, the church formulated some official provisions against homosexuality that were revealed and considered quite moderate. The first testimonies are those of the council of Elvira and the council of Ancira. The slower Latin interpretations made to precede the canons from a title in which was specified the fact that who had practised **bestiality** or sodomy, had lost sense of reason—were "out of their minds." Another testimony of the church's position against homosexuality could be found in the **penitentials**. These texts were widespread throughout the Middle Ages, and homosexuality was assigned a very important place in them. The prescribed punishments for such sin varied between three and twenty years of penitence.

The theological objections to homosexual acts in the early Middle Ages can be linked to the idea of the "seed" (semen) being wasted, as in not emitted through the act of **marriage**—heterosexual intercourse. The term "sodomy" was applied indifferently to all nonprocreative sexual acts. Homosexuality was reduced to a simple form of fornication. **Peter Damian**, in the eleventh century, wishing the reform of the customs of the clergy, fought with strength against the practice of homosexuality. To this purpose he wrote the *Liber Gomorrhianus* devoting it to Pope Leo IX, confiding in the reforming wish of the pontiff. In this brochure, Peter Damian did a detailed analysis of, according to him, the "terribly guilty," using such audacious and severe terms that they embarrassed the pontiff, who wanted to mitigate his severity. In the twelfth century Bernard of Chiaravalle, following Damian's example, fought against homosexual practice among the clergy. In the thirteenth century, **Thomas Aquinas** strongly condemned sodomy as a sin against nature, defining it as the most serious sexual sin, after bestiality. Catherine of Siena and Bonaventure of Bagnoregio also harshly denounced sodomy, above all in the clergy, in their writings. The canons of the councils and the town statutes reflect this conception, inflicting severe punishments against sodomites, such as burning at the stake or perpetual exile. In the fifteenth century, when preaching, **Bernardino of Siena** crusaded against sodomy. *See also* Anal and Intercrural Sex; Homosexuality, Male; Pederasty.

Further Reading: Boswell, John. *Christianity, Social Tolerance, and Homosexuality: Gay People in Western Europe from the Beginning of the Christian Era to the Fourteenth Century*. Chicago: University of Chicago Press, 1980; Bullough, Vern L., and James A. Brundage, eds. *Sexual Practices and the Medieval Church*. Buffalo, NY: Prometheus Books, 1982; Goodich, Michael. *The Unmentionable Vice: Homosexuality in the Later Medieval Period*. Santa Barbara, CA: ABC-Clio, 1979.

Elvio Ciferri

SOREL, AGNES (c. 1422–1450). The daughter of Catherine de Maignelais and Jean Soreau, Lord of Coudun, Agnes was born at the Castle of Fromenteau, Touraine, or Froidmantel, Picardy, circa 1422. Agnes joined the retinue of Isabelle of Lorraine, the wife of Rene of Anjou, serving them at a court noted for its patronage of chivalric love. In 1443, the court traveled to Saumur to meet Charles VII and his Queen Marie, Rene's sister. Agnes was probably introduced to the king by Pierre de Brézé, the seneschal of Normandy, capturing his attention with her beauty and wit. In the summer of 1444, Agnes gave birth to the first of her three daughters by the king, Marie, Charlotte, and Jeanne. Charles VII named her official mistress, the first woman to be publicly acknowledged as such.

Agnes formed the center of a political group around the king, including de Brézé, Jacques Coeur, the superintendent of finance, and Etienne Chevalier, the Treasurer of France. They pushed Charles VII to prosecute the Hundred Years' War, recover France from the occupying English, and subdue his fractious nobles. Agnes attended council sessions and placed members of her family in key positions within the royal household, bodyguard, and the church, securing her uncle Geoffroy the bishopric of Nimes. Charles VII was extraordinarily generous to Agnes, providing her with lavish gowns that set a fashion for décolletage and long trains, jewelry and land, giving her the Chateau de Beauté on the Marne River. Agnes's chief rival at the court was the king's son, the Dauphin Louis, who resented her influence and ability to discover his challenges to royal authority. Others, like chronicler George Chastelain, criticized Agnes's dresses, wantonness, and her exercise of political power.

Agnes died suddenly during a miscarriage on February 9, 1450. Shattered, the king ordered monuments at Loches and Jumiges inscribed *mites simplexque columba* (gentle, guileless dove). In his grief, the king believed rumors that Coeur poisoned Agnes, and allowed him to be exiled and bankrupted. Because her mausoleums were badly damaged in the French Revolution, the only surviving images of Agnes are in Etienne Chevalier's *Book of Hours*, and a diptych by Jean Fouquet, in which she poses with one bare breast as the Virgin Mary.

Further Reading: Cleugh, James. *Chant Royal*. Garden City, NY: Doubleday, 1970; Kemp-Welch, Alice. *Of Six Medieval Women*. Williamstown, MA: Corner House Publishers, 1972; Vale, M.G.A. *Charles VII*. Berkeley: University of California Press, 1974.

Margaret Sankey

SUFISM. Sufism (*tasawwuf*) is the mystical practice of Islamic members of Sufi orders (*sufiya*). "Sufi" comes from the Arabic word *suf* for wool. *Suf* refers to the rough wool garment worn by many Sufi ascetics. Sufism appeared early in the history of **Islam**. Sufis see their practices beginning with Mohammad's mystical experiences as reported in the Qur'an and the Hadiths. Mohammad is the starting point for all the Sufi orders (*taruq*). Sufi orders are usually named after a founding person who was directly linked to Mohammad or spiritually linked to him in some cases by chains (*silsilas*) of masters and disciples handed down orally in the Middle Ages, but eventually written down. Each Sufi order has a current master to whom disciples are joined. Some Sufi orders have permanent lodges where they live or meet.

A key verse in the Qur'an for Sufis is *Surah 17*, *ayah* 1, which says that Mohammed, in a night vision, was transported to Jerusalem. From there he rode on a mystical horse (which left its hoofprint on the Dome of the Rock) and ascended (Mi'raj) to see and hear from Allah directly. The actions of leaving temporal distractions behind, journeying toward Allah, to see and hear directly the ultimate reality are key actions in Sufi philosophy and practice. Islam is a religion of extreme monotheism. It stresses the unity of Allah (*tawhid*). Anything that assigns partners to Allah is idolatry and a terrible evil (*shirk*). For Sufis the way to avoid temptations that lead to *shirk* is to purify the heart.

A Sufi master is a spiritual guide (*murshid*). His teachings (*tariqas*) help disciples to work at purging distractions that keep them from entering the presence of Allah. These practices vary among the different Sufi orders. Among the most important mystical practices aiding those traveling on the Sufi path (*suluk*) are asceticism, praying (*du'a*) at the tomb of a Sufi saint (*wali*), poetry, music, and singing. These are believed to purify the heart (*tasfiyat al-qalb*) and to enable the refinement of the soul (*tazkiyat al-nafs*). These are acts of devotion (*'amal*) which are believed to lead to a pure love of Allah and to remembering (*dhiker*) him always.

The greatest of the Sufi masters of the Middle Ages who wrote love poetry was Jalal al-Din **Rumi** (1207–1273). Born in Khurasan (now in Afghanistan) he fled with his family to Konya (an area then called Rum, now in Turkey) when the Mongols invaded. The son of a famous Sufi Rumi met a mysterious dervish, Shams-i-Tabrizi. After a two-year association Rumi was transformed spiritually, but then Shams vanished mysteriously. In grief Rumi developed the religious dance or whirling of the Whirling Dervishes. In addition Rumi wrote great volumes of poetry. Much of it was love poetry. In some poems love for Shams is understood to be love for Allah.

Sufis from Persia and Afghanistan developed several musical styles designed to arouse passionate emotional states so devotees could draw close to Allah (*sama'*). These musical practices developed a wide following in **India** after the Muslim invasions. Throughout the Middle Ages Sufism was a part of the popular culture. Political leaders and the wealthy would endow Sufi lodges or places of practice and give other support to Sufi adepts. Being popular among the people many were initiated into several Sufi orders.

Further Reading: Algar, Hamid. *Sufism: Principles and Practices*. Oneonta, NY: Islamic Publications International, 1999; Arberry, A. J. *Sufism: An Account of the Mystics of Islam*. Mineola, NY: Dover Publications, 2002; Ernst, Carl W. *The Shambhala Guide to Sufism*. Boston: Shambhala Publications, 1997.

Andrew J. Waskey

SUKAYNA BINT AL-HUSAYN (fl. seventh century). Sukayna bint al-Husayn plays an ambivalent role in the Islamic tradition as an outstanding example of feminine self-confidence in the early days of **Islam**. She was a granddaughter of Ali b. Abi Talib and Fatima, the daughter of the prophet Mohammad. On her father's side, Sukayna stands not only for the inner circle of the prophet's family, but also for their tragic destiny. Her father Husayn became the outstanding Shiite martyr with his death at Karabala in the year 680. On her mother's side, Sukayna stemmed from one of the most illustrious Arab-Muslim clans. Her grandfather, a military leader of the tribe of Kalb, is said to have sworn an oath of allegiance to Muhammad's second successor, Umar b. al-Khattab.

In the year 686, Sukayna married Mus'ab b. az-Zubayr, at that time governor of Iraq, who was killed in 691. She returned to her place of origin, Medina, where she remarried twice. Sukayna was a strong personality and her mother had instilled in her a pronounced taste for intellectual matters. The sources portray her as a beautiful woman of illustrious lineage, a courageous person of caustic repartee, and an unapproachable feminist with a scorn for (traditionalist) men. She died in Medina in 736.

Throughout her life, Sukayna refused to wear a **veil**. Moreover, she underlined the beauty of her face with a special hairstyle named after her. However, not only her personal fashions and styles singled her out among contemporary women. In Medina, she maintained a literary salon where poets, singers, and literary men met, and where she acted as a patroness for young talents and actively engaged in debates. For this reason, Sukayna helped to bring about new forms of literary gatherings, of love poetry (**ghazal**), and of musical settings that were to become a dominant feature of urban society in later Islamic times.

Further Reading: Sanni, A. "Women Critics in Arabic Literary Tradition with Particular Reference to Sukayna Bint al-husayn." *British Society for Middle Eastern Studies Bulletin*, 1991, 358–64; Vadet, Jean Claude. *Une personnalitè fèminine du higaz au Ier/VIIe siècle: Sukayna, petite-fille de 'Ali. Arabica* 4 (1957): 261–87.

Susanne Enderwitz

SUN SIMIAO (581–682). Dubbed the "King of **Medicine**," Sun Simiao was one of the most influential figures in Chinese medicine. He was said to be versed in Confucian and Daoist classics at a young age, and was offered official court positions by emperors from both the Sui dynasty (581–617) and the Tang dynasty (618–907). Nevertheless, Sun declined these honors and chose medicine as his lifelong calling.

Sun Simiao's biggest contribution was the compilation of an encyclopedia for clinical practice, *Prescriptions Worth a Thousand Pieces of Gold for Every Emergency* (*Beiji qianjin yaofang*). First printed in 652, the book consists of thirty chapters and 4,500 formulas. Sun not only recorded prescriptions he collected from famous physicians of the past as well as his contemporaries, but also provided his theories regarding each topic/symptom. His work set the clinical standard in the literate tradition between the Tang dynasty and the Song dynasty (960–1279). In 682, Sun published his second book, *Rare Prescriptions Worth a Thousand Pieces of Gold* (*Qianjin yifang*). The book, with thirty volumes, 2,000 formulas, and a focus on folk remedies, embodied his thirty years of experience treating patients after the publication of his first book.

Sun Simiao's theory of medicine was strongly influenced by *The Book of Change*, Laozi, and the *yin-yang* philosophers. In medically describing the female, for example, Sun wrote the following: "The Classic says: women are a gathering place for yin influences, dwelling in dampness. From the age of fourteen on, their yin *qi* wells up and a hundred thoughts run their minds, damaging their organ system within and ruining their beauty without." Sun, thus, believed that there should be separate prescriptions for women. In fact, the first five chapters of the *Prescriptions Worth a Thousand Pieces of Gold for Every Emergency* are devoted to providing advice and treatments for **menstruation**, irregular feminine discharge, intercourse, conception, birth control, miscarriage, **abortion**, prenatal care, and postpartum. Because of his emphasis on specific therapies for women, Sun Simiao was long regarded the pioneer of Chinese gynecology and obstetrics. Sun's dedication to reproductive medicine reflected an effective response to the political and social stability, and to the growth in economy as well as population during the early period of the Tang dynasty.

Further Reading: Furth, Charlotte. *A Flourishing Yin: Gender in China's Medical History, 960–1665.* Berkeley: University of California Press, 1999; Unschuld, Paul U. *Medicine in China: Historical Artifacts and Images.* New York: Prestel, 2000.

Ping Yao

SYPHILIS. *See* Sexually Transmitted Diseases

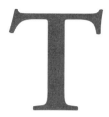

TACHIKAWA-RYŪ. The Tachikawa Sect (i.e., Tachikawa-ryū) was a branch of the esoteric Japanese Buddhist school Shingon that adopted Daoist yin-yang teachings (*omyōdō*) and male-female metaphors that were probably acted out in sexual rituals. Mainstream Shingon leaders regarded it a pernicious influence during the years it was active, between the twelfth and seventeenth centuries, because of its doctrine that enlightenment could be achieved through male-female sexual intercourse.

There are few extant Tachikawa-ryū texts or reliable historical documents on it. A source commonly used for understanding its history is the *Hōkyōshō* ("Compendium of the Jeweled Mirror"), written by Yūkai (1345–1416), a high-ranking Shingon priest critical of Tachikawa-ryū. According to the *Hōkyōshō*, Tachikawa-ryū started when the Shingon priest Ninkan (d. 1114), after being exiled to Izu for treason and shortly before committing suicide, taught Shingon to a yin-yang master (*onmyōji*) from Tachikawa (near present-day Tokyo). Although secretive, it gained in popularity and probably reached its peak in the early fourteenth century with Monkan (a.k.a., Kōshin 1278–1357), who became the head of the eminent Shingon temple Daigo-ji in Kyoto and is thought to have systematized Tachikawa-ryū's doctrine. After Monkan, Tachikawa-ryū's influence waned. In the fifteenth century the military government banned it as a vulgar religion and many of its texts were destroyed. By the seventeenth century it was extinct.

In Tachikawa-ryū doctrine, male-female imagery was widely employed, with semen and female blood described as the basic fluids of life. Male-female categories were also used for classifying basic Shingon ideas and objects. For example, the two mandala of Shingon, the Taizōkai ("Womb Realm") and the Kongkai ("Diamond Realm"), were seen as female and male, respectively. The use of male-female sexual imagery was not unique to Tachikawa-ryū and can be found in other interpretations of Shingon symbols. Some scholars, for example, have read the "wisdom-fist" gesture (*chiken-in* mudra), held by the Buddha Mahāvairocana in the Diamond Mandala, in which the left index finger is enclosed in the right fist, as having sexual connotations.

The most infamous sexual practice associated with the Tachikawa-ryū is the secretive skull ritual. It is described in *Juhō yōjinshū* ("On the Circumspect Reception of the Dharma," c. 1270) by Shinjō, a Shingon priest who regarded Tachikawa-ryū as heretical. For this ritual, Shinjō writes that the practitioner "must have sexual intercourse with a beautiful and willing woman, and must repeatedly wipe the liquid product of this action onto the skull until it reaches 120 layers." This, apparently, was thought to give greater power to the skull, which was set up as a main object of worship.

Tachikawa-ryū's practices echo some of those found in Indian **Tantric Buddhism**, but no link has been established. Its doctrines, while widely regarded as unorthodox, in part may be seen as related to a particular interpretation of the Mahayana nondualistic teaching that "desires are enlightenment" (*bonnō soku bodai*). *See also* Buddhism; Japan.

Further Reading: Sanford, James H. "The Abominable Tachikawa Skull Ritual." *Monumenta Nipponica* 46 (1991): 1–20; Yamasaki Taikō. *Shingon: Japanese Esoteric Buddhism*. Boston: Shambhala, 1988.

Clark Chilson

TANTRIC BUDDHISM. Tantric **Buddhism** is also known as Vajrayana Buddhism. In Sanskrit the word *tantra* means "loom" or "weaving". It is a metaphor for weaving together the various elements of the cosmos. These include both the fundamental energies and the personality of a tantric devotee with other elements. Tantric Buddhist writings are *tantras* ("weavings") rather than *sutras* (dialogues). *Vajrayana* is a compound of the word *vajra* (Sanskrit; *dorje*), which means "diamond, or adamantine," and *yana*, the Sanskrit word for "path" or "vehicle." Vajrayana means the Diamond or Indestructible Path. A *vajra*, a small ritual scepter, is often used in Vajrayana practice.

Tantric Buddhism developed during the Pala period in **India** (eighth–twelfth centuries) partly as a reaction to the material success of wealthy Buddhist monasteries. It was also a layperson's spiritual protest against privilege and scholastic elitism. Many scholars believed Buddhism was introduced to the people of the high Himalayas in the middle of the eighth century by Guru Rinpoche (also called Padmasambbhava). It developed into Tantric Buddhism when it combined *tantric* beliefs and practices that may have existed even at the time of the earthly life of the Buddha, with Mahayana Buddhism and elements of pre-Buddhist religion—such as Shamanism, belief in **magic**, demons, and deities. Tantric Buddhism became the official religion of **Tibet**, Bhutan, and beyond. Tantric Buddhism was a religious practice among the rulers of the Uddyana Kingdom (after 600) and the Pala dynasty in Bengal (750–1150). It was also planted in the Middle Ages in **China**, **Japan**, Java, and Mongolia, but was suppressed in India after the Muslim invasions.

Tantric Buddhism developed within Mahayana Buddhism. However, instead of using asceticism as the path to enlightenment, it seeks to use the natural energies of the cosmos to serve humanity. Instead of liberation from this world by ascetic denial, Vajrayana seek liberation through indulgence, especially through the bliss of delight between *lotus* (vagina) and *vajra* ("thunderbolt" or penis). Tantra rejects the paths of meditation and asceticism whether of Jain, Hindu, Mahayana, or other origin.

The metaphor of a spiritual path in Buddhism takes several names. In Vajrayana the "Diamond Path" is divided into progressive states that are called *lamrim*. A teacher (*lama*) leads a student through the path of Theravada and Mahayana. When the student is ready for advanced lessons *tantras* are taught. The *tantras* develop practice in visualizing, using mantras, prayer, and esoteric traditions. The goal is to develop a personality capable of harnessing spiritual energy. Using the imagination to harness the energy either possessed by or symbolized by the deities of Tantric Buddhism is one of the practices of this form of Buddhism. The devotee practices visualization to imagine the various deities and their consorts as well, even in sexual embrace. Instead of abandoning the self to the transcendent tantric practitioners, they abandon self to the whole cosmos. In some schools of Tantric Buddhism there is a denial of a difference between *samsara* (the world as it appears) and *nirvana*. To be liberated means that there is no difference between kindness and murder, chastity and **rape**, **incest** and abstinence.

In some forms of Tantric Buddhism ritual sexual intercourse (with orgasm) between individuals developed into a sacred practice. In more elaborate situations ritual group orgies would be performed. Sexual union and orgasm was seen as an extension of the self rather than gratification. Tantric Buddhist iconography in sculpture often depicts the "father-mother" union (in Tibetan, *yab-yum*). A divine couple sits face-to-face in embrace with the goddess sitting in a position to receive the god's penis. These types of sculptures are not erotic art, but understood as symbols of the union of insight (the goddess) and compassion (the god).

Tantric Buddhist paintings of the *yab-yum* also depict sexual union but with both male and female being expressed as emanations of the Buddha. The couple's bliss represents the bliss of Buddhahood. Another image of sexual union is the "churner and the churned." When the *vajra* or diamond scepter of the male churns the female partner, it produces the nectar of Buddhahood.

Further Reading: Chang, Garma C. C. *Teachings and Practice of Tibetan Tantra*. Mineola, NY: Dover Publications, 2004; Murthy, K. Krishna. *Sculptures of Vajrayana Buddhism*. Delhi, India: Classics India Publications, 1989; Ray, Reginald A. *Secret of the Vajra World: The Tantric Buddhism of Tibet*. Boston: Shambhala, 2002; Sarkar, Anil Kumar. *The Mysteries of Vajrayana Buddhism: From Atisha to Dalai Lama*. New Delhi: South Asian Publications & Research Institute, 1993; Subrahmanyam, B. *Vajrayana Buddhist Centers in South India*. Delhi, India: Bharatiya Kala Prakashan, 2001.

Andrew J. Waskey

TEMPLARS, TRIAL OF. *See* Trial of the Templars

THEODORA (c. 500–548). Born around 500, Theodora was the daughter of Acacius, bear-keeper for the "Green" faction at the Constantinople hippodrome. After his death left them destitute, his daughters sought support from the rival "Blue" faction and began performing at the hippodrome themselves. Theodora became famous for the "Leda and the Swan" dance in which a trained bird pecked grain off her body. After a short time as the mistress of a provincial governor, Theodora met Justinian, nephew of the Emperor Justin and heir to the throne. Their relationship horrified the emperor and the nobility, who expected Justinian to marry a woman of appropriate rank. In 524, Justinian spearheaded a change in the law permitting "repentant" former actresses to marry patricians, something that allowed not only Theodora to marry him in 525, but also her sisters and an illegitimate daughter to make rich matches as well.

In 527, Justinian acceded to the Byzantine throne and had Theodora crowned as Augusta. Oaths taken by imperial officials were, significantly, to both the emperor and empress. Theodora patronized the Blue faction of the city, remembering them from childhood, and protected the heretical Monophysite sect of Christianity in her own palace, providing dissidents a link to the imperial government. In response to criticism of her past, Theodora endowed a convent for the rehabilitation of actresses and prostitutes and championed laws protecting the property and rights of

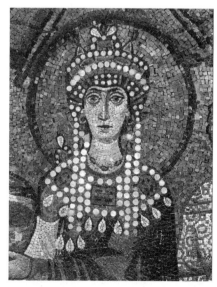

A 6th century mosaic representation of the Empress Theodora from Basilica San Vitale, Italy. © The Art Archive/Dagli Orti (A).

women and children. On two occasions, the Nike Riots of 532 and Justinian's brush with smallpox in 542, Theodora's cool head and decisive action steadied the throne and proved her a capable and intelligent coruler.

Although many imperial consorts had been powerful and important in deciding religious issues, Theodora stood out for her influence over Justinian, extending even into the selection of his heir, a nephew Justin II married to Theodora's niece Sophia. She was also a key link to the empire's most successful general, Belisarius, through her friendship with his wife Anastasias. Even so, Theodora could never entirely escape her past, which court-historian Procopius recorded with relish in his *Secret History*, tarring her as a harlot and heretic. Theodora died in 548, probably of cancer, and Justinian ruled until 565, always mourning her death and a far weaker emperor for her absence. *See also* Byzantium; Monophysite Churches; Prostitution.

Further Reading: Cesaretti, Paolo. *Theodora*. New York: Vendome, 2004; Diehl, Charles. *Theodora*. New York: F. Ungar, 1972; Evan, James. *Theodora*. Austin: University of Texas Press, 2002.

Margaret Sankey

THEOPHYLACTUS OF OCHRID (c. 1050–c. 1110). Theophylactus Hephaiston (of Ochrid or Ohrid) is also known as Theophylact or Theophylactos of Bulgaria. He was born on the island of Euboea, probably at Euripus, about the year 1050. He studied in Constantinople where he became a deacon in the Orthodox Church at the Basilica Hagia Sophia. Around 1078 Theophylactus was elected Bishop of Achrida in Bulgaria (now Ohrid in the Former Yugoslav Republic of Macedonia), then ruled by the Bulgars. Among his numerous writings are commentaries on the Gospels, Acts, and the Minor Prophets. Some of his sermons and orations have also survived as has his *Life of Clement of Orchrida* (the first Slavonic Bishop), and 130 of his letters.

Theophylactus wrote *In Defense of Eunuchs* (*Logos*) at the request of his brother Demetrios, a **eunuch**. The occasion was a Byzantine controversy over the gender of eunuchs. The controversy arose within the historic Greek understanding that men were hard, dry, and strong, while women were soft, wet, and weak. To which category did eunuchs belong? Were they to be identified by sex or by gender? Some contemporary opinion included them in a "third category." Secular opinion tended to center upon this conclusion. Theophylactus argued that eunuchs were neither a third gender nor a third sex. They were simply men.

The *Defense of Eunuchs* is organized as a debate between a noneunuch and a eunuch. The noneunuch argues that **castration** is in opposition to the Creator, the law of Moses, the teachings of the Apostles, the church fathers, and Justinian's laws, and has negative consequences. The eunuch responds that castration is not contrary to the Creator's will, the law of Moses, or Justinian's laws, and is supported as right by church musicians including **John Chrysostom**. Moreover, castration can lead to great improvements in careers, character, and moral purity. Castration was not a negative action upon the soul because there had been saints, patriarchs, bishops, and priests who had been eunuchs. Moreover children who became court eunuchs were a benefit to their families.

Further Reading: Mullet, Margaret. "Theophylact of Ochrid's *In Defence of Eunuchs*." In *Eunuchs in Antiquity and Beyond*, edited by Shaun Tougher. London: Gerald Duckworth, 2002; *Works of Theophylactus* (Greek and Latin). 4 vols. 2nd ed. Venice: J. F. B. M. de Rossi, 1754–1763.

Andrew J. Waskey

THEORIES OF SEXUAL DIFFERENCE. Medieval Europe inherited three main traditions on sexual difference from antiquity. From the Scripture it took the story of the creation of Adam and Eve and the hierarchy of male and female. From Greek and Roman antiquity it took Hippocratic-Galenic medical theories on the homology (physical similarity) of male and female. This has been termed the "one-sex" model. Also from Greek antiquity came Aristotle's works on animals and his argument for radical differences between male and female. This tradition, however, was not well known until Latin translations of Aristotle's works were made from the early thirteenth century, and then were mostly confined to an intellectual elite.

In Genesis God created Adam as the first human being, shaping him from the earth. Deciding that Adam needed a helper "fit" for him God shaped Eve from Adam's left rib. Although both were "in God's image," Adam was created first, indicating man's priority and superiority over woman. His creation from earth was a sign of his greater physical strength and solidity. Woman was created from man in order to serve him. She was soft because she was made from Adam's marrow. She was associated with the left—inferior—side, and many theories of generation contended that a girl was conceived in the left chambers of the womb, boys in the right, and **hermaphrodites** in the middle. **Thomas Aquinas** (d. 1274), however, wrote that woman's creation from Adam's rib rather than his head or feet showed that woman was to be man's companion rather than his master or slave.

Parts of the fifth-century-BCE Hippocratic treatises were available in medieval Latin copies, or refracted through early medieval authors. Emphasis was on the four humors of blood (hot and wet), choler (hot and dry), phlegm (cold and wet), and melancholy (cold and dry). All people were perceived to have all four humors to varying degrees, but women were dominated by wet and cold humors where men had a prevalence of hot and dry ones. Male and female were not radically different; rather they were variations on a theme. Both were thought to produce a "seed" that made an active contribution to conception, requiring the man's and woman's orgasm. The primary defining characteristic of the female was the presence of the uterus, and many "diseases of women" were explained as defects in uterine function. The Roman doctor Galen (d. c. 200 CE) produced a modified view, influenced by Aristotle. While his works were only partially available before the sixteenth century, they were filtered through Arab texts translated into Latin from the twelfth century onward. Male and female bodies were essentially the same, but the female, because colder, was inferior. Her genitals were closed within the body where his greater heat pushed his genitals outside. Man was more perfect; woman was less developed, like a child. Where the uterus defined the female the penis defined the male, and the vagina was understood as the neck of the uterus rather than a separate organ. Testicles and ovaries were homologous. The clitoris and breasts were rarely mentioned as markers of sex difference. Both male and female contributed a seed to conception, but the female seed was weaker and played less of a formative role. Females experienced greater pleasure in intercourse, partly because they at once emitted and received seed into their wombs.

Aristotle's (d. c. 322 BCE) works on animals were available to intellectuals in the universities and some monasteries by the thirteenth century, and were also filtered through translations of Arab treatises. Aristotelian philosophy emphasized a radical difference of male and female, based on degrees of "heat," or vital energy. A widely repeated doctrine in later medieval, medical, and encyclopedic works was that "the hottest woman is colder than the coldest man." Heat was assumed superior to cold. In Aristotle's words, woman's coldness made her a "defective male." Woman's coldness made her smooth, soft, weak, impressionable, suited to a sedentary life, inconstant, and needing guidance, while man's heat made him hard, brawny, decisive, intelligent, of sound judgment, and fit to lead. Woman's coldness explained **menstruation**: unable to burn up her excess humors, she was purged of them once a month. Menstruation was a reminder of Eve's sin and the Fall. Women lived longer than men (according to **Albertus Magnus**, d. 1280) despite their inferiority of heat, because of their monthly purgation, because sexual intercourse did not take so much of their vital energy, and because they worked less. Men's heat explained their beard and higher levels of sweat and body hair: their heat opened their pores and pushed excess humors out in the form of hair and perspiration. Masculine women might also produce such hair, while feminine men had little beard. Many authors acknowledged that some men possessed feminine character traits—such as malice, flexibility, or prudence—and some women had masculine qualities.

Aristotelian views were widely taken up by medical writers, even appearing in works available to the literate laity such as the "**Trotula**" texts that repeated the "hot/cold" dichotomy. Aristotelian theories of conception were more controversial. The male alone contributed an active and formative substance to generations through his semen, because his greater heat "cooked" or concocted his humors into active, white foamy semen. The colder woman contributed only passive matter through her menses. The existence and role of female seed was hotly debated from the thirteenth to late fifteenth centuries, and finally most settled on a form of Galenism: both male and female contributed active seed, but the female's was weaker and less formative than the male's. *See also* Medicine; Scholastic Philosophy.

Further Reading: Cadden, Joan. *The Meanings of Sex Difference in the Middle Ages: Medicine, Science, and Culture.* Cambridge: Cambridge University Press, 1993; Jacquart, Danielle, and Claude Thomasset. *Sexuality and Medicine in the Middle Ages.* Translated by Matthew Adamson. Princeton, NJ: Princeton University Press, 1988.

Kim M. Phillips

THOUSAND AND ONE NIGHTS. *Alf Laylah wa Laylah, The Thousand and One Nights,* commonly known as the Arabian Nights, is a collection of Indian, Persian, Arabic, and Egyptian folktales. Abu abd-Allah Muhammed el-Gahshigar of the ninth century was the first Arabic compiler. Stories of Indian origin were added to the Persian work, *Hazar Afsana* (thousand tales) in the tenth century by al-Jahshiyari of Iraq. The endless additions from different sources and developing through centuries, the Arabian Nights became a composite work with many forms.

The setting of the stories is somewhere between India and **China** with a temperamental sultan named Shahrayar, who was betrayed by his first wife. She and her servants were found having affairs with the slaves. Believing wrongly in the infidelity of women, he had taken a vow to behead a new wife in the morning after sleeping together in the night. His cruel operation continued for three years. When there was death of virgins, it was the turn of the Wazir's daughter to become the sacrificial lamb. The elder daughter, Shahrazad, well versed in history and biographies of the kings, volunteered for **marriage** to the sultan. She went to the palace along with her sister Dunyzad. The resourceful woman bemused the sultan by telling him different stories each night for 1,001 days.

The subject matters of each story varied: tales of scandal with a tinge of bawdiness, amorous affairs of unfaithful wives, love stories, tragedies, comedies, and fables and stories pertaining to **magic**, famous palaces, jinns, and Islamic religious legends.

Geography, historical characters, and important places were also dealt with. The Khalifa Harun al-Rashid occupied a central position. Apart from the Aladdin and the Wonderful Lamp, Sindbad the Sailor, and the tale of Ali Baba and the Forty Thieves, there were many stories like The Fisherman and the Jinni, The Porter and the Three Ladies of Baghdad, The Tale of the Bull and the Ass, Kalandar's Tale, Tale of Nur Al-Din Ali and His Son Badr Al-Din Hasan, The Eldest Lady's Tale, etc. The beautiful and resourceful Shahrazad triumphed over the king, giving him three sons, and Shahrayar ended the vow of killing a bride after being convinced of her loyalty.

Through the medium of stories, intrepid Shahrazad saved her own life and those of other women and thus put herself in an exalted position. She emerged from the stories as an intelligent woman fighting for survival through the art of storytelling. *See also* Islamic Society.

Further Reading: Irwin, Robert. *The Arabian Nights: A Companion.* London: Allen Lane, 1994; Lane, Edward William, trans. *Stories from Thousand and One Nights (The Arabian Nights' Entertainments).* The Harvard Classics. Vol. 16. New York: P.F. Collier & Son, 1909–1914; Mahdi, Muhsin. *The Thousand and One Nights.* New York: Brill, 1995.

Patit Paban Mishra

TIBET. Tibetan society has traditionally been relatively open sexually, with a great diversity of **marriage** practices and less oversight of sexual behavior. Perhaps in part for this reason, Tibet was the most receptive premodern Asian society to the dissemination of the most sexually oriented form of **Buddhism, Tantric Buddhism.**

LOVE AND MARRIAGE. Three forms of marriage were common in Tibet. Monogamy was widespread, but most common in the region of Amdo in the Northeast. **Polygamy** was less common, the prerogative of the wealthy. Polyandry was the most common form of marriage, found in both farming and nomadic communities. Normally fraternal polyandry was practiced. A single woman would be the wife of a group of brothers, who would participate in the economic maintenance of the estate and raise their children collectively. Given the marginal nature of most Tibetan farmland, this was a sensible practice, as it prevented the division of farming estates into nonviable units and kept the population at a sustainable level. It also facilitated a division of labor, with brothers responsible for various aspects of the household economy, such as farming, animal husbandry, and trade. Brothers who refused to participate in the marriage were not entitled to a division of the estate. These men typically became monks or traders.

Polyandry placed women in a position of considerable power and probably contributed to the relative autonomy of Tibetan women. A woman in a polyandrous marriage, however, would have the difficult task of negotiating good relations with all her husbands, in spite of the fact that she might have a greater preference for one of them.

Unlike many surrounding societies, Tibetan society typically did not place great value on female **virginity**. Among nomadic groups, sexual relations among unmarried young people was condoned, and pregnancy in an unmarried young woman could make her a desirable candidate for marriage, as it demonstrated her fertility. While women typically would not inherit property, they were entitled to a dowry, usually consisting of jewelry, that would remain their property. When a family had no sons, the eldest daughter could inherit property. She would then marry a man who would assume her family name. **Adultery** was condoned in parts of Tibet.

RELIGION AND SEXUALITY. The dominant religion in Tibet was Buddhism, which became the officially established religion during the eighth century. Prior to the eighth century, the pre-Buddhist religion, Bon, appears to have had no problem with marriage and sexuality. Buddhism has traditionally focused on celibate monasticism. However, the form of Buddhism imported into Tibet, Tantric Buddhism, celebrated sexuality as a potentially liberating practice. During the eighth century, the pivotal figures in the transmission of Buddhism to Tibet included a celibate monk and a noncelibate yogi. The former was Shantarakita (725–788 CE), a monk invited by King Trisongdetsen (742–c. 797 CE) to build the first monastery in Tibet. However, according to Tibetan legendary accounts, the temple could not be built without the supernatural power of Padmasambhava. According to his biographies, Padmasambhava had several consorts, including the Indian princess Mandarava and the Tibetan princess Yeshe Tsogyal (757–817 CE).

Padmasambhava needed consorts because he was a practitioner of Tantric Buddhism, many traditions of which call for the practice of sexual yogas. These practices typically involve the movement of vital energies into the central channel of the subtle body while engaged in sexual union. Several Tibetan traditions allow religious specialists to marry. The married lamas can turn to the legends of great figures such as Padmasambhava in order to legitimize their noncelibate lifestyle.

In spite of these legitimizing myths, there have been several attempts in Tibetan history to reform Buddhist practice to strengthen celibate monasticism, seen as the foundation of the Buddhist religion. These include the efforts of the kings of western Tibet to invite the great Indian saint Atisha (982–1054 CE) to Tibet in the early eleventh century in order to reform the monastic orders. Tsongkhapa (1357–1419 CE), the founder of the Geluk school of Tibetan Buddhism, was likewise concerned with the establishment of strict celibate monasticism. Celibate monasticism is practiced in all the traditions of Tibetan Buddhism, as well as in the Bon tradition, which borrowed this institution from the Buddhists. In spite of its prevalence, there have also been many transgressions of the monastic rules governing sexuality. Several powerful monks had mistresses, and homosexual love was widely believed to occur periodically within the monastic walls.

Further Reading: Aziz, Barbara. *Tibetan Frontier Families*. Chapel Hill: University of North Carolina Press, 1978; Goldstein, Melvyn, and Cynthia Beall. *Nomads of Western Tibet*. Berkeley: University of California Press, 1990; Stein, R. A. *Tibetan Civilization*. London: Faber and Faber, 1972.

David B. Gray

TRANSGENDERISM AND CROSS-DRESSING. Cross-dressing and the adoption of a social gender different from one's biological sex, temporarily or permanently, took place for many reasons in medieval societies. Some societies allowed an institutional place for transgendered individuals, as did **India** with its male-to-female community of **hijras**, but in most transgendered or cross-dressed people were isolated individuals.

Condemnation of cross-dressing and other forms of transgendered behavior goes back in the Jewish and Christian traditions as far as the book of Deuteronomy. Latin Europe's hostility to the cross-dresser drew on this tradition, but was also specifically aimed at European paganism. Cross-dressing was sometimes associated with classical and Germanic pre-Christian pagan rituals (although it was also forbidden in some pre-Christian German law codes). Although church law condemned all transgendered behavior, there was ambivalence toward biologically female cross-dressers. Female cross-dressing, whether accompanied by the adoption of a male social identity or not, was associated with a desire to move up in society, particularly in religious or military careers. The best-known female-to-male cross-dressers in medieval Europe were political and religious leaders, including **Joan of Arc** and one figure of legend, "**Pope Joan.**" In both cases, their adoption of male garb led to a bad end after a run of successes.

Female-to-male transgenderism was also part of the life, or legend, of some recognized saints of the church. Female saints like Pelagia and Euphrosyne supposedly cross-dressed to live as members of male monastic communities, successfully concealing their biological sex for many years, sometimes until death. (The legends of most of these saints originated in the Greek Mediterranean during the early centuries of Christian monasticism.) Hagiographers presented their impersonations as heroically chaste rather than perverse. Female-to-male cross-dressing also received some positive treatment in more secular literature. In a few narratives, such as the French epic *Tristan de Nanteuil*, a heroine's disguise as a male was validated by engagement or **marriage** to a woman and a magical or miraculous transformation into a man. This plot, which also appears in classical Greek and Latin as well as Arabic and Indian writings, would not have been completely incredible, as it was received medical opinion that it was possible for some women to spontaneously transform into men. The reverse was not considered possible and appeared far less often in literature.

Women outside Europe also cross-dressed as men to play traditionally male roles, such as military leadership. The Muslim equivalent of Joan of Arc was Sultana Raziya of the Delhi Sultanate, who reigned from 1236 to 1240. Designated as heir by her father to the exclusion of his sons, Raziya dressed as a man and appeared without a **veil**, although this strategy was as ultimately unsuccessful for Raziya as it was for Jeanne. The legendary Chinese heroine Mulan, whose story dates as far back as the Tang dynasty, also cross-dressed to serve as a soldier, although her story differs from Jeanne's and Raziya's in that she actually passed as a man and served as a common soldier rather than a leader.

A more playful and erotic form of female-to-male cross-dressing was based on the idea that it enhanced a woman's appeal to men. This practice among the Arabs was associated with a story of Zubayda, wife of the Caliph Harun-ar-Raschid. Concerned about her son, the future Caliph Al-Amin, and his sexual preference for young **eunuchs**, she had slave women with boyish figures put on male clothes and haircuts and brought before him. This led to a fashion for "boy-girls" in Baghdad society, which lasted for many decades and spread down the social scale from the Caliphal court to tavern society. The "boy-girls" even went so far as to paint mustaches on their faces.

Cross-dressed men appear less frequently in medieval European writings than do women. Male cross-dressing was seldom associated with the adoption of a female gender role. Rather it was an illicit means for men to gain access to women normally forbidden to them. In **Marie de France**'s *lai* of Yonec, for example, a knight with shape-changing abilities flew as a hawk into the tower where a jealous husband has imprisoned his wife, and, changing into his own form, announces that he loves her. When the woman hesitates, because she cannot be sure that he is a Christian, the knight volunteers to demonstrate this by taking communion from her chaplain. To fool the chaplain, the knight takes the form of the lady. Marie does not condemn this behavior. Male-to-female cross-dressing played little role in the European male homosexual world, which followed the classical model in being based on relationships differentiated by age rather than by gender roles. **China** followed a similar pattern, with little association between male cross-dressing and homosexuality outside the theatrical world where biological males played female roles.

By the later Middle Ages, the theater was also an area of sanctioned male-to-female cross-dressing and role play in Europe. Women were forbidden to appear on stage, so female roles had to be played by men or boys.

Further Reading: Bullough, Vern L., and Bonnie Bullough. *Cross-Dressing, Sex and Gender*. Philadelphia: University of Pennsylvania Press, 1993.

William E. Burns

TRIAL OF THE TEMPLARS (1307–1308). The destruction of the Order of the Temple by King Philip IV "the Fair" (r. 1285–1314) of France in 1307–1308 was an early example of the linking of charges of demon worship with charges of sexual deviance, a linkage that would become particularly prominent in the late medieval and early modern witch hunt. The Order was an organization of knights under religious vows, originally founded in the crusader states of the Middle East with the purpose of fighting the Muslims to defend Christian possessions there. With the loss of the last Christian outpost in 1291, the Order had less justification for its existence, but it remained vastly rich and powerful. Philip's motivation for his attack on the Order was in all likelihood simply the seizure of its wealth and the destruction of its political power. In order for the legal assault on a religious order to work, though, Philip claimed to be acting at the behest of an Inquisitor, and the charges were that the Order had violated its vows. Philip's agents charged the Templars with using an initiation ceremony requiring novices to deny Christ, spit on the cross, strip naked, and submit to three "**kisses of infamy**" from the master, on the buttocks, navel, and mouth, and sometimes another kiss on the penis (or to kiss the master in the same fashion.) The Templars were charged with universal **sodomy** as well as orgies with female demons, and worshipping an idol called Baphomet and a demonic cat who they kissed beneath the tail. It was claimed that new Templars took a vow binding them to never refuse to engage in homosexual acts with another Templar. (In fact, as a monastic order the Temple required that new recruits take a vow of chastity.) Assent to these charges was won from Templars who were tortured into confession, with the use of strappado, the rack, and holding the suspect's feet to a fire. Templars judged guilty were burned at the stake as heretics. The last Commander of the Order, Jacques de Molay, was burned in 1314, protesting his and the Order's innocence. Modern historians of the Templars regard the charges as false, although in the all-male environment of the Temple there may have been some basis to the charges of homosexuality.

Philip got away with this because the Papacy, which was supposed to oversee the Temple, was weak and dependent on French power. French pressure forced the pope to dissolve the order in 1312. The satanic and sexual charges against the Temple differed from those made against other groups of medieval heretics like the Cathars in that they were made by the French secular government rather than by the church. This is the earliest example of a secular government involving itself in such things, setting a precedent for the witch hunt. *See also* Witches and Witch-Hunting.

Further Reading: Barber, Malcolm. *The Trial of the Templars*. Cambridge: Cambridge University Press, 1978; Cohn, Norman, *Europe's Inner Demons: The Demonization of Christians in Medieval Christendom*, Rev. ed. Chicago: University of Chicago Press, 2000.

William E. Burns

TRISTAN. The legendary hero Tristan (Tristran, Tristram, etc.) was the nephew of King Mark of Cornwall and a Knight of the Round Table. He is most famous for his love affair with his uncle's wife, Iseut (or Isolde, in a common Germanic spelling).

Oral versions of *Tristan and Iseut* were circulating on the continent by the middle of the twelfth century. **Marie de France** bases her short but elegant *Chevrefoil* (c. 1165) on a clandestine rendezvous between the two lovers. In the introduction to *Cligés* (c. 1170), Chrétien de Troyes tells us that he created another tale, now lost, about "King Mark and Iseut the Blonde." Two Old French **romance**s develop the story in greater detail. The first was composed by Thomas of England and is known as the "courtly version" (c. 1172–1175). The second, "common version," was written by Béroul (c. 1179–1180). Eilhart von Oberg compiled a German *Tristrant* in the late twelfth century, which has not survived, and Gottfried von Strassburg formulated a lengthy and complex—although incomplete—adaptation of the love story around 1210.

In Béroul's account, Tristan goes to Ireland in order to bring back Iseut, who has been betrothed to King Mark. Secretly, Iseut's mother prepares a love potion for her daughter's wedding night and stows it within the ship. During the sea-crossing to Cornwall, however, the hot weather causes Tristan and Iseut to become thirsty. Mistaking the potion for wine, they ingest it and fall passionately in love. (The potion removes any intentionality in the lovers' actions; Béroul portrays them as victims of a force that is beyond their control.) Iseut marries Mark but continues to love Tristan, and the king's advisors try endlessly to trap the lovers and prove their **adultery**. Eventually, they flee to the forest. In a very touching scene, Mark discovers the two sleeping side by side, fully clothed, with Tristan's sword between them. Driven by anger, he is prepared to kill them both, but when he sees what appears to be the pure state of their union, he is overtaken by pity and love for his nephew and wife. He repents and forgives them, and as a sign of reconciliation, he places his own sword between the couple. As he is doing this, King Mark takes his glove and holds it above his wife's cheek, to shade her pale skin from the burning sun.

Gottfried's *Tristan* significantly expands upon the Old French sources. It is divided into two parts. The first recounts the love of Tristan's parents, Riwalin and Blanscheflor; the second—which is significantly longer—focuses on the escapades of Tristan and Isolde. For Gottfried, the protagonists' love exists on a higher plane. He explains in the prologue to his work that true lovers must suffer from excruciating anguish in order to become truly noble. Isolde exemplifies this paradigm when she refuses the gift of a magical bell that hangs around the neck of a dog (Petitcreiu) that Tristan wins for her. The person who hears the music of the bell will no longer experience any pain. Isolde, however, prefers to suffer and demonstrate her love for Tristan. The couple is discovered by the jealous King Mark, and Tristan must leave Cornwall. During his exile, he meets another princess, also named Isolde (of the White Hands). When the story breaks off, Tristan is torn between the two women. Later continuations—including those by Ulrich von Türheim (c. 1240) and Heinrich von Freiburg (c. 1290)—recount Tristan's **marriage** to Isolde of the White Hands. Despite his commitment, he never forgets his one, true love, Isolde the Blonde.

Most of the *Tristan* legends end with the hero's death. Having received a mortal wound, he sends messengers to summon his uncle's wife. The men devise a signaling system for Tristan to denote whether Iseut is on board or not as they make their way back into port. If she is with them, the sail will be white; if she cannot come, it will be black. Too ill to rise from bed, Tristan relies on his wife to watch for the ship. When it arrives and she sees the white sail, out of jealousy, she informs him it is black. Tristan breathes his last. Isolde arrives and, in turn, dies of grief in his arms.

Different versions of the legend survive in many medieval European languages. These include the thirteenth-century Scandinavian *Tristam Saga og Isonde* and the anonymous fourteenth-century Middle English *Sir Tristrem*. Tristan and Iseut's "Liebestod" (i.e., "story of love and death") was an extraordinarily popular and much beloved tale. *See also* Arthurian legend; Saga Literature.

Further Reading: Béroul. *The Romance of Tristan. The Tale of Tristan's Madness*. Translated by Alan S. Fedrick. New York: Penguin Classics, 1978; Hardman, Phillipa, ed. *The Growth of the Tristan and Iseut Legend in Wales, England, France, and Germany*. Studies in Medieval Literature 24. New York: Edwin Mellen Press, 2003.

K. Sarah-Jane Murray and Hannah Zdansky

TROBAIRITZ. Alongside the **troubadours**, there existed in the latter half of the twelfth and the opening decades of the thirteenth centuries several female poet-composers who also dealt with the theme of fin'amors—"fine" or "purified" love. These were the *trobairitz*. They wrote in *langue d'oc*, the vernacular of southern France. They tended toward less structurally intricate and more immediate poetry than that typically created by the troubadours, who often wrote complex stanzas voiced in the *persona* of a knight. Moreover, while the troubadours "idealized" love, the trobairitz usually wrote critically of the manner in which love was professed to them. A true picture of the times seems to require both perspectives.

Fewer than twenty names of the trobairitz survive and only twenty-three lyrics. Moreover, only a single song comes to us with a melody—"A chantar m'er de so qu'ieu non volria" ("To sing I must of what I would not")—of the Comtessa de Dia. (On musicological grounds, this melody might easily be a revision of her original, since it seems closer to the later style of the northern *trouvère*.)

The earliest of the trobairitz was likely Tibors, the sister of the troubadour Raimbaut d'Aurenga as well as the wife of Bertran de Baux, a major troubadour patron. Other important trobairitz are Maria de Ventadorn, Almucs de Castelnau, Garsenda, and Guillelma de Rosers.

A surprisingly large percentage of their surviving songs are *tensons*—putatively authored by two poet-composers in "dialogue." Nearly all these are cast as debates with male troubadours, although one—"Bona domna, tan vos ai fin coratge" ("Good lady, how deep for you is my care")—is a conversation between a married lady and an unmarried maiden.

Eleanor of Aquitaine deserves mention here for her important role in the diffusion of the new vernacular song. She was a patron of the art, and through her **marriage**s to Louis VII of France and later Henry II of England, she brought it north, thus planting seeds for the *trouvères* and, in time, the **minnesinger**. *See also* Bieris da Romans.

Further Reading: Bogin, Meg. *The Women Troubadours*. New York: W.W. Norton, 1980; Coldwell, M. V. "Jongleresses and Trobairitz: Secular Musicians in Medieval France." In *Women Making Music: The Western Art Tradition, 1150–1950*, edited by J. Bowers and J. Tick, pp. 39–61. Urbana: University of Illinois Press, 1986.

Edward Green

TROTULA (c. 1097–?). The Italian physician Trotula was one of the most famous physicians at the medical school in Salerno in southern Italy, the first Latin Christian medical school in southern Italy, although her existence remains a subject of scholarly debate to the present day. According to the legend, she both practiced and taught **medicine** at Salerno. Trotula married fellow physician John Platearius, and the two had two children. She collaborated with her husband on the medical encyclopedia *Regimen Sanitatis*.

Trotula focused primarily on women's health. Her most noted book is *Passionibus Mulierum Curandorum*, or *The Diseases of Women*. This work consists of sixty-three chapters with topics ranging from conception, pregnancy, and **childbirth** to various diseases and treatments. Contemporary physicians particularly appreciated her knowledge of gynecology. She revealed a method to ascertain the sex of an unborn baby. This procedure consisted of placing the mother's blood into a glass of water. If the blood sank to the bottom of the glass, the baby would be a boy.

Trotula especially sought to alleviate women's suffering in childbirth. She often used the drug opium to dull the pain. She also advocated the use of herbs, scented oils, and baths rather than surgery. Throughout her medical career at Salerno, Trotula also developed methods to cure sterility, acne, and other common ailments. One of her remedies for sterility was to have the patient eat the powdered testicles of a boar. If a woman wanted to induce sterility, however, Trotula advised her to carry a dried goat uterus in her pocket.

One of Trotula's colleagues at Salerno makes continued references to her groundbreaking work. Bernard of Provins reveals Trotula's manuscripts being studied by other Salerno faculty and nuns in the area. By the thirteenth century, John XXI (pope, 1276–1277) extensively quoted from Trotula's work in his *Thesaurus Pauperum*. Later physicians frequently praised Trotula's work. One even believed her to be among the seven most famous physicians at Salerno. She was also known by several other names including Trotta, Dame Trot, and Trocta.

Further Reading: Brooke, Elisabeth. *Women Healers: Portraits of Herbalists, Physicians, and Midwives*. Rochester, VT: Healing Arts Press, 1995; Hurt-Mead, Kate Campbell. "Trotula." *Isis* 14, no. 2 (October, 1930): 349–67.

Nicole Mitchell

TROUBADOURS. Throughout the twelfth and thirteenth centuries in southern France (Occitania), poet-composers created a new form of vernacular literature and planted the seeds for the future of Western songwriting. These were the troubadours. They wrote in Provençal, the *langue d'oc*. Their poetry tended toward intricacy of rhyme scheme and metric design, was overwhelmingly secular in emphasis, was almost always voiced in first-person singular, and had as its primary theme the radically new notion of *fin'amors*—"fine" or "purified" love.

In earlier medieval thought, it was love for God that elevated a person. Now it is love for a fellow human being. Many scholars have traced modern notions of "romantic" love to this conception.

Since most troubadours were male (female troubadours, such as the Comtessa de Dia, were called ***trobairitz***), there arose a cluster of literary tropes expressing the adoration of, and unquestioning service to, a *dompna*—his "lady." She was nearly always married and of a higher social class. While **adultery** was thus "in the air," it may be questioned how far it was actually advocated. In the same courts in which troubadours sang so openly on this theme, adultery was harshly punished. It is probable, therefore, something less bodily, and more spiritual, was most often being advocated.

The term "**courtly love**" was not used at the time. A late nineteenth-century coinage, it points to the fact that the troubadours wrote for an aristocratic audience. Sometimes, they were aristocrats themselves. The first known troubadour, **William IX** (1071–1127) was Duke of Aquitaine, and others—Jaufré Rudel, Bertran de Born, Arnaut Daniel, and Peire Cardenal—appear to have been, to varying degrees, of the nobility. According to the biographical *vidas* accompanying the manuscript evidence of

TROUBADOURS

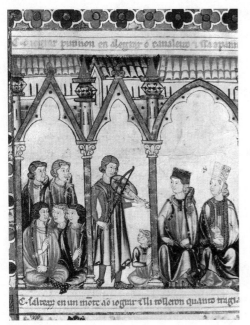

Troubadour playing for two princesses. From the *Canticles of Saint Mary*, a 13th century manuscript by Alfonso X, King of Castile and Leon. © The Art Archive/Real biblioteca de lo Escorial/Dagli Orti.

their work (all put down decades, if not centuries, after their deaths), some were so taken by the new art that they broke religious vows to become troubadours—Peire d'Alvernhe among these.

Most, however, were men of the lower classes whose artistic talent gained them aristocratic patronage. Some may have been *joglars*—singer-entertainers who served the Occitanian courts. (The word derives from the Latin for "juggler.") This may have been the case with **Marcabru**, one of the greatest of troubadours, and the earliest whose melodies survive.

We have approximately 2,600 troubadour lyrics, yet only 250 melodies. All in all, the names of 460 troubadours are known. Among the greatest (with those already mentioned) were Bernart de Ventadorn, Girault de Bornelh, and Peire Vidal. Guiraut Riquier, often called "the last troubadour," died in 1292. Due to the ravages of the Albigensian Crusades, the art died out in the land of its birth, but soon spread to northern Italy (eventually reflected in the poetry of **Dante Alighieri**), as well as to northern France (the *Trouvères*) and, through the **Minnesingers**, into German-speaking territory. Etymologically, troubadour and trouvre imply the concept of "finding"—poetry as discovery. Minnesinger means "singer of love."

The origins of troubadour song are complex and under scholarly dispute. Likely there was significant Arabic influence. Among the principal genres of their song (all monophonic) were the *vers, canso, pastorela, sirventes* (a sharply satiric song), *planh* (a song of lament), and the *tenso*—a song of debate, with the participation (real or implied) of two troubadours.

Further Reading: Akehurst, F.R.P., and Judith M. Davis, eds. *A Handbook of the Troubadours.* Berkeley: University of California Press, 1995; Briffault, Robert. *The Troubadours.* Translated and edited by Lawrence Koons. Bloomington: Indiana University Press, 1965; Rosenberg, Samuel, Margaret Switten, and Gérard Le Lot, eds. *Songs of the Troubadours and Trouvères: An Anthology of Poems and Melodies.* New York: Garland Publishing, 1998.

Edward Green

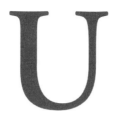

UDHRITE LOVE. Udhrite love, an elegiac and chaste love, is so called after the name of the Banu Udhra, a tribe of Yemenite origin that settled in the northern part of Hijaz. In the Umayyad period an amatory genre of poetry emerged among the Banu Udhra, giving birth to what the Arabic tradition calls udhrite love. This is considered the counterpart of the realistic and frivolous erotic poetry of the Hijazi school, whose main representative is **Umar Ibn Abi Rabia**. The Banu Udhra are depicted in the Arabic tradition as "people who, when they love, die," the same words mentioned by Heinrich Heine in his poem "Der Asra," through which they became famous in European literature.

The main features of udhrite love are chastity (in the sense that the lovers refrain from illicit love), faithfulness until death, passion for a unique woman, and absolute devotion to the beloved. It is a noble and sentimental love, born even before the birth of the two lovers, extolled by suffering and resignation, a perennial pact that ties the lovers until death. Dying of love is in fact compared to martyrdom.

Udhrite poetry develops the tradition of the pre-Islamic nasib (amatory prelude of the ode) in its emotional appeal by speaking of a present love, in contrast to the past love of the nasib. Its tone is introspective and imbued with melancholy and longing for the beloved whose beauty is often referred to, but without any detailed description. Love transcending death, the idea that the two souls will meet beyond the grave, is often found in the verses of udhri poets. The bedouin origins of udhrite poetry (in contrast to the urban roots of hijazi poetry) are stressed by the use of traditional meters and a conventional style and patterns of composition, even if the archaic language of the bedouin tradition is abandoned in favor of one more simple and immediate.

The best-known udhrite poet is Jamil (d. 701), whose love for Buthayna is represented in elegiac and spontaneous verses. In the early Abbasid period they were transformed into romantic heroes and their story gave birth to a very popular legend. The same can be said of other famous udhri poets and their beloved, as Majnun and Layla or Kuthayyir and Azza. The stories that circulated about them soon became a literary topos following this pattern: the two heroes, who grew up together, fall in love and want to marry, but the family prevents them from **marriage**, or eventually obliges them to **divorce**. The woman is married to another man, but nevertheless the two lovers remain faithful until death, or die of sorrow. Whatever change the idea of udhrite love has undergone during the ages, it has always been identified with bedouin and chaste as opposed to urban and frivolous love. *See also* Courtly Love.

Further Reading: Blachere, Regis. *Histoire de la litterature arabe des origines a la fin du XVe siecle*. Paris: A. Maisonneuve, 1952–1966; Giffen, Lois Anita. *Theory of Profane Love among the Arabs: The Development of the Genre*. New York: New York University Press, 1971.

Antonella Ghersetti

UMAR IBN ABI RABIA (644–712/721). Umar ibn Abi Rabia was a famous Arab love poet of the Umayyad period, perhaps the most known representative of the Hijazi poetic school. Information about his life is scanty. We know that he belonged to a rich family of the Meccan aristocracy and that he spent long periods of his life in Medina. The toponyms he often quotes in his poems do not constitute proof of the journeys that some traditions attribute to him but rather constitute imaginative settings. He often came back to Mecca, in particular during the pilgrimage periods, an opportunity for mischief and amorous adventures. Although his life is generally depicted as dissolute, one tradition claimed he repented at the end of his life, and even died as a martyr during a shipwreck while he was going to fight the holy war.

Umar played an important role in the urban society of the Hijaz, which saw the emergence of a leisured aristocracy: he was the esteemed companion of poets and musicians. His poetry testifies to the amorous adventures he had with many ladies of rank belonging to the noble families of the Hijaz, including the family of the Caliph. His diwan consists of 333 poems and 109 fragments. Although it includes exemples of panegyric, tribal pride, and elegy, his poems are mostly erotic. Both forms of classical erotic poetry can be recognized in Umar's poetry: the lengthy one, polythematic (a sequence of themes), and the short one, monothematic (love poetry). The latter one was probably conceived to be sung. His poetry, written in simple and direct language, was highly appreciated during his life and his contemporaries called him "the best poet of love." The characteristic features of his poetic production are the light-hearted and sometimes frivolous tone, the vividness in the description of love encounters (typically very concrete and not at all platonic), the extensive use of dialogue, remarkable psychological insight, and the active role played by women in their relationships. A frequent use of parody of both the themes of the literary tradition and himself must also be stressed. With his use of dialogue and insertion of individual elements, he made an important contribution toward the development of Arabic erotic poetry.

Further Reading: Blachere, Regis. *Histoire de la litterature arabe des origines a la fin du XVe siecle*. Paris: A. Maisonneuve, 1952–1966.

Antonella Ghersetti

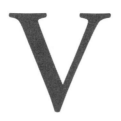

VEIL. The veil has never been as popular as it was during the late Middle Ages when it was in vogue both in western Europe and the Muslim lands. It was introduced to Muslims in the tenth century through assimilation of Byzantine and Persian customs. Initially, Muslims adopted the veil to represent social status; only later did the veil symbolize modesty. While the Islamic injunction to dress modestly has a wide range of interpretations, by the sixteenth century *yashmak* (veil) had become obligatory in the Ottoman empire.

Veiling serves both cultural and functional needs. Nomadic life imposed certain functional requirements on clothing. Desert life meant people needed clothing that protected them against the scorching sun, cold winds, and blowing sand—thus, the need for a cloak to protect the face and head from the sun and sand, and the headdress that serves as hat, veil, and shawl. Basic patterns have remained unchanged despite advances in manufacturing, tailoring, and increased selection in cloth. While veiling practices vary widely, they all need at least one of the following basic elements: a scarf, headband, overdress, cloak, and face mask.

When the Roman empire fell, the only large power left in Europe was the Church. Europeans were concerned with survival and clothing had to be functional. Women were expected to cover their hair after **marriage** with a veil. This sign of Christian chastity and modesty is still evident in some parts of Europe today.

By the ninth century, clothing began to change because of the increase in trade. The first Crusade captured Jerusalem in 1099, introducing Europe to sumptuous fabrics and better weaving techniques. Initially sheering scissors were used for cloth. The Crusades brought back smaller scissors made exclusively for fabric, which contributed to improvements in construction techniques. Women wore wimples, cloth veils draped over the head, around the neck and up to the chin. The barbette (a crown-type accessory) secured the wimple.

By the thirteenth century a prosperous merchant class was rising as was their disposable income. One way they displayed wealth was through clothing. At that time hair was braided and worn in buns over the ears. Hair nets woven from silk and gold held the buns in place. This style gave way to an entire fashion of elaborate headdresses. One of these is the butterfly, which incorporated a hair cap and wires with sheer fabric draped over it. The steeple-shaped hennin (cone-shaped hat with long trailing veil) and horned veil were also popular during this time. They both completely covered the hair. Given the preparation time and restrictions these veils placed on the wearer, these styles could only be maintained by the rich.

While veiling practices are influenced by other cultures and earlier eras, there was no "wholesale" adoption. Cultural developments in human history occur by processes of independent innovation and through assimilation and syncretism. Veiling practices carry multiple layers of meaning in diverse contexts. Each region in the different eras used the same or similar elements in different ways and gave veiling a different meaning unique to its customs and traditions. *See also* Islamic Society; Seclusion of Women.

Further Reading: Ahmed, Leila. *Women and Gender in Islam: Historical Roots of a Modern Debate.* New Haven, CT: Yale University Press, 1992; Cosgrave, Bronwyn. *The Complete History of Costume & Fashion: From Ancient Egypt to the Present Day.* New York: Checkmark Books, 2001; Eicher, Joanne, ed. *Dress and Ethnicity: Change across Space and Time.* Oxford: Berg, 1995; Norris, Herbert. *Medieval Costume and Fashion.* Mineola, NY: Dover Publications, 1999; Stowasser, Barbara. *Women in the Qur'an, Traditions and Interpretation.* New York: Oxford University Press, 1994.

Muhammed Hassanali

VIRGIN MARTYRS. Since the initial spread of Christianity, there have been women who have risen to prominence marked by the seal of **virginity**, a symbol of their special relationship with God, and their readiness to surrender their lives for Him. Their martyrdom usually came about because they were the objects of desire for men, who wanted to take the place of Jesus, the Bridegroom, and take their virginity. These martyrs were the protagonists of an exceptional cult of the Middle Ages.

Among the most well-known virgin martyrs were Lucy of Siracusa, Catherine of Alexandria, Agatha of Catania, Margaret of Antiochia, Agnes, Emerenziana of Rome, and others. Sometimes the tyrant previously described was a stepfather, as in the story of Christine of Bolsena or Barbara; however, the common factor is the refusal to be subjugated by the wishes of a domineering man. For the virgin Apollonia this act brought her to the point of suicide, throwing herself in the fire to escape the sexual desires of her persecutors, the only case qualified from church history to be acknowledged as martyrdom and justified by Saint **Augustine** himself.

Tortures suffered by the virgins usually centered on sexually attractive parts of the body, like the cut breasts of Agatha of Catania, the ripped eyes of Lucy of Siracusa, or the eradicated teeth of Apollonia. These body parts in turn became what the martyrs were considered the patron saints of, protecting each respective part of the body. However, Catherine of Alexandria was summoned by young girls, asking help to find a husband.

The Middle Ages added to the number of the legendary virgin martyrs, who inflamed the fervid imagination of devotees, with fictional women like Ursula and her 11,000 virgins, followers, and many others, whose dead bodies were found in catacombs, churches, and caves. Their relics are more sought after than others, because they were brides of Christ and therefore more able to obtain favor from the intercession of their Divine Bridegroom.

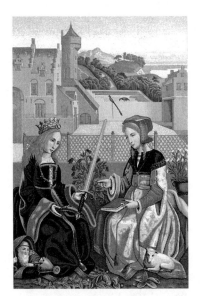

St. Catherine (left) and St. Agnes (right). Catherine of Alexandria, wearing a coronet representing royal descent, holds a sword and spiked wheel, instruments of her martyrdom in 307. Agnes, patron saint of virgins, is shown with her emblem, a lamb. © HIP/Art Resource, NY.

Martyred virgins differed from other martyrs in that they defended together with their faith, their chastity: their resistance was a virtue considered suitable to women. The woman who grants her virginity to this cause, testifies a noble and purer passion than sexual desire. The mystical-nuptial relationship, with the ability to make the supreme offer, was considered typical of female spirituality in which the senses are involved and transcended. The eschatological aspect made of the virgin's choice the sign of an exceptional strength of mind, so much as to overcome the division of the sexes. The virgin enters the shrine as bride of Christ realizing a superior state. Among the virgins and the church, an advantageous interchange was created. Women who escaped men, with martyrdom or later in the convents, were able to spiritually influence the church and the society. *See also* Catholicism; Joan of Arc; Wilgefortis, Saint.

Further Reading: *Bibliotheca Sanctorum.* 15 vols. Roma: Città Nuova Editrice, 1961–2000.

Elvio Ciferri

VIRGIN MARY. *See* Marianism

VIRGINITY. Virginity, closely associated with chastity, occupied an important place in medieval society, both spiritually and culturally. It was held in high regard by the Christian church, which praised young men and women for focusing their affection on the service of God rather than a baser, imperfect form of temporal love. In keeping with this ideology, the Christian clergy practiced **celibacy**. To theologians like St. **Bernard of Clairvaux**, the body of the virgin represented the Body of Christ—the church—faithfully awaiting her bridegroom, Christ. The most famous female virgin in the Christian world was Mary, mother of Jesus, to whom many cathedrals and churches were dedicated. Other chaste maidens were also venerated as saints, such as St. Agnes, the patron saint of virgins, who was martyred at age twelve or thirteen for refusing to marry and have sex. St. Lucy suffered a similar fate, as did the popular St. Foy, whose relics are enshrined at Conques (France) on the route to Compostela in Spain. The life of chastity was not solely reserved to young women, however; holy young men practiced sexual abstinence in imitation of Christ. For example, St. Alexis, a noble Roman youth, abandoned his bride on the night of their wedding, having recognized the incompatibility of loving her in the flesh and serving God. A rich body of religious poems, including the *Life of Saint Alexis* (c. 1040) and the *Song of St. Fides* (c. 1160–1180), were composed to commemorate such holy virgins.

Throughout the Islamic world, men and women were instructed to act modestly and remain chaste before **marriage** for the glory of Allah and the dignity of their family. The Eastern collection of tales known as the ***Thousand and One Nights*** attests to the importance of virginity before marriage in the Muslim world: King Shahriyar, torn and disgraced by the infidelity of his wife, henceforth takes a virgin in marriage to his bed every night, killing her the next morning so that she cannot commit **adultery**. Lifelong virginity, however, was neither promoted as a pious duty nor common. According to **Islam**, marriage is God's gift to his people. The conception and bearing of children is therefore considered a form of service to God. This ideology is reflected in the married status of many Islamic saints.

In both the East and the West, the physical intactness of unmarried women was highly valued. Tests were developed to prove a maiden's virginity. Sometimes a string was passed through the vagina to verify that the hymen was not broken. Physicians could also examine the woman's urine: she was declared a virgin if it was pure and clear. Cases are recorded of young women being given a variety of ground-up flowers to ingest. If the maiden urinated immediately afterward, she was considered corrupt.

The importance placed on physical intactness caused many women to resort to extreme treatments in order to feign chastity on their wedding night, such as applying leeches to the vagina. Albertus Magnus recounts the story of a maiden who, stricken with guilt after giving in to **lust**, attempts suicide on three occasions. When she cuts open her stomach, a sympathetic divine virgin appears and reestablishes the young woman's virginity.

Medieval women frequently sought to recapture their virginity by submitting themselves to a variety of treatments, including the inhaling of ill-smelling vapors and the application of foul pomades to their sexual organs. This concern was closely related to the fear of a disease named *suffocation matrices*, thought to cause women to suffocate if they had once been sexually active and later abstained. Widows were considered particularly susceptible to the illness. Christian widows could, however, reclaim their spiritual virginity by accepting God as their new bridegroom and living a life of faithful service and chastity.

The theme of virginity is reflected in many medieval legends. It is said, for example, that the magical unicorn can be taken by no hunter but will willingly lay his head on a virgin's lap. In the pan-European stories associated with *Tristan and Iseut*, the queen Iseut asks her virgin chambermaid, Brangein, to take her place in the nuptial bed, for fear that King Mark will discover that she is not physically intact. And in Chrétien de Troyes's *Cligés*, the heroine preserves her virginity for her lover by giving her husband a **magic** potion on their wedding night. Henceforth, the king dreams that he sleeps with his wife every night although in reality he never touches her. *See also* Chastity in Marriage.

Further Reading: Bernau, Anke, Ruth Evans, and Sarah Salih, eds. *Medieval Virginities*. Toronto, ON: University of Toronto Press, 2003; Coyn, Kathleen. *Performing Virginity and Testing Chastity in the Middle Ages*. New York: Routledge, 2000; Winstead, Karen A., ed. *Chaste Passions*. London: Cornell University Press, 2000.

Jamie A. Gianoutsos and K. Sarah-Jane Murray

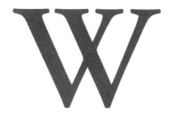

WALLADA BINT AL-MUSTAKFI (1011–1091). Wallada bint Al-Mustakfi was an Andalusian poet whose life and poetry were characterized by stormy love affairs. The daughter of the Caliph of Cordoba, Al-Mustakfi Billah (r. 1023–1031), and an Ethiopian Christian slave, she became fabulously rich at the age of thirty and led an independent life. Cordoba, the Jewel of the World, on the banks of the Guadalquivir was a cosmopolitan city of scholars and poets. Wallada opened her literary salon in the city, where poets, musicians, and ladies from aristocratic families gathered. The poetry of Wallada blossomed in this environment and her defiant attitude against conventions led her to walk the streets unveiled and with her own Arabic verses embroidered on her dress. One proclaimed that she deserved greatness and followed her path with pride. Another gave her cheek to her lover and her kisses to anyone longing for them. Wallada became a symbol of emancipation of women of her times. She was open in her sexual behavior and had passionate love affairs. Wallada became famous for her love toward another eminent poet, Ibn Zaydun (1003–1071).

Wallada had met Ibn Zaydun in her salon during a poetry recital. A passionate love affair followed. Their tempestuous and uninhibited affair included public displays of togetherness, scandals, court intrigues, condemnation from conservative forces, and above all love poems from both poets that enriched Arabic poetry. Wallada wrote that she would conceal Ibn Zaydun in the pupil of her eyes until the Day of Judgment in spite of her fear. When she discovered that Ibn Zaydun was making love to her favorite slave girl, she castigated him in a poem telling him that he chose a dark planet instead of a shining moon. Her scorn was more bitter with abusive poetry bordering on vulgarity, when she caught him in an affair with a man. The intrigue of the Caliph's Wazir, Abi Amer ibn Abdus, resulted in the banishment of Ibn Zaydun from the kingdom and Wallada coming under the protection of the Wazir. The love between the two poets has been immortalized in the sculpture of two hands reaching toward each other in a plaza of Cordoba.

Further Reading: Fletcher, Richard. *Moorish Spain*. Berkeley: University of California Press, 1993; Irwin, Robert, ed. *Night and Horses and the Desert: An Anthology of Classical Arabic Literature*. Woodstock, NY: Overlook Press, 2000; Menocal, Maria Rosa. *The Ornament of the World: How Muslims, Jews and Christians Created a Culture of Tolerance in Medieval Spain*. Boston: Little, Brown, 2002.

Patit Paban Mishra

WEDDING RITUALS. The rituals associated with **marriage**, expressed in a formal wedding ceremony, varied across cultures during the Middle Ages. In the Christian context marriage became a sacrament, which, in uniting husband and wife, reflected the union between Christ and his church. Medieval wedding rituals exhibited ceremonial, legal, and economic aspects.

From the early Middle Ages, Christian marriage involved symbolic rituals: the blessing by a priest, the presentation of a ring by the bridegroom to his bride (placed on the third finger of her left hand as a solemn promise of faithfulness), and the covering of the couple with a nuptial **veil**. In some cases vows and the ring were exchanged in a ceremony of betrothal (an undertaking to marry in future) with the wedding itself following later. Other familiar elements of the wedding ceremony that were known in the Middle Ages include the giving away of the bride by her father (or by friends or family) and the kiss between the bride and the groom. Not all medieval marriages took place in church. Secular weddings were celebrated in private homes or at other venues. Older secular practices (feasting; the giving of gifts) retained their popularity. But increasingly the legitimacy of marriage depended on participation in Christian rituals.

As ecclesiastical control over marriage became more entrenched from approximately the eleventh century, wedding rituals involved confirmation of the legal validity of marriage under **canon law** (the law of the church). Two important twelfth-century collections of church rulings, Gratian's *Decretum* and Peter Lombard's *Sentences*, clarified church teachings on what made a marriage valid. Gratian emphasized the need for freely expressed consent between the marrying couple, reinforced by consummation in the sexual act. Lombard refined this stance by insisting that consent needed to be exchanged in words of the present tense (*verba de presenti*) rather than being simply a promise to marry in future (*verba de futuro*). Thus the exchange of present consent became a central element of the marriage ceremony and reflected the desire of church authorities to ensure that the decision to marry was taken freely by the couple themselves, rather than being forced upon them by fathers and families (although the latter was often still the case).

Another requirement which became enshrined in canon law was that weddings should be celebrated publicly. The "reading of the banns" (an announcement that marriage would soon take place) was to occur thrice in the weeks preceding the ceremony, allowing anyone who knew of potential impediments to the marriage to come forward. The ceremony itself was conducted in public at the church door, where witnesses were able to observe proceedings. By the late Middle Ages a fixed liturgy laid out the order of ceremonies: reading of the banns, questioning of the couple by the priest, and exchanging of vows all at the church door, before the celebration of mass inside. The formal ceremony would end with the blessing of the marriage bed.

Despite the emphasis on consent and openness, economic considerations also influenced the rituals associated with marriage. Exchanges of gifts or property between the marriage partners themselves or between their families remained important throughout the Middle Ages, although the value of these exchanges tended to shift in favor of husbands rather than wives. Germanic societies of the earlier medieval period generally practiced a system of payments by the husband: either a "brideprice" (payment made to the bride's family) or a "morning gift" (*morgengabe*—payment to the bride herself as a settlement for her **virginity**). By the early part of the second millennium the practice of dowry had become more prevalent. In this case the bride or her family would offer wealth or property to the husband. The two forms of exchange were not mutually exclusive. Later medieval marriages often entailed both a dowry (or "marriage portion") from the bride's family and a dower: an allocation of wealth or land promised by the husband from his own resources as a means of support for his bride in the event of her widowhood. In practice husbands tended to retain control of both dowry and dower during their lifetimes, but the provision of dower allowed widows some independence if the rest of the husband's property passed to his children.

In the Orthodox Church, Byzantine wedding ceremonies retained a strong memory of Roman civil tradition along with Christian spiritual elements. Ornamentation of the nuptial chamber, the wearing of white clothing, the coronation of the couple, and an exchange of rings represented the union of husband and wife. Jewish weddings reflected the idea of marriage as both a spiritual and a legal event. Rabbinic tradition considered marriage an ideal state for man and woman, whereas in Western Christianity it was a compromise for those unable to fulfill the ideal of virginity or **celibacy**. All that was required for a valid marriage in **Judaism** was the presence of two witnesses and a document outlining financial arrangements (the *ketubah*), but more elaborate rituals became commonplace. These included blessing by a rabbi, public celebration, and the entry of the bride into her husband's house (often represented symbolically in the form of a canopy, the *chuppah*). Over time common practice separated the wedding into two parts, a betrothal (*erusin*) and a "completion" (*nisuin*). Islamic weddings were more legal than sacramental in nature. They required the confirmation of a witnessed document (the *'aqd nikah*), outlining each partner's rights and obligations (including the allocation of a dower by the husband), and were marked by the groom's questioning of his bride's intentions and her formal consent. This procedure was followed by familial celebrations and the exchange of gifts.

Further Reading: Broyde, Michael J., ed. *Marriage, Sex, and Family in Judaism.* Lanham, MD: Rowman and Littlefield, 2005; d'Avray, David. *Medieval Marriage: Symbolism and Society.* Oxford: Oxford University Press, 2005; Murray, Jacqueline, ed. *Love, Marriage, and Family in the Middle Ages: A Reader.* Peterborough, ON: Broadview Press, 2001; Sheehan, Michael M. *Marriage, Family, and Law in Medieval Europe: Collected Studies.* Toronto, ON: University of Toronto Press, 1996.

Lindsay Diggelmann

WILGEFORTIS, SAINT. The legendary St. Wilgefortis was the patron saint of young women who wished to disencumber themselves of an unwanted husband or suitor. Wilgefortis was frequently called upon by victims of **rape**, **incest**, and sexual abuse, as well as those seeking relief from specifically female medical problems, such as irregular **menstruation**, difficult pregnancies or deliveries, and infertility. Furthermore, it was believed that anyone who invoked Wilgefortis before dying would leave this world without anxiety. Her name is derived from either "hilge vratz" ("holy face") or "virgo fortis" ("strong virgin").

Wilgefortis's story was first written down in the early fifteenth century. She is said to be a Portuguese princess and to have had nine sisters, all born at one birth. When her father promised her hand in **marriage** to the pagan king of Sicily, Wilgefortis, who had taken a vow of chastity, prayed to God that she be disfigured in some way. In answer to her prayers, Wilgefortis miraculously sprouted a beard, causing her suitor to reject her. Her father became so outraged that he commanded that Wilgefortis be crucified.

The cult of St. Wilgefortis probably developed around a crucifix in the cathedral of Lucca (Italy). The figure, known as the *Volto Santo* ("holy face") and attributed to Nicodemus, represents Christ with a beard and long hair, wearing a crown, and clothed in a full-length regal robe. Such depictions of the crucifixion were not uncommon during the early Middle Ages. By the eleventh century, however, they had become exceedingly rare. In most cases, Christ's long robe had been replaced by a simple loincloth. It is hardly surprising therefore that the many reproductions of the *Volto Santo*, carried throughout western Europe by medieval pilgrims, were mistaken for the figure of a mysterious crowned and martyred woman, wearing a dress and strangely endowed with a beard.

Wilgefortis is known by many names, including Librada (Spain), Libertata (Portugal), Kümmernis (Germany), Uncumber (England), Ontkommer or Ontkommena (Low Countries), and Livrade (France). Her story is closely linked to those of St. Galla of Rome (d. 550) and Paula of Avila (fourteenth century), who also miraculously grew long beards so as to be less attractive to men. In iconography, Wilgefortis is typically represented as a young girl crucified. At other times, she is depicted as throwing her golden boot to a musician. This is in keeping with another legend according to which a destitute fiddler played before the virgin's martyred body. Wilgefortis gave him one of her golden boots. The fiddler, unjustly accused of stealing the boot, was sentenced to death. When he requested to play in front of Wilgefortis a second time, she kicked off the other boot and established his innocence in front of numerous witnesses. The feast of St. Wilgefortis is celebrated on July 20.

Further Reading: Friesen, Ilse E. *The Female Crucifix: Images of St. Wilgefortis since the Middle Ages*. Ontario, Canada: Wilfred Laurier University Press, 2001.

Jennifer Boulanger and K. Sarah-Jane Murray

WILLIAM IX, DUKE OF AQUITAINE AND GASCONY, COUNT OF POITIERS (1071–1126).

William IX was an important **troubadour** poet, the first whose work has been preserved. The thirteenth-century biographical sketch (*vida*) about him states: "The Count of Poitiers was one of the most courtly men in the world, and one of the greatest deceivers of women, and a good knight-at-arms and generous in his love life; and he was well able to compose and sing songs. And for a long time he traveled about the world in order to seduce women." He is described in clerical sources as "the enemy of all chastity and all feminine virtue," a supreme entertainer but at the same time a buffoon who turned everything—including divine Providence—into a joke.

William married in 1094 and had, altogether, two sons and five daughters. From 1099 to 1101 he participated in the First Crusade, but the army only got as far as Heraclea (modern Turkey) where it was annihilated by the Turks. William survived, reached Jerusalem as a pilgrim, and then returned home. In 1112 he began an affair with Dangerosa-Maubergeonne, the wife of a neighboring viscount, and was excommunicated—for the second time in his life—because of it. According to William of Malmesbury, he vowed to have her image engraved on his shield, to show that he supported her in battle just as she supported him in bed. His wife Philippa-Mathilde fruitlessly petitioned the pope for redress; in around 1117 she withdrew to the women's abbey of Fontevrault, whose foundation (by Robert of Arbrissel) William had mocked by declaring that he would found his own abbey of whores. Later (1120–1123), after he had stopped composing songs, William fought successfully against the Moors in Spain. He died in 1126, the year after the birth of his granddaughter, Eleanor of Aquitaine, future queen of France and queen of England.

Eleven lyric poems in Old Provençal constitute William's surviving *œuvre*. Love and sex—together with what William calls *foudatz* "folly, foolish love"—are major topics. So are politics, social pretences, and poetic craft itself. The poet generally courts the favor of the aristocratic *pro* or *bona gent* "high society" to which the noble Duke of

Aquitaine indeed belonged. Keen ironic wit, machismo, a high degree of self-awareness, and at times self-mockery characterize William's poetic persona. Some of his poems are fairly conventional celebrations of **courtly love** (*fin'amors*); others are more vulgar (as when he represents his choice between two ladies as deciding which of two horses to ride), or more personal. One poem compares the composition of poetry, and the act of love (the poet claims to be "Perfect Master" of both), to a game of chance with loaded dice; another exemplifies *foudatz*, relating how the poet-protagonist is set upon by two sexually insatiable so-called "ladies" and their scratching cat; a third (*Faray un vers de dreit niën* "I shall compose a poem about nothing at all") concerns the poet's lady-friend whom he has never seen, nor does he mean to. Some scholars view the last poem as a satire on the whole genre of courtly love poetry. Others argue it is meant quite seriously—though the unseen lady may not have a life outside William's poetic imagination, she is whole and beloved within it, and perhaps she satisfied him in a way that his real-life conquests could not.

Further Reading: Bond, Gerald A., ed. and trans. *The Poetry of William VII, Count of Poitiers, IX Duke of Aquitaine*. New York: Garland, 1982.

Matthieu Boyd

WITCHES AND WITCH-HUNTING. As the great witch hunt got under way in late medieval Europe, witchcraft became more strongly linked with sex. Sex between humans and demons played a large role in both demonological theory and actual witch trials. It was the ultimate form of physical interaction between the witch and the Devil, whether Satan himself or a lesser demon. The bond between devils and female witches was particularly likely to be conceptualized as sexual. This claim appears for the first time in a witch trial in 1324, when **Alice Kyteler** was tried in Ireland. However, the Kyteler case was not immediately followed by other sex-based witch cases, and the close linkage of witchcraft and sex was delayed until the fifteenth century and the beginnings of large-scale witch-hunting.

This immediately brought up the problem of how a material human body could have sex with an immaterial spirit. This was mainly a problem for intellectuals—for ordinary people, the relationship of spiritual devils to carnal intercourse was no mystery since they thought of devils as material beings anyway. The theoretical question of how demons could have intercourse with people was handled by claiming that devils, while ultimately spirits, could create a "body" out of compacted air. The artificial nature of the demonic body was particularly useful intellectually in explaining how women could conceive children by demons. The standard explanation, going back to **Thomas Aquinas**, was that the demon first formed and inhabited a female body as a succubus, had intercourse with a human male, and preserved the semen. It then formed and inhabited a male body as an incubus, ejaculating the preserved semen into a human woman's vagina. Thus the actual father of the woman's child was the human male. Despite this fact, many argued that the children conceived by demonic intercourse were more likely to become witches themselves, and to be especially powerful ones.

One curious aspect of human-demon sex as envisioned in medieval Europe was that it was hardly ever same-sex. The influential fifteenth-century demonologist and Inquisitor Heinrich Kramer, author of the *Malleus Maleficarum*, was among many who emphasized the horror even demons felt at the unnatural vice of **sodomy**. The goal of this distinction was not to palliate the sinfulness of the witch, but to emphasize that of the sodomite, who could be portrayed as worse than demons. Men were also believed to be able to gain favor with demons in ways other than sex.

Witchcraft was also associated with promiscuous sex between humans, opposite sex or same sex. Sexual orgies were closely associated with the idea of the sabbat, the meeting of witches presided over by the Devil or a lesser demon. The idea of the sabbat emerged in the mid-fifteenth century in writings such as the Dominican professor Johannes Nider's *Formicarius*, probably written between 1435 and 1438. Early descriptions of the sabbat including Nider's closely resemble medieval accounts of gatherings of heretics in featuring the **kiss of infamy** and group sex. *See also* Misogyny in Latin Christendom.

Further Reading: Cohn, Norman. *Europe's Inner Demons: The Demonization of Christians in Medieval Christendom*. Rev. ed. Chicago: University of Chicago Press, 2000; Stephens, Walter. *Demon Lovers: Witchcraft, Sex, and the Crisis of Belief*. Chicago: University of Chicago Press, 2002.

William E. Burns

WU ZETIAN (627–705). Wu Zetian, or Empress Wu, was the only official female ruler in Chinese imperial history. Born to an aristocratic family in Taiyuan of northern **China** as Wu Zhao, she was selected by the court as a low-ranking consort of the emperor Taizong (r. 627–649) during her early teens. After the emperor died, Wu Zhao was ordained as a Buddhist nun, a customary arrangement for those childless consorts, and was expected to spend the rest of her life in a monastery. However, Wu's charm caught the attention of the new emperor, Gaozong (r. 649–683), who visited her monastery in 650 to commemorate the emperor Taizong's anniversary. Wu was called back to the palace, first as a consort of the emperor Gaozong, and later as his empress, whereupon she took the title Zetian (655). It was said that her ascent to the position was accomplished by framing the reigning empress for the death of her daughter, a murder she herself committed.

The emperor Gaozong suffered a stroke in 660, and for more than three decades, Empress Wu ruled the dynasty on behalf of her husband and her son, the emperor Ruizong (r. 684–710). To consolidate her power and build her support base, Empress Wu demoted the officials who opposed her to provincial posts or had them executed on false charges. She promoted the Civil Service Examination to recruit high-ranking officials and carried out a series of reforms that promoted agriculture and reduced taxes. Unsatisfied with her position as an empress dowager, Wu Zetian demoted the emperor Ruizong to Emperor Expectant, declared herself the emperor in 690, and changed the name of the dynasty to Zhou (690–705).

To legitimize her rule, Empress Wu elevated **Buddhism** to the state religion. As a result, the membership of Buddhist temples and monasteries increased dramatically, as did the numbers of monks and nuns. Women's position improved significantly during her rule. At her urging, for example, the Tang court issued an edict to extend the mourning period for a mother to three years, the same as for one's father. She also employed scholars to write biographies of famous women.

Confucian historians often depicted Wu Zetian as a vicious and ruthless usurper. However, it is undeniable that the period of her dominance paved the way for the unprecedented political stability and economic wealth of the High Tang era.

Further Reading: Guisso, R.W.L. *Wu Tse-t'ien and the Politics of Legitimation in T'ang China*. Bellingham: West Washington University Press, 1978; Twitchett, Denis, and Howard J. Wechsler. "Kao-tsung (reign 649–83) and the Empress Wu: The Inheritor and the Usurper." In *The Cambridge History of China*, edited by Denis Twitchett and John K. Fairbank, 242–89. Vol. 3, part 1. Cambridge: Cambridge University Press, 1979.

Ping Yao

Y

YANG GUIFEI (719–756). Yang Guifei was the consort of the Emperor Xuanzong (r. 712–756) of the Tang dynasty in **China** (618–907). Her given name was Yuhuan; Guifei, or Precious Consort, was her rank in the imperial palace. Born to an official family, Yang Guifei was said to be exceptionally beautiful and talented in dance and music. In 736, she was selected by the imperial house to be the wife of Xuanzong's eighteenth son, Prince Shou. However, her beauty and charm captivated Xuanzong, and she was ordained a Daoist nun and moved into a monastery. This arrangement allowed her to leave her **marriage** with Prince Shou and paved the way for her to be remarried. In 745, Yang Guifei entered the palace and became the Precious Consort of Xuanzong.

The emperor's infatuation with Yang Guifei was evident. In her companionship, he neglected state affairs and showed no interest in the thousands of women in his **harem**. During their thirteen years together, Yang Guifei's family gained unprecedented influence. The emperor promoted her sisters to nobility and her male relatives to important offices. Among them was her cousin Yang Guozong, a prime minister, and her adopted son, An Lushan, a general of Turkic origin.

In 755, a power struggle over control of the central government broke out between Yang Guozong and An Lushan. An Lushan's army captured the capital and the imperial palace was completely ransacked. The An Lushan Rebellion (755–763) was the turning point of Tang history; the dynasty never recovered. As the royal entourage fled to Sichuan in southern China, the imperial army refused to march and demanded the execution of Yang Guifei and Yang Guozong. The helpless emperor relented and Yang Guifei hung herself in a Buddhist shrine. She was thirty-seven.

The Xuanzong-Guifei love story was brilliantly recaptured by the renowned Tang literatus, Bo Juyi (772–846), in his "Song of Lasting Regret." For over a thousand years, the poem was revered as an enduring masterpiece of beauty and passion, and Xuanzong-Guifei's vow, "to be on Earth as linked branches, in Heaven as one-winged birds," became a virtual manifesto of love in Chinese literary history.

Further Reading: Chen, Fan-pen. "Problems of Chinese Historiography as Seen in the Official Records on Yang Kuei-fei." *T'ang Studies* 8–9 (1990–1991): 83–96; Kroll, Paul W. "Po Chü-i's 'Song of Lasting Regret': A New Translation." *T'ang Studies* 8–9 (1990–1991): 97–104.

Ping Yao

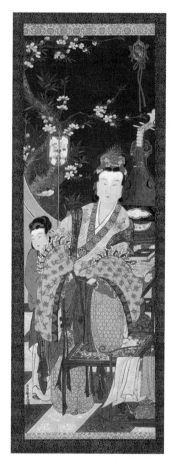

Yang Guifei was a symbol of beauty in women in East Asian cultures for many centuries after her death. This image is the work of the Japanese artist Kano Yoshinobu (18th–19th c.). HIP/Art Resource, NY.

ZHANG BODUAN (983–1082). Zhang Boduan was an influential Daoist alchemist. According to his biography in the *Complete Biographies of the Immortals* (*lie xian quan zhuan*) and Chinese government records, he was born in Tiantai, a city in eastern **China** in Zhejiang province. He was well educated and served as a military advisor to a high official of the Song dynasty. In 1069 CE, he traveled to Sichuan province to study alchemy with a master named Liu Haichan, who taught him the secrets of compounding the elixir. He also formed a close friendship with a Buddhist monk named Dinghui. According to his biography, both he and Dinghui possessed magical powers, such the power to travel long distances in meditative states. Following this study, he changed his name to Pingshu ("Peaceful Younger Brother") and took on the title of Ziyang ("Purple Yang"). He died at age ninety-nine at Jinhu. Following his death, his followers erected a temple in his honor and established the Ziyang "Purple Yang" school of Daoist alchemy.

His most important work, *Awakening to Truth* (*wu zhen pian*), was composed between 1075 and 1078. According to his biography, he gave it to his disciple Chu Hou, stating that it represents the entirety of his knowledge of alchemy. A classic of the tradition of inner alchemy, it is a cryptic text written in the style of Daoist alchemical poetry. The current version of the text contains ninety-nine poems, although an early district record states that the work consisted of eighty-one poems, which may indicate that the current text is an expansion of a shorter original work now lost. *Awakening to Truth* is a work of dualistic alchemy, advocating the union of feminine and masculine energies, *yin* and *yang*. These are coded by complex imagery that makes reference both to minerals such as mercury and lead, animals such as tigers and dragons, rabbits and crows, and celestial bodies such as the moon and the sun. Despite the references to minerals, it is generally understood as a work of internal alchemy, using symbols to refer to meditative exercises conducted within one's own body. While the text also poetically evokes male and female sexual union, this is understood by the commentators as referring to an internal alchemical process of union. In other words, it does not advocate the sexual cultivation practiced by some Daoists. It became very well known and has been commented upon by several prominent Daoists. *See also* Daoism.

Further Reading: Baldrian-Hussein, Farzeen. "Review of *Understanding Reality* by Thomas Cleary." *Harvard Journal of Asiatic Studies* 50, no. 1 (1990): 335–41; Cleary, Thomas. *Understanding Reality: A Taoist Alchemical Classic by Chang Po-tuan.* Honolulu: University of Hawaii Press, 1987; Davis, Tenny L., and Chao Yün-ts'ung. "Chang Po-Tuan of T'ien-T'ai, His

Wu Chen P'ien, Essay on the Understanding of the Truth." *Proceedings of the American Academy of Arts and Sciences* 73 (1939): 97–117.

David B. Gray

ZHANG ZHUO (c. 660–740). Zhang Zhou, courtesy name Wencheng, was a literati official of the Tang dynasty (618–907). He was known for his eight consecutive successes in the Civil Service Examinations and broad literary works. A *Jinshi* (Advanced Scholar) degree holder, Zhang Zhou took several court-official positions, with the highest being a Vice Director of the Transit Authorization Bureau. Three Tang literary works were attributed to him: *Stories of Government and the People* (*Chaoye qian zai*), *Rulings of Dragon Muscle Phoenix Marrow* (*Longji fengsui pan*), and *The Dwelling of Playful Goddesses* (*You xianku*). The first, *Stories of Government and the People*, recorded anecdotes, mysteries, and many of his personal encounters during the early period of the Tang dynasty. The book was widely cited by later scholars of Tang history. *Rulings of Dragon Muscle Phoenix Marrow* was a collection of Zhang Zhuo's essays on hypothetical legal cases and was one of the most valuable sources for study of medieval Chinese legal history and Chinese legal philosophy.

Zhang Zhuo's *The Dwelling of Playful Goddesses* was lost in **China** but preserved in **Japan** and had a profound influence on Japanese culture for more than a thousand years. Considered the first novelette and the earliest work of the "scholar and beauty" (*caizi jiaren*) romance genre, the story tells of the accidental encounter between a young official, Scholar Zhang, and a divinely beautiful woman, Shiniang. Scholar Zhang met Shiniang, who lived with her sister-in-law in a secluded mansion on the Jishi Mountains, during an official trip. Thanks to various schemes of the mischievous sister-in-law, Scholar Zhang and Shiniang were immediately attracted to each other and their affection grew rapidly. After an extended banquet and many games that often involved exchanging erotic poems, the two spent a long and passionate night together.

Further Reading: Levy, Howard S., trans. *The Dwelling of Playful Goddesses*. Tokyo: Dai Nippon Insatsu, 1965.

Ping Yao

Bibliography

Abbot, Elizabeth. *A History of Celibacy*. New York: Scribner, 2000.
Abdalati, Hammudah. *Islam in Focus*. Kuala Lumpur, Malaysia: Islamic Book Trust, 2001.
Abdullah, Achmed. *Lute and Scimitar*. New York: Payson & Clarke, 1928.
Abrahams, Israel. *Jewish Life in the Middle Ages*. Philadelphia: Jewish Publication Society of America, 1896.
Agrimi, Jole. *Ingeniosa scientia nature. Studi sulla fisiognomica medievale*. Florence: Sismel-Edizioni del Galluzzo, 2002.
Ahmed, Leila. *Women and Gender in Islam: Historical Roots of a Modern Debate*. New Haven, CT: Yale University Press, 1993.
Akehurst, F.R.P., and Judith M. Davis, eds. *A Handbook of the Troubadours*. Berkeley: University of California Press, 1995.
Albertus Magnus. *Man and the Beasts* (*De animalibus*, books 22–26). Translated by James J. Scanlan. Binghampton, NY: Medieval & Renaissance Texts & Studies, 1987.
Aldhouse-Green, Miranda J. *Celtic Goddesses: Warriors, Virgins and Mothers*. London: British Museum Press, 1995.
Alfonso X. *Cantigas de Santa Maria*. Madrid: Castalia, 1986.
Algar, Hamid. *Sufism: Principles and Practices*. Oneonta, NY: Islamic Publications International, 1999.
Ali, Abdullah Yusuf, trans. *The Holy Qur'an*. Indianapolis, IN: American Trust Publications, 1977.
Ali, Maulana Muhammad. *A Manual of Hadith*. 2nd ed. Lahore, Pakistan: The Ahadiyyha Anjuman Ishaat Islam, 2001.
Allen, Peter L. *The Art of Love: Amatory Fiction from Ovid to "The Romance of the Rose."* Philadelphia: University of Pennsylvania Press, 1992.
Anand, Margo. *The Art of Sexual Ecstasy*. Los Angeles: Jeremy P. Tarcher, 1989.
Andreas Capellanus. *On Love*. Translated by P. G. Walsh. London: Duckworth, 1982.
Aquinas, Thomas. *Summa Theologiae*. Translated by the Fathers of the English Dominican Province. Westminster, MD: Christian Classics, 1981.
Arberry, A. J. *Sufism: An Account of the Mystics of Islam*. 1950. Reprint, Mineola, NY: Dover Publications, 2002.
Arberry, A. J., ed. *Persian Poems: An Anthology of Verse Translations*. New York: Dutton, 1964.
Archer, W. G. *The Loves of Krishna: In Indian Painting and Poetry*. 1957. Reprint, Mineola, NY: Dover Publications, 2004.
Archibald, Elizabeth. *Incest and the Medieval Imagination*. Oxford: Oxford University Press, 2001.
Arden, Heather M. *The Romance of the Rose*. Boston: Twayne, 1987.
Arjava, Antti. *Women and Law in Late Antiquity*. Oxford: Oxford University Press, 1996.
Arntzen, Sonja, trans. *Ikkyu and the Crazy Cloud Anthology: A Zen Poet of Medieval Japan*. Tokyo: University of Tokyo Press, 1986.

Atiya, Aziz S. *A History of Eastern Christianity*. Notre Dame, IN: University of Notre Dame Press, 1968.

Augustine of Hippo. *On Christian Doctrine*. Translated by D. W. Robertson Jr. Upper Saddle River, NJ: Prentice Hall, 1997.

Awde, Nicholas, ed. and trans. *Women in Islam: An Anthology from the Qur'an and Hadiths*. New York: St. Martin's Press, 2000.

Ayalon, David. *Eunuchs, Caliphs and Sultans: A Study in Power Relationships*. Jerusalem: Magnes Press, Hebrew University, 1999.

Aziz, Barbara. *Tibetan Frontier Families*. Chapel Hill: University of North Carolina Press, 1978.

Babras, Vijaya G. *The Position of Women during the Yadava Period: 1000AD to 1350 AD*. Mumbai, India: Himalaya Publishing House, 1996.

Badawi, Jamal. *Gender Equity in Islam: Basic Principles*. Indianapolis, IN: American Trust Publications, 1995.

Bakalian, Ellen Shaw. *Aspects of Love in John Gower's "Confessio Amantis."* New York: Routledge, 2003.

Baldick, Julian. *Animal and Shaman: Ancient Religions of Central Asia*. New York: New York University Press, 2000.

Baldrian-Hussein, Farzeen. "Review of *Understanding Reality* by Thomas Cleary." *Harvard Journal of Asiatic Studies* 50, no. 1 (1990): 335–41.

Baldwin, John W. *The Government of Philip Augustus: Foundations of French Royal Power in the Middle Ages*. Berkeley: University of California Press, 1986.

Baldwin, John W. *The Language of Sex: Five Voices from Northern France around 1200*. Chicago: University of Chicago Press, 1997.

Bano, Afsar. *Status of Women in Islamic Society*. Vols. 1 and 2. New Delhi: Anmol Publicatons, 2003.

Barber, Malcolm. *The Cathars: Dualist Heretics in Languedoc in the High Middle Ages*. New York: Longman, 2000.

Barber, Malcolm. *The Trial of the Templars*. Cambridge: Cambridge University Press, 1978.

Baumgarten, Elisheva. *Mothers and Children: Jewish Family Life in Medieval Europe*. Princeton, NJ: Princeton University Press, 2004.

Bell, Joseph Norment. *Love Theory in Later Hanbalite Islam*. Albany: State University of New York Press, 1979.

Berger, Sidney E. "Sex in the Literature of the Middle Ages." In *Sexual Practices and the Medieval Church*, edited by Vern L. Bullough and James A. Brundage, 162–75. Buffalo, NY: Prometheus Books, 1982.

Bernard of Clairvaux. *On Loving God*. Translated by Emero Stiegman. Kalamazoo, MI: Cistercian Publications, 1995.

Bernau, Anke, Ruth Evans, and Sarah Salih, eds. *Medieval Virginities*. Toronto, ON: University of Toronto Press, 2003.

Béroul. *The Romance of Tristan: The Tale of Tristan's Madness*. Translated by Alan S. Fedrick. New York: Penguin Classics, 1978.

Besteiro, J. M. Forneas, and C. Alvarez de Morales. *Kitab al-Kulliyyat fi l-tibb*. Madrid: Escuela de Estudios Arabes de Granada, 1987.

Bey, Hakim. *O Tribe That Loves Boys*. Amsterdam: Entimos Press, 1993.

Bhattacharya, S. K. *Krsna-cult in Indian Art*. New Delhi: M.D. Publications, 1996.

Bhyani, H. C., ed. *Vasudevahindi Majjimakhando*. Lalbhai Dalpatbhai Series 99. Ahmedabad: Lalbhai Dalpatbhai Institute of Indology, 1979.

Bibliotheca Sanctorum. 15 vols. Roma: Città Nuova Editrice, 1961–2000.

Bierhorst, John, ed. *A Nahuatl-English Dictionary and Concordance to the Cantares Mexicanos*. Stanford, CA: Stanford University Press, 1985.

Bierhorst, John, trans. *Cantares Mexicanos: Songs of the Aztecs*. Stanford, CA: Stanford University Press, 1985.

Biller, Peter. "Cathars and Material Women." In *Medieval Theology and the Natural Body*, edited by Peter Biller and A. J. Minnis, 61–107. Rochester, NY: York Medieval Press, 1997.

Biller, Peter. "Childbirth in the Middle Ages." *History Today* 36 (1986): 42–49.

Birrell, Anne M., trans. *New Songs from a Jade Terrace: An Anthology of Early Chinese Love Poetry*. London: George Allen & Unwin, 1982.

Blachere, Regis. *Histoire de la litterature arabe des origines a la fin du XVe siecle*. Paris: A. Maisonneuve et Larose, 1952–1966.

Blamires, Alcuin, ed. *Woman Defamed and Woman Defended: An Anthology of Medieval Texts*. Oxford: Oxford University Press, 1992.

Bloch, R. Howard. *The Anonymous Marie de France*. Chicago: University of Chicago Press, 2003.

Bloch, R. Howard. *Medieval Misogyny and the Invention of Western Romantic Love*. Chicago: University of Chicago Press, 1991.

Boccaccio, Giovanni. *The Decameron*. Translated by G. H. McWilliam. Harmondsworth, UK: Penguin Books, 1972.

Bogin, Meg. *The Women Troubadours*. New York: W.W. Norton, 1980.

Bond, Gerald A., ed. and trans. *The Poetry of William VII, Count of Poitiers, IX Duke of Aquitaine*. New York: Garland, 1982.

Bondeson, Jan. *The Two-Headed Boy, and Other Medical Marvels*. Ithaca, NY: Cornell University Press, 2000.

Bonebakker, Seeger Adrianus. "'*Adab* and the Concept of Belles-Lettres." In *'Abbasid Belles-Lettres*, edited by Julia Ashtiany et al., 16–30. The Cambridge History of Arabic Literature series. Cambridge: Cambridge University Press, 1990.

Bornstein, Diane. *The Lady in the Tower: Medieval Courtesy Literature for Women*. Hamden, CT: Archon, 1983.

Boswell, John. *Christianity, Social Tolerance, and Homosexuality: Gay People in Western Europe from the Beginning of the Christian Era to the Fourteenth Century*. Chicago: University of Chicago Press, 1980.

Boswell, John. *Rediscovering Gay History: Archetypes of Gay Love in Christian History*. London: Gay Christian Movement, 1982.

Boswell, John. *Same Sex Unions in Pre-Modern Europe*. New York: Villard, 1994.

Bouchard, Constance B. "Consanguinity and Noble Marriages in the Tenth and Eleventh Centuries." *Speculum* 56 (1981): 268–87.

Boureau, Alain. *The Lord's First Night: The Myth of the Droit de Cuissage*. Translated by Lydia G. Cochrane. Chicago: University of Chicago Press, 1998.

Bowden, Muriel. *A Reader's Guide to Geoffrey Chaucer*. New York: Farrar, Straus, 1964.

Bowring, Richard, ed. *The Diary of Lady Murasaki*. New York: Penguin, 1996.

Boyle, Elizabeth Heger. *Female Genital Cutting*. Baltimore: Johns Hopkins University Press, 2002.

Bradbury, Jim. *Philip Augustus*. London: Longman, 1998.

Brakke, David. *Athanasius and the Politics of Asceticism*. New York: Oxford University Press, 1995.

Branca, Vittore. *Boccaccio: The Man and His Works*. Translated by Richard Monges and Dennis J. McAuliffe. New York: New York University Press, 1976.

Briffault, Robert. *The Troubadours*. Translated and edited by Lawrence Koons. Bloomington: Indiana University Press, 1965.

Brody, Heinrich. *Selected Poems of Jehudah Halevi*. Translated by Nina Salaman. Philadelphia: Jewish Publication Society of America, 1924.

Brooke, Elisabeth. *Women Healers: Portraits of Herbalists, Physicians, and Midwives*. Rochester, VT: Healing Arts Press, 1995.

Brown, Percy. *Indian Architecture*. Mumbai, India: Taraporevala, 1959.

Brown, Peter. *The Body and Society: Men, Women, and Sexual Renunciation in Early Christianity*. New York: Columbia University Press, 1988.

Brown, Peter. *The Rise of Western Christendom: Triumph and Diversity*. Oxford: Blackwell, 1996.

Browne, E. G. *A Literary History of Persia*. Vol. 3. London: Cambridge University Press, 1920.

Brown-Grant, Rosalind. *Christine de Pisan and the Moral Defense of Women.* Cambridge: Cambridge University Press, 1999.

Broyde, Michael J., ed. *Marriage, Sex, and Family in Judaism.* Lanham, MD: Rowman and Littlefield, 2005.

Bruckner, Matilda Tomaryn, Laurie Shepard, and Sarah White, eds. *Songs of the Women Troubadours.* New York: Garland Publishing, 1995.

Brundage, James A. "Intermarriage between Christians and Jews in Medieval Canon Law." *Jewish History* 3 (1988): 25–40.

Brundage, James A. *Law, Sex, and Christian Society in Medieval Europe.* Chicago: University of Chicago Press, 1987.

Brynteson, William E. "Roman Law and Legislation in the Middle Ages." *Speculum* 41 (1996): 420–37.

Bullough, Vern L. *Sexual Variance in Society and History.* New York: John Wiley and Sons, 1976.

Bullough, Vern L., and James A. Brundage, eds. *Handbook of Medieval Sexuality.* New York: Garland Publishing, 1996.

Bullough, Vern L., and James A. Brundage, eds. *Sexual Practices and the Medieval Church.* Buffalo, NY: Prometheus Books, 1982.

Bullough, Vern L., and Bonnie Bullough. *Cross-Dressing, Sex and Gender.* Philadelphia: University of Pennsylvania Press, 1993.

Burgess, Glyn S. *The "Lais" of Marie de France: Text and Context.* Athens: University of Georgia Press, 1987.

Burke, James. "Virtue and Sin, Reward and Punishment in the Cantigas de Santa Maria." In *Studies on the Cantigas de Santa Maria: Art, Music, and Poetry*, edited by Israel Kats and John E. Keller, 247–52. Madison, WI: Hispanic Seminar on Medieval Studies, 1987.

Burkhart, Louise. *The Slippery Earth: Nahua and Christian Moral Dialogue in Sixteenth-Century Mexico.* Tucson: University of Arizona Press, 1989.

Byland, Bruce E., and John M. D. Pohl. *In the Realm of 8 Deer.* Norman: University of Oklahoma Press, 1994.

Bynum, Carolyn. *Holy Feast and Holy Fast.* Berkeley: University of California Press, 1987.

Cadden, Joan. *Meanings of Sex Difference in the Middle Ages: Medicine, Science, and Culture.* Cambridge: Cambridge University Press, 1993.

Cahill, Thomas. *How the Irish Saved Civilization.* New York: Anchor Books, 1995.

Campenhausen, Hans von. *Men Who Shaped the Western Church.* New York: Harper and Row, 1964.

Cesaretti, Paolo. *Theodora.* New York: Vendome, 2004.

Chakraborthy, Kakolee. *Women as Devadasis: Origin and Growth of the Devadasi Profession.* Delhi: Deep & Deep, 2000.

Chaliand, Gerard. *Nomadic Empires: From Mongolia to the Danube.* Translated by A. M. Berret. New Brunswick, NJ: Transaction Publishers, 2003.

Chandra, Moti. *Gita Govinda.* Lalit Kala Series Portfolio No. 3. New Delhi: Lalit Kala Akademi, 1972.

Chandra, Satish. *Medieval India: From Sultanat to the Mughals.* Delhi: Har Anand, 1998.

Chang, Garma C. C. *Teachings and Practice of Tibetan Tantra.* Mineola, NY: Dover Publications, 2004.

Chejne, A. *Ibn Hazm.* Chicago: Kazi Publications, 1982.

Chen, Fan-pen. "Problems of Chinese Historiography as Seen in the Official Records on Yang Kuei-fei." *T'ang Studies* 8–9 (1990–1991): 83–96.

Clark, Victoria. *Why Angels Fall: A Journey through Orthodox Europe from Byzantium to Kosovo.* New York: St. Martin's Press, 2000.

Clark, W. B., and M. T. McMunn. *Beasts and Birds of the Middle Ages: The Bestiary and Its Legacy.* Philadelphia: University of Pennsylvania Press, 1989.

Cleary, Thomas. *Understanding Reality: A Taoist Alchemical Classic by Chang Po-tuan.* Honolulu: University of Hawaii Press, 1987.

Clendinnen, Inga. *Aztecs*. Cambridge: Cambridge University Press, 1991.

Cleugh, James. *Chant Royal*. Garden City, NY: Doubleday, 1970.

Clifford, John J. "The Ethics of Conjugal Intimacy according to St. Albert the Great." *Theological Studies* 3 (1942): 1–26.

Cohn, Norman. *Europe's Inner Demons: The Demonization of Christians in Medieval Christendom*. Rev. ed. Chicago: University of Chicago Press, 2000.

Coldwell, M. V. "Jongleresses and Trobairitz: Secular Musicians in Medieval France." In *Women Making Music: The Western Art Tradition, 1150–1950*, edited by J. Bowers and J. Tick. Urbana: University of Illinois Press, 1986.

Cole, Peter, trans. *Selected Poems of Solomon Ibn Gabirol*. Princeton, NJ: Princeton University Press, 2000.

Colville, Jim. *Poems of Wine and Revelry: The Khamriyyat of Abu Nuwas*. London: Kegan Paul, 2004.

Conner, Randy P. "Sexuality and Gender in African Spiritual Traditions." In *Sexuality and the World's Religions*, edited by David W. Machacek and Melissa M. Wilcox, 3–30. Santa Barbara, CA: ABC-Clio, 2003.

Cooper, Helen. *The English Romance in Time*. New York: Oxford University Press, 2004.

Cosgrave, Bronwyn. *The Complete History of Costume & Fashion: From Ancient Egypt to the Present Day*. New York: Checkmark Books, 2001.

Cotterell, Arthur. *A Dictionary of World Mythology*. New York: G. P. Putman's Sons, 1980.

Coulson, N. J. *A History of Islamic Law*. 1964. Reprint, Edinburgh: University of Edinburgh Press, 1999.

Cowan, James. *A Troubadour's Testament*. Boston: Shambhala Publications, 1998.

Coyn, Kathleen. *Performing Virginity and Testing Chastity in the Middle Ages*. New York: Routledge, 2000.

Cuesta, Angel Martìnez. "Maddalene." In *Dizionario degli Istituti di Perfezione*. Vol. 5. Roma: Edizioni Paoline, 1978, pp. 801–812.

da Crispiero, Massimo. *Il matrimonio cristiano*. Torino: Edizioni Marietti, 1976.

da Crispiero, Massimo. *Teologia della sessualità. approfondimenti sui temi del matrimonio e della verginità*. Bologna: Edizioni Studio Domenicano, 1994.

Dalarun, Jacques. "The Clerical Gaze." Translated by Arthur Goldhammer, chapter 1. In *A History of Women in the West: Silences of the Middle Ages*, edited by Christiane Klapisch-Zuber. Cambridge, MA: Belknap Press of Harvard University, 1992.

Dalla, Danilo. "Ubi Venus mutatur." *Omosessualitàe diritto nel mondo romano*. Milano: Giuffrè, 1987.

Davis, Tenny L., and Chao Yün-ts'ung. "Chang Po-Tuan of T'ien-T'ai, His Wu Chen P'ien, Essay on the Understanding of the Truth." *Proceedings of the American Academy of Arts and Sciences* 73 (1939): 97–117.

d'Avray, David. *Medieval Marriage: Symbolism and Society*. Oxford: Oxford University Press, 2005.

De, Sushil Kumar. *Ancient Indian Erotics and Erotic Literature*. Kolkata, India: Firma K.L. Mukhopadhyay, 1959.

de Weever, Jacqueline. *Sheba's Daughters: Whitening and Demonizing the Saracen Women in Medieval French Epic*. New York: Garland, 1998.

Debby, Nirit Ben-Aryeh. *Renaissance Florence in the Rhetoric of Two Popular Preachers: Giovanni Dominici (1356–1419) and Bernardino of Siena (1380–1444)*. Turnhout, Belgium: Brepols, 2001.

Deegan, Marilyn. "Pregnancy and Childbirth in the Anglo-Saxon Medical Texts." In *Medicine in Early Medieval England: Four Papers*, edited by Marilyn Deegan and D. G. Scragg, 17–26. Manchester: Manchester Centre for Anglo-Saxon Studies, 1989.

Deguilhem, Randi, and Manuela Marin, eds. *Writing the Feminine: Women in Arab Sources (The Islamic Mediterranean)*. London: I.B. Tauris, 2002.

Dev, Usha. *The Concept of Sakti in the Puranas*. New Delhi: Nag Publishers, 1987.

Devadhar, Chintaman Ramachandra. *Amaruśatakam with Sringaradîpika of Vemabhpâla*. Poona: Oriental Book Agency, 1959.
Devadhar, Chintaman Ramachandra. *Meghaduta of Kalidasa*. Delhi: Motilal Banarsidass, 1985.
Devereau, R. "XIth Century Muslim Views on Women, Marriage, Love, and Sex." *Central Asiatic Journal* 11 (1966): 134–40.
Diehl, Charles. *Theodora*. New York: F. Ungar, 1972.
Dowman, Keith, trans. *The Divine Madman: The Sublime Life and Songs of Drukpa Kunley*. Clearlake, CA: Dawnhorse Press, 1980.
Dronke, Peter. "Andreas Capellanus." *Journal of Medieval Latin* 4 (1994): 51–63.
Duby, Georges, ed. *A History of Private Life: Revelations of the Medieval World*. Cambridge, MA: Harvard University Press, 1988.
Duby, Georges. *The Legend of Bouvines: War, Religion, and Culture in the Middle Ages*. Berkeley: University of California Press, 1990.
Dudbridge, Glen. *The Tale of Li Wa: Study and Critical Edition of a Chinese Story from the Ninth Century*. London: Oxford University Press, 1983.
Ebrey, Patricia Buckley. *Women and the Family in Chinese History*. London: Routledge, 2003.
Eckenstein, Lina. *Woman under Monasticism*. Cambridge: Cambridge University Press, 1896.
Eicher, Joanne, ed. *Dress and Ethnicity: Change across Space and Time*. Oxford: Berg, 1995.
Eidelberg, Shlomo. *The Responsa of Rabbenu Gershom Meor Hagolah*. New York: Yeshiva University, 1955.
Elliott, Dyan. *Spiritual Marriage: Sexual Abstinence in Medieval Wedlock*. Princeton, NJ: Princeton University Press, 1993.
Ellis, Steve. *Chaucer: An Oxford Guide*. New York: Oxford University Press, 2005.
Enderwitz, Susanne. *Liebe als Beruf: al-'Abbas ibn al-Ahnaf und das Ghazal*. Stuttgart: Franz Steiner Verlag, 1995.
Epstein, Louis M. *Sex Laws and Customs in Judaism*. New York: Ktav Publishing House, 1967.
Ernst, Carl W. *The Shambhala Guide to Sufism*. Boston: Shambhala Publications, 1997.
Eskildsen, Stephen. *Asceticism in Early Taoist Religion*. Albany: State University of New York Press, 1998.
Evan, James. *Theodora*. Austin: University of Texas Press, 2002.
Evans, G. R. *The Mind of St. Bernard of Clairvaux*. New York: Oxford University Press, 2000.
Fakhry, Majid. *A History of Islamic Philosophy*. New York: Columbia University Press, 1983.
Fakhry, Majid. *Ibn Rushd (Averroes): His Life, Works and Influence*. Oxford: Oneworld, 2001.
Falk, Ze'ev W. *Jewish Matrimonial Law in the Middle Ages*. Scripta Judaica 6. London: Oxford University Press, 1966.
Farmer, Sharon A., and Carol Braun Pasternack. *Gender and Difference in the Middle Ages*. Minneapolis: University of Minnesota Press, 2003.
Faure, Bernard. *The Red Thread: Buddhist Approaches to Sexuality*. Princeton, NJ: Princeton University Press, 1998.
Flanagan, Sabina. *Hildegard of Bingen*. London: Routledge, 1989.
Flandrin, Jean Louis. *Il sesso e l'Occidente*. Milano: Mondadori, 1983.
Fletcher, Richard. *Moorish Spain*. Berkeley: University of California Press, 1993.
Förster, Richard, ed. *Scriptores physiognomonici graeci et latini*. 2 vols. Lipsiae: Teubner, 1893.
Foster, Kenelm. *Petrarch: Poet and Humanist*. Edinburgh: University of Edinburgh Press, 1984.
Frakes, Robert M. "Item Theodosianus? (Observations on Coll. V. 3. 1)," *Quaderni Urbinati di Cultura Classica* n. s. 71 (2002): 163–68.
Fraser, James. *The Golden Bough: A Study in Magic and Religion*. 3rd ed., parts 1–2. London: Macmillan, 1963.
Freitag, Barbara. *Sheila-na-Gigs: Unravelling an Enigma*. London: Routledge, 2004.
French, R. M., trans. *The Way of a Pilgrim and the Pilgrim Continues His Way*. San Francisco: HarperCollins, 1965.
Frend, W.H.C. *The Rise of the Monophysite Movement: Chapters in the History of the Church in the Fifth and Sixth Centuries*. Cambridge: Cambridge University Press, 1972.

Friedman, Clarence William. *Prefigurations in Meistergesang: Types from the Bible and Nature*. New York: AMS Press, 1970.
Friesen, Ilse E. *The Female Crucifix: Images of St. Wilgefortis since the Middle Ages*. Ontario, Canada: Wilfred Laurier University Press, 2001.
Furth, Charlotte. *A Flourishing Yin: Gender in China's Medical History, 960–1665*. Berkeley: University of California Press, 1999.
Gambero, Luigi. *Mary and the Fathers of the Church: The Blessed Virgin Mary in Patristic Thought*. Translated by Thomas Buffer. San Francisco: Ignatius Press, 1999.
Gambero, Luigi. *Mary in the Middle Ages: The Blessed Virgin Mary in the Thought of Medieval Latin Theologians*. Translated by Thomas Buffer. San Francisco: Ignatius Press, 2005.
Gaunt, Simon, Ruth Harvey, and Linda Paterson. *Marcabru: A Critical Edition*. Cambridge: D.S. Brewer, 2000.
Gernet, Jacques. *Daily Life in China on the Eve of the Mongol Invasion, 1250–1276*. Stanford, CA: Stanford University Press, 1970.
Gies, Frances, and Joseph Gies. *Marriage and the Family in the Middle Ages*. New York: Harper and Row, 1987.
Giffen, Lois Anita. *Theory of Profane Love among the Arabs: The Development of the Genre*. New York: New York University Press, 1971.
Gilbert, Jane. "The Practice of Gender in *Aucassin and Nicolette*." *Forum for Modern Language Studies* 33, no. 3 (1977): 217–28.
Gillespie, Jeanne. *Saints and Warriors: Tlaxcalan Perspectives on the Fall of Tenochtitlan*. New Orleans, LA: University Press of the South, 2004.
Gilson, Etienne. *The Mystical Theology of Saint Bernard*. Translated by A.H.C. Downes. New York: Sheed and Ward, 1955.
Goldberg, P.J.P. "Pigs and Prostitutes: Streetwalking in Comparative Perspective." In *Young Medieval Women*, edited by Katherine J. Lewis, Noel James Menuge, and Kim M. Phillips, 172–93. Thrupp, Stroud, UK: Sutton Publishing, 1999.
Goldstein, Melvyn, and Cynthia Beall. *Nomads of Western Tibet*. Berkeley: University of California Press, 1990.
Gonsette, J. *Pierre Damien et la culture profane*. Louvain: Publications Universitaires & Paris: Béatrice-Nauwelaerts, 1956.
Goodich, Michael. *The Unmentionable Vice: Homosexuality in the Later Medieval Period*. Santa Barbara, CA: ABC-Clio, 1979.
Graef, Hilda. *Mary: A History of Doctrine and Devotion*. Vol. 1, *From the Beginnings to the Eve of the Reformation*. New York: Sheed and Ward, 1963.
Gray, David. *The Cakrasamvara Tantra: A Study and Annotated Translation*. New York: American Institute of Buddhist Studies, 2006.
Gray, David. "Disclosing the Empty Secret: Textuality and Embodiment in the *Cakrasamvara Tantra*." *Numen* 52, no. 4 (2005): 417–44.
Gray, E. T. *The Green Sea of Heaven*. Ashland, OR: White Cloud Press, 1995.
Greilsammer, Myriam. "The Midwife, the Priest, and the Physician: The Subjugation of Midwives in the Low Countries at the End of the Middle Ages." *Journal of Medieval and Renaissance Studies* 21 (1991): 285–329.
Gross, Jo-Ann. *Muslims in Central Asia: Expressions of Identity and Change*. Durham, NC: Duke University Press, 1992.
Grossman, Avraham. "Medieval Rabbinic Views on Wife-Beating, 800–1300." *Jewish History* 5, no. 1 (1991): 53–62.
Guisso, R.W.L. *Wu Tse-t'ien and the Politics of Legitimation in T'ang China*. Bellingham: West Washington University Press, 1978.
Gupte, Ramesh Shankar, and B. D. Mahajan. *Ajanta, Ellora and Aurangabad Caves*. Mumbai, India: Taraporevala, 1962.
Gybbon-Monypenny, G. B., ed. *Libro de Buen Amor Studies*. London: Tamesis, 1970.

Haines, Roy Martin. *King Edward II: Edward of Caernarfon, His Life, His Reign, and Its Aftermath, 1284–1330.* Montreal, Canada: McGill Queens University Press, 2003.

Hambly, Gavin. *Women in the Medieval Islamic World: Power, Patronage, and Piety.* New York: St. Martin's Press, 1998.

Hanan, Patrick, trans. *The Carnal Prayer Mat, Li Yu.* Honolulu: University of Hawaii Press, 1996.

Hanawalt, Barbara A. *The Ties That Bound: Peasant Families in Medieval England.* New York: Oxford University Press, 1986.

Hardman, Phillipa, ed. *The Growth of the Tristan and Iseut Legend in Wales, England, France, and Germany.* Studies in Medieval Literature 24. New York: Edwin Mellen Press, 2003.

Hardy, Friedhelm. *Viraha Bhakti: The Early Development of Krsna Devotion in South India.* Oxford: Oxford University Press, 1981.

Harvey, Ruth. *The Troubadour Marcabru and Love.* London: Westfield Publications, 1989.

Hasan, Masudul. *History of Islam.* Vol. 1. Delhi: Adam Publishers, 2002.

Hatto, Arthur T., ed. *Eos: An Enquiry into the Theme of Lovers' Meetings and Partings at Dawn in Poetry.* London: Mouton, 1965.

Heffening, W. "Mut'a." In *The Encyclopaedia of Islam.* Second ed., vol. 7, p. 759. Leiden: Brill, 1960.

Hellwarth, Jennifer Wynne. "'I wyl wright of women prevy sekenes': Imagining Female Literacy and Textual Communities in Medieval and Early Modern Midwifery Manuals." *Critical Survey* 14 (2002): 44–63.

Helmholz, R. H. "And Were There Children's Rights in Early Modern England? The Canon Law and 'Intra-Family Violence' in England, 1400–1640." *The International Journal of Children's Rights* 1 (1993): 23–32.

Helmholz, R. H. *Marriage Litigation in Medieval England.* London: Cambridge University Press, 1974.

Helminski, E. Kabir, ed. *The Rumi Collection: An Anthology of Translations of Mevlana Jalaluddin Rumi.* Boston: Shambhala Publications, 2000.

Hergemöller, Bernd-Ulrich, ed. *Sodom und Gomorrha. Zur Alltagswirklichkeit und Verfolgung Homosexueller im Mittelalter.* Hamburg: Männerschwarm Skript Verlag, 2000.

Herlihy, David. *Medieval Households.* Cambridge, MA: Harvard University Press, 1985.

Hewson, M. Anthony. *Giles of Rome and the Medieval Theory of Conception: A Study of the De formatione Corporis Humani in Utero.* London: Athlone Press, 1975.

Hollander, Robert. *Dante: A Life in Works.* New Haven, CT: Yale University Press, 2001.

Hopkins, Andrea. *The Book of Courtly Love: The Passionate Code of the Troubadours.* New York: HarperCollins, 1994.

Hreinsson, Víðar, ed. *The Complete Sagas of Icelanders Including 49 Tales.* 5 vols. Reykjavík, Iceland: Leifur Eiríksson Publishing, 1997.

Hull Walton, Alan. *Love Recipes Old and New: A Study of Aphrodisiacs throughout the Ages, with Sections on Suitable Food, Glandular Extracts, Hormone Stimulation and Rejuvenation.* London: Torchstream Books, 1956.

Hunt, Mary, Patricia B. Jung, and Radhika Balakrishnan, eds. *Good Sex: Feminist Perspectives from the World's Religions.* New Brunswick, NJ: Rutgers University Press, 2001.

Hurt-Mead, Kate Campbell. "Trotula." *Isis* 14, no. 2 (October 1930): 349–67.

Hyamson, Moses. *Collatio Legum Mosaicarum et Romanarum.* Oxford: Oxford University Press, 1913.

Ibn Hazm, Ali ibn Ahmad. *The Ring of the Dove: A Treatise on the Art and Practice of Arab Love.* Translated by A. J. Arberry. New York: AMS Press, 1981.

Irwin, Robert. *The Arabian Nights: A Companion.* London: Allen Lane, 1994.

Irwin, Robert, ed. *Night & Horses & the Desert: An Anthology of Classical Arabic Literature.* Woodstock, NY: Overlook Press, 2000.

Jackson, W.T.H. *Medieval Literature: A History and a Guide.* New York: Collier Books, 1967.

Jacobi, Hermann, ed. *Samaraiccakaha.* Kolkata, India: Asiatic Society of Bengal, 1926.

Jacquart, Danielle, and Claude Thomasset. *Sexuality and Medicine in the Middle Ages.* Cambridge: Polity Press, 1988.

Jaffrey, Zia. *The Invisibles: A Tale of the Eunuchs of India.* New York: Pantheon, 1996.

Jahiz, Abu Uthman Amr b. Bahr al-. *The Epistle on Singing-Girls by Jahiz.* Edited and translated by A.F.L. Beeston. Warminster: Aris and Phillips, 1980.

Jahiz, Abu Uthman Amr b. Bahr al-. *Nine Essays of al-Jahiz.* Translated by William M. Hutchins. New York: Peter Lang, 1989.

Jain, Jagadish Chandra. *The Vasudevahindi: An Authentic Jain Version of the Brhatkath.* Lalbhai Dalpatbhai Series 59. Ahmedabad, India: Lalbhai Dalpatbhai Institute of Indology, 1977.

Jaini, Padmanabh S. *The Jaina Path of Purification.* Berkeley: University of California Press, 1979.

Jha, Damodar, ed. *Vetalapancavimsati, with "Prakash" Hindi Commentary.* Varanasi, India: Chowkamba Vidyabhavan, 1968.

Joan Crow, ed. *Les quinze joyes de marriage.* Oxford: Blackwell, 1969.

Jochens, Jenny. *Old Norse Images of Women.* Philadelphia: University of Pennsylvania Press, 1996.

Johnson, Penelope Delafield. *Equal in Monastic Profession: Religious Women in Medieval France.* Chicago: University of Chicago Press, 1991.

Jones, Prudence, and Nigel Pennick. *A History of Pagan Europe.* London: Routledge, 1995.

Jong, Mayke de. "To the Limits of Kinship: Anti-Incest Legislation in the Early Medieval West (500–900)." In *From Sappho to de Sade: Moments in the History of Sexuality,* edited by Jan Bremmer, 36–59. London: Routledge, 1989.

Jordan, Mark D. *The Invention of Sodomy in Christian Theology.* Chicago: University of Chicago Press, 1997.

Jordan, Michael. *Encyclopedia of Gods.* New York: Facts on File, 1993.

Jordan, William Chester. *Europe in the High Middle Ages.* New York: Penguin, 2004.

Kai Ka'us ibn Iskandar. *A Mirror for Princes.* New York: Dutton, 1951.

Kaiser, Wolfgang. *Die Epitome Iuliani.* Frankfurt am Main: Vittorio Klostermann, 2004.

Kale, Moreswar Ramachandra. *Uttararamacarita of Bhavabhuti.* Mumbai, India: Gopal Narayan, 1934.

Kanitkar, Hemant. *Kalidas's Abhijnana Shakuntala.* Mumbai: Popular Prakashan, 1984.

Karras, Ruth Mazo. *Sexuality in Medieval Europe: Doing unto Others.* New York: Routledge, 2005.

Katz, Marion Holmes. *Body of Text: The Emergence of the Sunni Law of Ritual Purity.* Albany: State University of New York Press, 2002.

Kausar, Zinat. *Muslim Women in Medieval India.* Patna, India: Janaki Prakashan, 1992.

Kayser, Rudolf. *The Life and Time of Judah Halevi.* New York: Philosophical Library, 1949.

Keen, Maurice. *The Penguin History of Medieval Europe.* New York: Penguin, 1991.

Kelly, James Martin. *Female Genital Mutilation: A Search for Its Origins.* Ann Arbor: University of Michigan Press, 1993.

Kelly, J.N.D. *Golden Mouth: The Story of John Chrysostom—Ascetic, Preacher, Bishop.* Ithaca, NY: Cornell University Press, 1998.

Kelly, J.N.D. *Jerome: His Life, Writings and Controversies.* London: Duckworth, 1975.

Kemp-Welch, Alice. *Of Six Medieval Women.* Williamstown, MA: Corner House Publishers, 1972.

Kennedy, Philip F. *The Wine Song in Classical Arabic Poetry: Abu Nuwas and the Literary Tradition.* Oxford: Clarendon Press, 1997.

Kilpatrick, H. "Some Late Abbasid and Mamluk Books about Women: A Literary Historical Approach." *Arabica* 42 (1995): 56–78.

Kiple, Kenneth F., ed. *The Cambridge World History of Human Disease.* Cambridge: Cambridge University Press, 1993.

Klostermaier, Klaus K. *A Survey of Hinduism.* New York: State University of New York Press, 1994.

Kristjánsson, Jónas. *Eddas and Sagas: Iceland's Medieval Literature.* Translated by Peter Foote. Reykjavík, Iceland: Hið íslenska bókmenntafélag, 1997.

Kroll, Paul W. "Po Chü-i's 'Song of Lasting Regret': A New Translation." *T'ang Studies* 8–9 (1990–1991): 97–104.
Krueger, Roberta, ed. *The Cambridge Companion to Medieval Romance*. New York: Cambridge University Press, 2000.
Kruger, Steven F. "Conversion and Medieval Sexual, Religious, and Racial Categories." In *Constructing Medieval Sexuality*, edited by Karma Lochrie, Peggy McCracken, and James A. Schultz, pp. 158–79. Minneapolis: University of Minnesota Press, 1997.
Kuefler, Mathew. "Male Friendships and the Suspicion of Sodomy in Twelfth Century France." In *The Boswell Thesis; Essays on Christianity, Social Tolerance and Homosexuality*, edited by Mathew Kuefler, 179–214. Chicago: University of Chicago Press, 2006.
Laboa, Juan Maria, ed. *The Historical Atlas of Eastern and Western Christian Monasticism*. Collegeville, MN: Liturgical Press, 2003.
Laing, Ellen Johnston. "Chinese Palace-Style Poetry and the Depiction of A Palace Beauty." *Art Bulletin* 72, no. 1 (March 1990): 284–95.
Lal, Kanwar. *The Religion of Love*. New Delhi: Arts & Letters, 1971.
Lal, K. S. *Muslim Slave System in Medieval India*. New Delhi: Aditya Prakashan, 1994.
Lambert, Malcolm. *The Cathars*. Malden, MA: Blackwell, 1999.
Lane, Edward William, trans. *Stories from Thousand and One Nights (the Arabian Nights' Entertainments)*. The Harvard Classics 16. New York: P.F. Collier & Son, 1909–1914.
Lansing, Carol. *Power & Purity: Cathar Heresy in Medieval Italy*. New York: Oxford University Press. 1998.
Laqueur, Thomas W. *Solitary Sex: A Cultural History of Masturbation*. New York: Zone Books, 2003.
Layne, Gwendolyn. *Kadambari of Banabhatta: A Classic Sanskrit Story of Magical Transformations*. New York: Garland Publications, 1991.
Lazar, Moshe, and Norris J. Lacy, eds. *Poetics of Love in the Middle Ages: Texts and Contexts*. Fairfax, VA: George Mason University Press, 1989.
Lee, B. R. "A Company of Women and Men: Men's Recollections of Childbirth in Medieval England." *Journal of Family History* 27 (2002): 92–100.
Lemay, Helen Rodnite. *Women's Secrets: A Translation of Pseudo-Albertus Magnus's De Secretis Mulierum with Commentaries*. Albany: State University of New York Press, 1992.
Lerner, Gerda. *The Creation of Patriarchy*. Oxford: Oxford University Press, 1985.
Levin, Eve. *Sex and Society in the World of the Orthodox Slavs, 900–1700*. Ithaca, NY: Cornell University Press, 1989.
Levy, Howard S., trans. *The Dwelling of Playful Goddesses*. Tokyo: Dai Nippon Insatsu, 1965.
Lewis, C. S. *The Allegory of Love*. 1936. Reprint, New York: Oxford University Press, 1985.
Lightfoot-Klein, Hanny. *Prisoners of Ritual: An Odyssey into Female Genital Circumcision in Africa*. Binghamton, NY: Haworth Press, 1989.
Liu Fangru, ed. *Glimpses into the Hidden Quarters: Paintings of Women from the Middle Kingdom (Shinü hua zhi mei)*. Taipei: National Palace Museum, 1988.
Loewe, Raphael. *Ibn Gabirol*. London: Peter Halban, 1989.
Lopez Austin, Alfredo. *Tamoanchan, Tlalocan: Places of Mist*. Translated by Bernard Ortiz de Montellano and Thelma Ortiz de Montellano. Niwot: University Press of Colorado, 1997.
Maddocks, Fiona. *Hildegard of Bingen*. New York: Doubleday, 2001.
Mahdi, Muhsin. *The Thousand and One Nights*. New York: Brill, 1995.
Maimonides, Moses. *The Guide for the Perplexed*. Translated by M. Friedlander. 1881. New York: Dover Publishers, 1956.
Maimonides, Moses. *Maimonides "On Sexual Intercourse": Fi 'l-jima*. Brooklyn, NY: Rambash, 1961.
Manz, Beatrice, ed. *Central Asia in Historical Perspective*. Boulder, CO: Westview Press, 1994.
Marmon, Shaun. *Eunuchs and Sacred Boundaries In Islamic Society*. New York: Oxford University Press, 1999.

Martin, John. *Roses, Fountains, and Gold: The Virgin Mary in History, Art, and Apparition.* San Francisco: Ignatius Press, 1998.

Matarasso, P. *Aucassin and Nicolette and Other Tales.* Harmondsworth, UK: Penguin, 1971.

Mayer, Wendy, and Pauline Allen. *John Chrysostom.* London: Routledge Press, 1999.

McCullough, William H. "Japanese Marriage Institutions in the Heian Period." *Harvard Journal of Asiatic Studies* 27 (1967): 103–67.

McKinley, Kathryn L. *Reading the Ovidian Heroine: "Metamorphoses" Commentaries, 1100–1618.* Leiden: Brill, 2001.

McLaren, Angus. *A History of Contraception from Antiquity to the Present Day.* Cambridge: Basil Blackwell, 1990.

McLeod, Enid. *The Order of the Rose: The Life and Ideas of Christine de Pizan.* Totowa, NJ: Rowman and Littlefield, 1976.

McNamara, Jo-Ann, and Suzanne F. Wemple. "Marriage and Divorce in the Frankish Kingdom." In *The Chivalrous Society*, edited by Georges Duby, 112–22. Berkeley: University of California Press, 1977.

McNeill, John T., and Helena M. Gamer. *Medieval Handbooks of Penance: A Translation of the Principal "Libri poenitentiales" and Selections from Related Documents.* New York: Columbia University Press, 1990.

Menocal, Maria Rosa. *The Ornament of the World: How Muslims, Jews and Christians Created a Culture of Tolerance in Medieval Spain.* Boston: Little, Brown, 2002.

Mernissi, Fatima. *Beyond the Veil: Male-Female Dynamics in Modern Muslim Society.* London: Saqi Books, 2003.

Mews, Constant J. *Abelard and Heloise.* New York: Oxford University Press, 2005.

Mews, Constant J. *The Lost Love Letters of Heloise and Abelard.* New York: St. Martin's Press, 1999.

Meyer, Johann H. *Sexual Life in Ancient India.* New York: Barnes and Noble, 1953.

Michell, George. *The Penguin Guide to the Monuments of India.* Vol. 1. London: Viking, 1989.

Miller, Barbara Stoler. *Gita Govinda of Jayadeva: Love Song of the Dark Lord.* New Delhi: Motilal Banarsidass, 1996.

Mirza, Wahid. *Life and Works of Amir Khusrau.* Kolkata, India: Baptist Mission Press, 1935.

Mithal, Akhilesh. "The Power of Myth." *Deccan Chronicle* (Visakhapatnam), May 1, 2005.

Moffett, Samuel. *A History of Christianity in Asia.* Vol. 1, *Beginnings to 1500.* San Francisco: Harper San Francisco, 1992.

Moioli, Giovanni. "Per una rinnovata riflessione sui rapporti tra matrimonio e verginità" *La Scuola Cattolica* 95 (1967): 201–55.

Moore, R. I. *The Formation of a Persecuting Society: Power and Deviance in Western Europe, 950–1250.* Oxford: Basil Blackwell, 1987.

Mormando, Franco. *The Preacher's Demons: Bernardino of Siena and the Social Underworld of Early Renaissance Italy.* Chicago: University of Chicago Press, 1999.

Morris, Ivan. *The World of the Shining Prince.* New York: Alfred A. Knopf, 1964.

Mourad, Yousef. *La physiognomonie arabe et le Kitab al-firasa de Fakhr al-Din al-Razi.* Paris: Librarie Orientaliste Paul Geuthner, 1939.

Müller, Wolfgang P. "The Recovery of Justinian's *Digest* in the Middle Ages." *Bulletin of Medieval Canon Law* 20 (1990): 1–29.

Muni, Jinavijya, ed. *Kathakosa Prakarana of Jinesvara Suri.* Singhi Jain Grantha Mala 11. Mumbai, India: Bharatiya Vidya Bhavan, 1949.

Murata, S. *Temporary Marriage (Mut'a) in Islamic Law.* London: Muhammadi Trust, 1987.

Murray, Jacqueline, ed. *Love, Marriage, and Family in the Middle Ages: A Reader.* Peterborough, ON: Broadview Press, 2001.

Murstein, Bernard I. *Love, Sex and Marriage through the Ages.* New York: Springer, 1974.

Murthy, K. Krishna. *Sculptures of Vajrayana Buddhism.* Delhi: Classics India Publications, 1989.

Musacchio, Jacqueline Marie. *The Art and Ritual of Childbirth in Renaissance Italy.* New Haven, CT: Yale University Press, 1999.

Musallam, B. F. *Sex and Society in Islam: Birth Control before the Nineteenth Century.* Cambridge: Cambridge University Press, 1983.

Mvuyekure, Pierre-Damien. *West African Kingdoms, 500–1590.* Detroit, MI: Gale Group, 2004.

Nafzawi, Muhammad ibn Muhammad. *The Perfumed Garden of Sheykh Nefzawi.* Translated by Sir Richard Burton. New York: Castle Books, 1964.

Nallino, Carlo Alfonso. *La litterature arabe des origines a l' epoque de la dynastie umayyade.* Paris: G. P. Maisonneuve, 1950.

Nanda, Serena. *Neither Man nor Woman: The Hijras of India.* Belmont, CA: Wadsworth, 1990.

Nandgrikar, G. R., ed. *Meghdutam of Kalidas.* With English Translation and Notes. New Delhi: Asiatic Books, 2001.

Nederman, Cary, and Jacqui True. "The Third Sex: The Idea of the Hermaphrodite in Twelfth-Century Europe." *Journal of the History of Sexuality* 6 (1996): 497–517.

Newhauser, Richard, ed. *In the Garden of Evil: The Vices and Culture in the Middle Ages.* Toronto, ON: Pontifical Institute of Mediaeval Studies Press, 2005.

Nirenberg, David. *Communities of Violence: The Persecution of Minorities in the Middle Ages.* Princeton, NJ: Princeton University Press, 1996.

Nizami. *The Story of Layla and Majnun.* Translated by R. Gelpke. New Lebanon, NY: Omega Publications, 1978.

Noonan, John T., Jr. *Contraception: A History of Its Treatment by the Catholic Theologians and Canonists.* Cambridge, MA: Belknap Press, 1965.

Norris, Herbert. *Medieval Costume and Fashion.* Mineola, NY: Dover Publications, 1999.

Nuttall, Zelia, ed. *Codex Zouche-Nuttall: A Picture Manuscript from Ancient Mexico.* New York: Dover, 1975.

O'Carroll, Michael. *Theotokos: A Theological Encyclopedia of the Blessed Virgin Mary.* Wilmington, DL: M. Glazier, 1983.

O'Dwyer, Peter. *Mary: A History of Devotion in Ireland.* Dublin: Four Courts Press, 1988.

O'Rahilly, Cecile, ed. *Táin Bó Cúailnge.* Dublin: Dublin Institute for Advanced Studies, 1976.

Orchard, Andy. *Cassell's Dictionary of Norse Myth and Legend.* London: Cassell, 2002.

Oriel, J. D. *The Scars of Venus: A History of Venereology.* London: Springer-Verlag, 1994.

Orme, Nicholas. *Medieval Children.* London: Yale University Press, 2001.

Orr, Patricia. "Men's Theory and Women's Reality: Rape Prosecutions in the English Royal Courts of Justice, 1194–1222." In *The Rusted Hauberk: Feudal Ideals of Order and Their Decline,* edited by Liam O. Purdon and Cindy L. Vitto, 121–59. Gainesville: University Press of Florida, 1994.

Otis, Leah Lydia. *Prostitution in Medieval Society: The History of an Urban Institution in Languedoc.* Chicago: University of Chicago Press, 1985.

Pande, Susmita. *Medieval Bhakti Movement, Its History and Philosophy.* Meerut, India: Kusumanjali Prakashan, 1989.

Pardoe, Rosemary, and Darroll Pardoe. *The Female Pope: The Mystery of Pope Joan.* Guildford, Surrey: Thorsons Publishing Group, 1988.

Pathy, Dinanath, et al., eds. *Jayadeva and Gitagovinda in the Traditions of Orissa.* New Delhi: Harman Publishing, 1995.

Payer, Pierre J. *Book of Gomorrah: An Eleventh-Century Treatise against Clerical Homosexual Practices.* Waterloo, ON: Wilfrid Laurier University Press, 1982.

Payer, Pierre J. "Early Regulations Concerning Marital Sexual Relations." *Journal of Medieval History* 6 (1980): 353–76.

Payer, Pierre J. *Sex and the Penitentials.* Toronto, ON: University of Toronto Press, 1984.

Pearsall, Derek. *Arthurian Romance: A Short Introduction.* Malden, MA: Blackwell, 2003.

Pelikan, Jaroslav. *Mary through the Centuries: Her Place in the History of Culture.* New Haven, CT: Yale University Press, 1998.

Pellat, Charles. *The Life and Works of Jahiz: Translations of Selected Texts.* Translated from the French by D. M. Hawke. Berkeley: University of California Press, 1969.

Pennington, Kenneth. "Medieval Law." In *Medieval Studies: An Introduction*, edited by J. M. Powell, 333–52. Syracuse, NY: Syracuse University Press, 1992.

Penzer, N. M. *The Ocean of Story being C.H. Tawney's Translation of Somadeva's Kathasaritsagara*. New Delhi: Motilal Banarsidass, 1968.

Pernoud, Regine. *Joan of Arc by Herself and Her Witnesses*. Translated from the French by Edward Hyams. New York: Stein and Day, 1982.

Petrarca, Francesco. *Petrarch: The Canzoniere, or Rerum vulgarium fragmenta*. Translated by Mark Musa. Bloomington: Indiana University Press, 1996.

Phillips, Roderick. *Putting Asunder: A History of Divorce in Western Society*. London: Cambridge University Press, 1988.

Pincherle, Alberto. *Vita di Sant'Agostino*. Bari: Laterza, 1980.

Prentiss, Karen Pechilis. *The Embodiment of Bhakti*. New York: Oxford University Press, 1999.

Puette, William. *The Tale of Genji: A Readers' Guide*. Rutland, VT: Charles Tuttle, 1992.

Ramanujan, A. K. *Poems of Love and War from Eight Anthologies and Ten Long Poems of Classical Tamil*. New York: Columbia University Press, 1985.

Ranke-Heinemann, Uta. *Eunuchs for the Kingdom of Heaven: Women, Sexuality and the Catholic Church*. New York: Doubleday, 1990.

Ranking, G.S.A. "The Life and Works of Rhazes." *Proceedings of the Seventeenth International Congress of Medicine*. London, 1913, pp. 237–68.

Raven, W. "Ibn Dawud al-Isbahani and His Kitab al-Zahra." PhD diss., Leiden University, Amsterdam, 1989.

Rawcliffe, Carole. "Women, Childbirth, and Religion in Later Medieval England." In *Women and Religion in Medieval England*, edited by Diana Wood, 91–117. Oxford: Oxbow, 2003.

Ray, Hrudananda. *Śankara as a Romantic Philosopher*. Cuttack, India: Akash Publications, 1991.

Ray, Reginald A. *Secret of the Vajra World: The Tantric Buddhism of Tibet*. Boston: Shambhala Publications, 2002.

Rice, Edward. *Eastern Definitions: A Short Encyclopedia of Religions of the Orient*. New York: Doubleday, 1978.

Richards, Jefferey. *Sex, Dissidence and Damnation. Minority Groups in the Middle Ages*. London: Routledge, 1994.

Richey, M. F. *Essays on the Mediaeval German Love Lyric*. Oxford: Oxford University Press, 1942.

Riddle, John M. *Eve's Herbs: A History of Contraception and Abortion in the West*. Cambridge, MA: Harvard University Press, 1997.

Rider, Catherine. "Between Theory and Practice: Medieval Canonists on Magic and Impotence." In *Boundaries of the Law: Geography, Gender and Jurisdiction in Medieval and Early Modern Europe*, edited by Anthony Musson, pp. 53–66. Aldershot, UK: Ashgate, 2005.

Rieger, Angelica. "Was Bieiris de Romans Lesbian? Women's Relations with Each Other in the World of the Troubadours." In *The Voice of the Trobairitz: Perspectives on the Women Troubadours*, edited by William D. Paden, 73–94. Philadelphia: University of Pennsylvania Press, 1989.

Ringrose, Kathryn M. *The Perfect Servant: Eunuchs and the Social Construction of Gender in Byzantium*. Chicago: University of Chicago Press, 2003.

Rosenberg, Samuel, Margaret Switten, and Gérard Le Lot, eds. *Songs of the Troubadours and Trouvères: An Anthology of Poems and Melodies*. New York: Garland Publishing, 1998.

Rossiaud, Jacques. *Medieval Prostitution*. Translated by Lydia G. Cochrane. Oxford: Blackwell, 1988.

Ruan, Fang Fu. *Sex in China: Studies in Sexology in Chinese Culture*. New York: Plenum Press, 1991.

Ruggiero, Guido. *The Boundaries of Eros. Sex Crime and Sexuality in Renaissance Venice*. New York: Oxford University Press, 1987.

Ruggiero, Guido. "Sexual Criminality in the Early Renaissance: Venice, 1338–1358." *Journal of Social History* 8 (1975): 18–37.

Ruiz, Juan. *Libro de buen amor*. Madrid: Cátedra, 1992.

BIBLIOGRAPHY

Russell, Jeffrey Burton. *Witchcraft in the Middle Ages.* Ithaca, NY: Cornell University Press, 1972.

Sadasivan, K. *Devadasi System in Medieval Tamil Nadu.* Nagercoil, South India: CBH Publications, 1993.

Sahagun, Bernardino de. *Florentine Codex: General History of the Things of New Spain.* 13 vols. Edited by Arthur J. O. Anderson and Charles Dibble. Santa Fe, NM: School of American Research, 1950–1982.

Salisbury, Joyce E. *The Beast within: Animals in the Middle Ages.* New York: Routledge, 1994.

Sanford, James H. "The Abominable Tachikawa Skull Ritual." *Monumenta Nipponica* 46 (1991): 1–20.

Sanni, A. "Women Critics in Arabic Literary Tradition with Particular Reference to Sukayna Bint al-husayn." *British Society for Middle Eastern Studies Bulletin*, 1991, pp. 358–64.

Sarkar, Anil Kumar. *The Mysteries of Vajrayana Buddhism: From Atisha to Dalai Lama.* New Delhi: South Asian Publications & Research Institute, 1993.

Sautman, Canadé, and Pamela Sheingorn. *Same Sex Love and Desire among Women in the Middle Ages.* New York: Palgrave, 2001.

Sayce, Olive. *The Medieval German Lyric, 1150–1300.* Oxford: Oxford University Press, 1982.

Sayyid-Marsot, Afaf Lutfi, ed. *Society and the Sexes in Medieval Islam.* Malibu, CA: Undena Publications, 1979.

Schacht, Joseph. *An Introduction to Islamic Law.* Oxford: Clarendon Press, 1982.

Schimmel, Annemarie. *I Am Wind, You Are Fire: the Life and Work of Rumi.* Boston: Shambhala Publications, 1992.

Schimmel, Annemarie. *Look! This Is Love: Poems of Rumi.* Boston: Shambhala Publications, 1991.

Schipper, Kristofer. *The Taoist Body.* Berkeley: University of California Press, 1993.

Schulburg, Jane Tibetts. *Forgetful of Their Sex.* Chicago: University of Chicago Press, 1998.

Scott, George Ryley. *Phallic Worship: A History of Sex and Sex Rites in Relation to the Religions of All Races from Antiquity to the Present Day.* Twickenham, UK: Senate, 1996.

Shapiro, Norman. *The Comedy of Eros.* Urbana: University of Illinois Press, 1971.

Sharma, Satish Kumar. *Hijras, the Labelled Deviants.* New Delhi: Gian Publishing House, 1989.

Sharma, Tripat. *Women in Ancient India, from 320 AD to c. 1200 AD.* New Delhi: Ess Publications, 1987.

Shaw, Miranda. *Passionate Enlightenment: Women in Tantric Buddhism.* Princeton, NJ: Princeton University Press, 1994.

Sheehan, Michael M. *Marriage, Family, and Law in Medieval Europe: Collected Studies.* Toronto, ON: University of Toronto Press, 1996.

Shobha, Savitri Chandra. *Medieval India and Hindi Bhakti Poetry: A Socio-Cultural Study.* New Delhi: Har-Anand Publications, 1996.

Shonagon, Sei. *The Pillow Book of Sei Shonagon.* Translated and edited by Ivan Morris. New York: Columbia University Press, 1991.

Sigal, Gale. *Erotic Dawn-Songs of the Middle Ages: Voicing the Lyric Lady.* Gainesville: University Press of Florida, 1996.

Silberman, Lauren. "Mythographic Transformations of Ovid's Hermaphrodite." *Sixteenth Century Journal* 19 (Winter 1988): 643–52.

Singh, A. D. *Kaalidaasa: A Critical Study.* Columbia, MO: South Asia Books, 1977.

Smith, Susan L. *The Power of Women: A Topos in Medieval Art and Literature.* Philadelphia: University of Pennsylvania Press, 1995.

Soranus. *Soranus' Gynecology.* Translated by Owsei Temkin. Baltimore: Johns Hopkins University Press, 1956. Reprint 1991.

Soustelle, Jacques. *Daily Life of the Aztecs.* Mineola, NY: Dover Publications, 2002.

Southern, Richard W. *The Making of the Middle Ages.* New Haven, CT: Yale University Press, 1961.

Southern, Richard W. *Western Society and the Church in the Middle Ages.* New York: Penguin, 1990.

Speaker-Yuan, Margaret. *Women in Islam*. Detroit, MI: Greenhaven Press, 2005.
Spencer, Colin. *Homosexuality in History*. New York: Harcourt, Brace, 1995.
Spink, Walter. *Ajanta to Ellora*. Mumbai, India: Marg Publications for the Center for South and Southeast Asian Studies, University of Michigan, 1967.
Stanford, Peter. *The Legend of Pope Joan: In Search of the Truth*. New York: Henry Holt, 1998.
Stein, R. A. *Tibetan Civilization*. London: Faber and Faber, 1972.
Steinmann, Jean. *Saint Jerome and His Times*. Translated by Ronald Mathews. Notre Dame, IN: Fides Publishing, 1959.
Stengers, Jean, and Anne Van Neck. *Masturbation: The History of a Great Terror*. Translated by Kathryn A. Hoffmann. New York: Palgrave, 2001.
Stephens, Walter. *Demon Lovers: Witchcraft, Sex, and the Crisis of Belief*. Chicago: University of Chicago Press, 2002.
Stowasser, Barbara. *Women in the Qur'an, Traditions, and Interpretation*. New York: Oxford University Press, 1994.
Stuard, Susan Mosher, ed. *Women in Medieval Society*. Philadelphia: University of Pennsylvania Press, 1976.
Sturm, Sara. "The Presentation of the Virgin in the Cantigas de Santa Maria." *Philological Quarterly* 49 (January 1970): 1–7.
Subrahmanyam, B. *Vajrayana Buddhist Centers in South India*. Delhi: Bharatiya Kala Prakashan, 2001.
Sundaram, P. S., trans. *The Kural of Tiruvalluvar*. London: Penguin Books, 1991.
Swabey, Ffiona. *Eleanor of Aquitaine, Courtly Love, and the Troubadours*. Westport, CT: Greenwood Press, 2004.
Swarup, Ram. *Understanding the Hadith: The Sacred Traditions of Islam*. Amherst, NY: Prometheus Books, 2002.
Symonds, John Addington. *Wine, Women and Song*. New York: Cooper Square Publishers, 1966.
Tadgell, Christopher. *The History of Architecture in India*. London: Phaidon Press, 1990.
Taglia, Kathryn. "Delivering a Christian Identity: Midwives in Northern French Synodal Legislation, c. 1200–1500." In *Religion and Medicine in the Middle Ages*, edited by Peter Biller and Joseph Ziegler, 77–90. Rochester, NY: York Medieval Press, 2001.
Tanquerey, Adolfo. *Brevior synopsis theologiae moralis*. Torino: Marietti, 1934.
Taylor, Archer. *The Literary History of Meistergesang*. New York: Modern Language Association of America, 1937.
Taylor, Gordon Rattray. *Sex in History*. New York: Harper & Row, 1973.
Taylor, Julius Heyward. *Rhazes: The Greatest of the Arabians*. Charlotte, NC: Southern Medicine and Surgery, 1934.
Thapar, Romila. *Sakuntala: Text, Readings, Histories*. New Delhi: Kali for Women, 1999.
Theophylactus of Ochrid. *Works of Theophylactus* (Greek and Latin). 2nd ed. 4 vols. Venice: J. F. B. M. de Rossi, 1754–1763.
Thurston, Edgar, and K. Rangachari. *Castes and Tribes of Southern India*. Vol. 4. New Delhi: Asian Educational Services, 1987.
Tomarelli, Ubaldo. *San Vincenzo Ferreri apostolo e taumaturgo*. Bologna: Edizioni Studio Domenicano, 1990.
Torrey, C. C. "The History of al-'Abbas b. al-Ahnaf and His Fortunate Verses." *Journal of the American Oriental Society* 15 (1894): 43–70.
Trivedi, Prathibha, ed. *Sri Mahendra Suri Viracita Nammayasundari Kaha*. Mumbai, India: Bharatiya Vidya Bhavan, 1960.
Tsai, Shih-Shan Henry. *The Eunuchs in the Ming Dynasty*. New York: State University of New York Press, 1996.
Twitchett, Denis, and Howard J. Wechsler. "Kao-tsung (r. 649–683) and the Empress Wu: The Inheritor and the Usurper." In *The Cambridge History of China*, edited by Denis Twitchett and John K. Fairbank, 242–89. Vol. 3, part 1. Cambridge: Cambridge University Press, 1979.
Unschuld, Paul U. *Medicine in China: Historical Artifacts and Images*. New York: Prestel, 2000.

BIBLIOGRAPHY

Upadhye, A. N. *Kuvalayamala Katha Samksepa*. Mumbai, India: Bharatiya Vidya Bhavan, 1961.

Vadet, Jean Claude. *L'Esprit courtois en Orient dans les cinq premiers siëcles de l'Hègire*. Paris: G. P. Maisonneuve et Larose, 1968.

Vadet, Jean Claude. "Une personnalitè feminine du higaz au Ier/VIIe siècle: Sukayna, petite-fille de 'Ali." *Arabica* 4 (1957): 261–87.

Vale, M.G.A. *Charles VII*. Berkeley: University of California Press, 1974.

Van Gulik, Robert Hans, and Paul Rakita Goldin. *Sexual Life in Ancient China: A Preliminary Survey of Chinese Sex and Society from ca. 1500 BC till 1644 AD*. Leiden: Brill Academic Publishers, 2003.

Vanita, Ruth, ed. *Queering India: Same-Sex Love and Eroticism in Indian Culture and Society*. New York: Routledge, 2002.

Vanita, Ruth, and Saleem Kidwai, eds. *Same-Sex Love in India: Readings from Literature and History*. New York: St. Martin's Press, 2000.

Velsquez, Primo F., ed. "Leyenda de los soles." *Anales de Cuauhtitln. Cûdice Chimalpopoca*. Mexico: Imprenta Universitaria, 1945.

Venarde, Bruce L. *Women's Monasticism and Medieval Society: Nunneries in France and England, 890–1215*. Ithaca, NY: Cornell University Press, 1997.

Vine, Aubrey Russell. *The Nestorian Churches*. New York: AMS Press, 1980.

Waddell, Helen. *The Wandering Scholars*. 7th ed. London: Constable, 1947.

Walker, Barbara G. *The Woman's Encyclopedia of Myths and Secrets*. New York: HarperCollins, 1983.

Walther, Wiebke. *Women in Islam from Medieval to Modern Times*. Princeton, NJ: Markus Wiener Publishers, 1995.

Wang Ping. *Aching for Beauty: Footbinding in China*. Minneapolis: University of Minnesota Press, 2000.

Warner, Marina. *Alone of All Her Sex: The Myth and the Cult of the Virgin Mary*. 1976. Reprint, New York: Vintage, 1983.

Warren, Nancy Bradley. *Spiritual Economies: Female Monasticism in Later Medieval England*. Philadelphia: University of Pennsylvania Press, 2001.

Weis, J. Max. *Great Men in Israel: Sketches from Rabbinic and Medieval Jewry*. New York: Bloch, 1922.

Wheeler, Brannon. "Touching the Penis in Islamic Law." *History of Religions* 44 (2004): 89–119.

Wile, Douglas. *Art of the Bedchamber: The Chinese Sexual Yoga Classics, including Women's Solo Meditation Texts*. Albany: State University of New York Press, 1992.

Wilhelm, James J., ed. *The Romance of Arthur: An Anthology of Medieval Texts in Translation*. Exp. ed. New York: Garland Publishing, 1994.

Wilken, Robert. *John Chrysostom and the Jews: Rhetoric and Reality in the Late 4th Century Church*. Berkeley: University of California Press, 1983.

Willard, Charity. *Christine de Pizan: Her Life and Works*. New York: Persea Books, 1984.

Williams, Bernadette. "'She Was Usually Placed with the Great Men and Leaders of the Land in the Public Assemblies'—Alice Kyteler: A Woman of Considerable Power." In *Women in Renaissance and Early Modern Europe*, edited by Christine Meek, 67–83. Dublin: Four Courts Press, 2000.

Williams, Charles. *The Figure of Beatrice: A Study in Dante*. New York: Farrar, Straus and Cudahy, 1961.

Wilson, Peter Lambon, and Nasrollah Pourjavady, eds. *Drunken Universe: An Anthology of Persian Sufi Poetry*. Grand Rapids, MI: Phanes Press, 1987.

Winer, Rebecca Lynn. "Defining Rape in Medieval Perpignan: Women Plaintiffs Before the Law." *Viator: Medieval and Renaissance Studies* 31 (2000): 165–83.

Wines, Leslie. *Rumi, a Spiritual Biography*. New York: Crossroad Publishing Company, 2000.

Winkler, Gershom. *Sacred Secrets: The Sanctity of Sex in Jewish Law and Lore*. Northvale, NJ: Jason Aronson, 1998.

Winstead, Karen A., ed. *Chaste Passions*. London: Cornell University Press, 2000.

Yamamoto, Dorothy. *The Boundaries of the Human in Medieval English Literature*. Oxford: Oxford University Press, 2000.
Yamasaki Taik. *Shingon: Japanese Esoteric Buddhism*. Boston: Shambhala Publications, 1988.
Yarshater, Ehsan, ed. *Persian Literature*. Albany, NY: Bibliotheca Press, 1988.
Young, Serinity. *Courtesans and Tantric Consorts: Sexualities in Buddhist Narrative, Iconography, and Ritual*. New York: Routledge, 2004.
Zannad, Traki. *Le lieux du corps en Islam*. Paris: Publisud, 1994.
Zysk, Kenneth G. *Conjugal Love in India: Ratisastra and Ratiramana; Text, Translation, and Notes*. Leiden: Brill, 2002.

Index

Boldfaced page numbers indicate main entries.

Abbas ben al-Ahfnaf, al-', **3**
Abelard, Peter, **4**, 93, 164–65, 209
Ablution, 80
Abortion, **4–6**, 62
Abu Nuwas, **6**
Adab literature, **6–7**
Adam and Eve, 81, 82, 229
Adultery, **7–9**; definitions, 8; jurisdiction over cases of, 8; punishment for, 8–9. *See also* Arthurian legend; Extramarital love
Africa, **9–10**
Agnes, Saint, 242
Alain of Lille, **10–11**, 28
Albas, **11–12**
Albertus Magnus, **12–13**, 211–12
Allah, 214, 215
Amaru, 90
Amidism, 120
An Lushan, 251
Anal sex, **13–14**
Ananga Ranga, **14–15**
Andreas Capellanus (Andrew the Chaplain), **15–16**
Annulments, 70–71, 104
Anthony of Egypt, Saint, 165
Aphrodisiacs, **16–17**, 139
Aquinas, Thomas, **17**, 24, 42, 47, 82, 126, 151–52, 210
Arabia, pre-Islamic, 113
Arabian Nights. *See Thousand and One Nights*
Arabs, 29. *See also* Islam
Aristotle, **18**, 212, 229, 230

Arthur, King, 146. *See also* Arthurian legend
Arthurian legend, **18–19**, 41
Asceticism, Daoist, 68
Ashkenazi Jews, 81
Asia, xvii–xviii. *See also* Central Asia
Athanasius, Saint, 167
Aucassin and Nicolette, **20**
Augustine of Hippo, Saint, **20–21**, 82, 136, 148, 165–66, 209
Averroes. *See* Ibn Rushd
Avicenna. *See* Ibn Sina

Basil the Great, Saint, bishop of Caesarea, 165, 167
Bastardy. *See* Illegitimacy
Beatrice, 66–67
Beauty, 119–20
Bellemère, Gilles, 77–78
Benedict of Nursia, Saint, 166
Bernard of Clairvaux, **22–23**, 136, 145–46
Bernardino of Siena, **23**
Bestiality, **24**
Bestiary, **25**
Bhagavata Purana, 132
Bhakti, **25–26**, 91
Bhavabhuti, 91
Bieris de Romans, **26–27**
Bigamy, **27–28**. *See also* Polygamy
Bisexuality, **28–29**
Bo Xingjian, 29
Boccaccio, Giovanni, **30–31**
Bodhisattvas, 31, 32
Book of the Flower (Ibn Dawud), 98

Breviary of Love (Ermengaud), 75
Brigid, Saint, 164
Buddha Vajrasattva, 32
Buddhism, **31–33**, 45, 120; in Tibet, 231–32
Burton, Francis, 15
Byzantium, **33–34**, 75, 95, 176, 177

Caesarius of Arles, 135
Cakrasamvara Tantra, **35**
Canon law, **36–37**, 104–5, 110
Canterbury Tales, The (Chaucer), 48
Cantigas de Santa Maria, **37–38**
Castration, **38–39**. *See also* Eunuchs; Hijras
Cathars, 141–42
Catherine of Alexandria, Saint, 242
Catholic Europe, **39–42**; foundation, 39–40; love and, 41–42
Catholicism, **42–43**
Celibacy, **43–45**, 170. *See also* Clerical marriage
Centeotl, 159
Central Asia, **45–46**
Charlemagne (Charles the Great), 40
Charles VII, 221
Chastity in marriage, **47**
Chaucer, Geoffrey, **47**
Childbirth, **48–50**; roles of men, 50
China, **50–53**, 59, 75–76, 171; alternate sexualities, 53; love and marriage, 50–51; medical

INDEX

and religious views of heterosexuality, 51–53
Chinese paintings of elite women, 53–54
Chrétien de Troyes, 18–19, 65, 202–3
Christianity: sexual life and, xvi. *See also* Canon law; *specific topics*
Christine de Pisan, **54–55**
Chrysostom, John, **55–56**
Circumcision, 9, **56–57**
Cleanliness, 159
Clerical marriage, 34, 36. *See also* Celibacy
Clitoridectomy, 9, **57**
Collatio Legum Mosaicarum et Romanarum, **58**
Columbanus, St., 40
Concubinage, **58–60**
Confessio Amantis (Gower), 83, 84
Confession, 43, **60**
Confucius, xvii
Consanguinity, **61–62**
Consolamentum, 142
Constantinople, 175
Contraception, 5, **62–64**, 114, 154
Courtly love, **64–65**
Cross-dressing, 88. *See also* transgenderism
Crusades, 109

Dakinis, 35
Damian, Peter. *See* Peter Damian
Damiani, 13
Dante Alighieri, **66–67**
Daoism, 52, **67–68**
Decameron (Boccaccio), 30
Demons and demonology, 249
Devadasis, **68–69**
Devotional practices. *See* Bhakti
Divine Comedy, The (Dante), 66–67
Divorce, 37, **69–71**, 81; medieval, 69–70
Domestic violence, **71–72**; in the arts, 72; in church courts, 72; social hierarchy and, 71
Droit du seigneur, **72–73**
Dualism, 141–42

East Asia, sex and love in, xvii–xviii

Eastern Orthodox church. *See* Orthodox Christianity
Edward II, King of England, **74**
Ejaculation. *See* Orgasm, male
Eleanor of Aquitaine, 61–62
Elite women, Chinese paintings of, 53–54
Ermengaud, Matfre, **75**
Eunuchs, 38, **75–76**, 176–77, 219, 228. *See also* Hijras
Extramarital love, 91

Female genital mutilation. *See* Clitoridectomy
Ferrer, Vinente, **77**
Fertility, 154–55. *See also* Sterility
Feudal system, 219
Fifteen Joys of Marriage, **77–78**
Flamel, Nicolas, 16
Footbinding, 51
Fornication, 7–8
Freya/Frigg, **78–79**

Galen, 174, 229
Gaozong, 250
Gaveston, Piers, 74
Genital contact in Islamic law, **80–81**
Genital mutilation. *See* Circumcision; Clitoridectomy
Geoffrey of Monmouth, 18
Gershom ben Judah, **81**
Ghazals, 3, **82**
Ghilman, 219
Ghusl, 80
Giles of Rome, **82–83**
Gita Govindam (Jayadeva), 121
Goliard poets, **83**
Gopis, 133
Gottfried von Strassburg, 235
Gower, John, **83–84**
Gratian, 246
Guhyasamaja Tantra, 32
Guillaume de Lorris, 204
Guinevere, 18, 19

Hadith, 98
Hafiz, **85**
Hafsa Bint al-Hadjdj, **85–86**
Hakon Hakonarson, King, 207
Halevi, Judah, 86, 124
Harem, **86–87**

Heian period, 119–21
Heloise, **4**, 164–65
Herbalism and magic, 138–39
Hermaphrodites, **87–88**
Hermaphroditos, 87
Hermaphroditus, 87, 88
Hijras, **88–89**, 93. *See also* Eunuchs
Hilda, Saint, 164
Hildegard of Bingen, **89–90**
Hindu literature, **90–91**
Hinduism, 44, **92–93**, 108. *See also* Bhakti
Homosexuality, 53, 115, 175–76; female, 27, 53, **93–94**; male, 14, 53, **95–96**, 108, 115, 175–76, 219. *See also* Pederasty
Houris, **96–97**
Hugh of St. Victor, 209–10

Ibn Dawud al-Zahir, Muhammad, **98–99**
ibn Gabirol, Solomon, **99**
Ibn Hazm, Abu Muhammad Ali, **100**
Ibn Qayyim al-Jawziyya, **100–101**
Ibn Rushd, **101–2**
Ibn Sina, **102–3**
Illegitimacy, **103–4**
Impotence, 70, **104–5**. *See also* Eunuchs; Hijras
In Defense of Eunuchs (Theophylactus), 228
Incest, 61, 70, **105–7**, 149
India, **107–9**; homosexuality and "third gender" roles, 108. *See also* Hijras
Indian religion: sexuality and, 108–9. *See also specific religions*
Interconfessional sex and love, **109–11**
Intercrural sex, **13–14**
Interfemoral connection. *See* Intercrural sex
Islam, xvi–xvii, 44, 57, 62, 76, 95–97, **111–13**; Christian Empire and the threat of, 40–41; schools of, 215. *See also* Interconfessional sex and love
Islamic empire, non-Muslim communities in, 115–16
Islamic law, 5, 113; genital contact in, 80–81. *See also* Sharia
Islamic society, **113–16**

274

INDEX

Jahiz, Abu Uthman Amr b. Bahr al-, **117–18**
Jainism, **118**
Japan, **119–21**; rise of warrior class, 120–21
Japanese religion, 119, 120
Jayadeva, **121**
Jean de Meun, 204
Jerome, Eusebius Hieronymus, **122**
Jesus Christ, 42, 88, 164, 243, 247–48; humanity, 41. *See also* Marianism
Jews, 28, 72, 81, **122–24**. *See also* Judaism
Jing, 52
Joan, Pope. *See* Pope Joan
Joan of Arc, **124–25**
Joseph, husband of Mary, 47
Judaism, 44, 56–57, **125–27**. *See also* Jews

Kailasanath (Kailasha) Temple at Ellora, **128**
Kalidasa, xviii, **128–29**
Kama Sutra, 14, 15, **129–30**
Kansa, 132–33
Khajuraho temple complex, **130–31**
Kiss of infamy, **131–32**
Kitab al-zahra (Ibn Dawud), 98
Krishna, 108–9, **132–33**
Kuzari, The (Halevi), 86
Kyteler, Alice, **133–34**, 249

Labor: aid for mothers in, 49–50. *See also* Childbirth
Lancelot, 19, 65
Lancelot (Chrétien), 65
Lent, **135**
Leo XI, Pope, 177
Lesbianism. *See* Homosexuality, female
Li Wa zhuan (Bo Xingjian), 29
Literature, sex and love in, xviii
Lombard, Peter, 209, 246
Louis VII of France, King, 61
Love: defined, 15; degrees of, 22
Lover's Confession, The (Gower), 83, 84
Lust, 18, 21, **136–37**; types of, 17

Magic, **138–40**; religion and, 139–40

Mahayana Buddhism, 31–32, 226
Maidens. *See* Houris
Maimonides, Moses, 56–57, **140–41**
Malory, Thomas, 203
Manicheans, **141–42**
Marcabru, **142–43**
Margaret of Henneberg, **143–44**
Marianism, 41, **144–46**. *See also* Virgin Mary
Marie de France, **146–47**, 223
Marital affection, 149
Marital process, 149
Marriage, 34, 77–78, 122, **147–49**; canon law and, 37; chastity in, 47; in China, 50–51; clerical, 34, 36 (*see also* Celibacy); consanguineous, 61–62; consent theory, 148–49; influence of Christianity on, 148; in Islamic society, 113–14; Jewish, 122–23; *Mut'a*, 168–69; in Orthodox Christianity, 175–76; out of force or fear, 70; as public institution, 72; purpose, 209; roots of medieval, 147–48; as sacrament, 148–49; in Tibet, 231; under-aged, 70–71; virgin, 47. *See also* Remarriage
Marriageability, ages of, 149
Martin of Tours, Saint, 39
Martyred virgins. *See* Virgin martyrs
Mary, Mother of Jesus. *See* Marianism; Virgin Mary
Mary Magdalene, cult of, **149–50**
Masturbation, 114, **150–52**
Medb, **152**
Medicine, xviii, 48, **152–55**; background, 153; Islamic, 5–6; in Western Europe, 153–54
Meistersinger, **155–56**
Menstruation, 126, 154, **156–57**
Mesoamerica, **157–60**
Metamorphoses (Ovid), 179
Metta Sutta, The, 31
Midwives, 49, 159, **160–61**
Minnesinger, **161–62**
Misogyny in Latin Christendom, **162–63**
Monastic Buddhism, 31
Monasticism: Daoist, 68; female, **163–65**; male, **165–66**

Monophysite churches, **167**
Muhammed, Prophet, 190, 222
Muhammed of Ghur, 191
Murasaki Shikibu, **168**
Mut'a marriage, **168–69**

"Na Maria, pretz e fina valors" (Bieris de Romans), 26
Nestorian churches, **170–71**
New Life, The (Dante), 66
New Songs from a Jade Terrace, **171–72**
Niddah, 126
Nizami Ganjavi, Abu Muhammad ibn Yusif, xviii, **172**

Obstetrics, 48
On Love (Andreas Capellanus), 15–16
Orgasm: female, **173–74**; male, **174–75**
Oribasius, 214
Orthodox Christianity, **175–77**; historical background, 175; love and marriage, 175–76; sexual relations, 176
Orthodox Europe, **177–78**
Osculum infame. See Kiss of infamy
Ovidianism, **179–80**

Pagan Europe, **181–82**
Patriarchy and religion in Christian and Islamic lands, xv–xvi
Patrick, St., 39–40
Paul, Saint, 165, 166
Pederasty, 6, **182–83**, 219
Penitentials, 24, 36, **183–84**
Peter Damian, 151, **184–85**, 220
Peter of Abano, **185**, 212
Petrarch, Francesco, **185–86**
Petronilla of Meath, 133–34
Phallic worship, **186–87**
Phillip II Augustus, King of France, **187–88**
Phillip IV "the Fair," King, 234
Phyllis legend, 18
Physiognomics, **188–89**
Poetry, 37–38; love, 3, 46, 78–79, 90, 92, 171–72, 204 (*see also* Ghazals; Minnesinger; Poets); male homosexual, 6; udhrite, 239

275

INDEX

Poets, 6, 47–48, 75, 83–85, 98–99, 240. *See also* Kalidasa; Marie de France; Nizami; Rumi
Polygamy, 9, 81, **189–90**. *See also* Bigamy
Pope Joan, **191**
Pornography, **191–92**
Pregnancy: aid for mothers in, 49–50; sex during, 12–13
Premarital love, 91
Prithviraj III, **192–93**
Prostitution, 176, **193–95**; male, 176
Purdah, 210–11
Purification rituals, 80–81

Qiyan. *See* Singing girls

Radegunde, Saint, 164
Rape, **197–98**; as crime, 197–98; definition, 197
Razi, Abu Bakr Muhammad ibn Zakariya al-, **199**
Remarriage, **200–201**. *See also* Bigamy
Roman law, 58, **201–2**
Romance, **202–3**
Romance of the Rose, The (Guillaume de Lorris and Jean de Meun), 204, **204–5**, 212–13
Ruiz, Juan, **205**
Rumi, Maulana Jalaluddin, **206**, 222

Sachs, Hans, 155
Sadako, Empress, 217
Saga literature, **207–8**
Sakthism, **208–9**
Sanjukta, princess of Kannauj, 192–93
Sankara, 90
Scholastic philosophy, **209–10**
Science, xviii
Seclusion of women, **210–11**. *See also* Veil
Secrets of Women, **211–12**
Sex manuals, **212–13**
Sexual cultivation, 68
Sexual differences. *See* Theories of sexual difference
Sexual health, 154

Sexual morality: in Islamic society, 114–15. *See also* Sins
Sexual positions, 13
Sexually transmitted diseases, **213–14**
Shajarat ad-Durr, **214**
Shakti, 208
Sharia, 8, **214–16**
Shaving, 111
Sheela-na-gig, **216**
Shinto, 120
Shinü hua. *See* Chinese paintings of elite women
Shiva, 128, 131
Shonagon, Sei, **217**
Singing girls, **217–18**
Sins, 17, 37–38, 60
Sir Gawain and the Green Knight, 203
Slavery, 59, 114, 217–18, **218–19**
Sodomy, 13, 23, 95, 96, **220–21**
Songs. *See* Albas Bhakti; Minnesinger
Soranus, 63
Sorel, Agnes, **221**
South Asia, xvii. *See also* East Asia
Sterility, 101–2
Sufism, **222**
Sukayna bint al-Husayn, **222–23**
Sun Simiao, **223–24**

Tachikawa-ryu, **225–26**
"Tale of Li Wa" (Bo Xingjian), 29
Talmud, 81, 123, 125
Tantric Buddhism, 32–33, 35, 52–53, **226–27**
Taoism. *See* Daoism
Tawq al-hamama (ibn Hazm), 100
Templars, Trial of. *See* Trial of the Templars
Theodora, **227–28**
Theophylactus of Ochrid, **228**
Theories of sexual difference, **229–30**
Thousand and One Nights, The, **230–31**
Tibet, **231–32**; love and marriage, 231; religion and sexuality, 231–32

Tlazoteotl (Divine Eater of Filth), 159
Transgenderism, 88–89, **232–34**
Trial of the Templars, 132, **234**
Tristan, 203, **234–36**
Trobairitz, **236**. *See also* Bieris de Romans
Troilus and Criseyde (Chaucer), 48
Trotula, **236–37**
Troubadours, 11, **237–38**
Tuizhi. *See* Bo Xingjian

Udhrite love, **239**
Umar ibn Abi Rabia, **240**

Veil, **241–42**. *See also* Seclusion of women
Venus, 30
Vice against nature: types of, 17. *See also* Sins
Violence: against children, 71. *See also* Domestic violence
Virgin marriage, 47
Virgin martyrs, **242–43**
Virgin Mary, 37–38, 41–42, 47, 163, 203. *See also* Marianism
Virginity, 17, 21, 72, 102, 122, **243–44**

Wallada bint Al-Mustakfi, **245**
Washing, 80
Wedding rituals, **246–47**
Wilgefortis, Saint, **247–48**
William I, 103
William IX, Duke of Aquitaine and Gascony, Count of Poiters, **248–49**
Witches and witch-hunting, 133, **249–50**. *See also* Magic
Wu Zetian, **250**
Wudu, 80

Yang Guifei, **251**
Yin and yang, 52, 67
Yogas, sexual, 33
Yoginis, 35

Zhang Boduan, **252**
Zhang Zhuo, **253**
Zhu Xi, 51
Zhuo, Zhang, xviii

About the Editor and Contributors

Bethany Hope Allen is a graduate student in medieval history at the University of New Hampshire. She holds a BA from this university in both history and classics.

Stephen A. Allen received a master's degree in medieval studies from the University of Notre Dame, Indiana, and is currently a graduate student at the University of Illinois at Chicago. His research has focused on canon law and church history.

Lara C. W. Blanchard is Henry Luce assistant professor of East Asian art at Hobart and William Smith Colleges in Geneva, New York. Her doctoral dissertation was titled "Visualizing Love and Longing in Song Dynasty Paintings of Women" (2001). Her research interests include Song dynasty paintings, text-image relationships, the construction of gender in China, and Chinese theories of representation.

Jennifer Boulanger is a student at the Baylor University Honors College, Texas, specializing in English and the great texts of the Western tradition. Her research interests include comparative literature and women's studies. Jennifer's current research explores the portrayal of medieval women in religious and vernacular writings of the eleventh through the fourteenth centuries.

Matthieu Boyd is a graduate of Princeton University, Stumdi (a language institute for Breton), and University College Dublin. He is a presidential scholar of the Graduate School of Arts and Sciences and a PhD student in Celtic languages and literatures at Harvard University.

Emiliano J. Buis is a PhD candidate and lecturer in Greek language and literature and in Roman law at the University of Buenos Aires, Argentina. He completed his postgraduate studies at the University of Paris 1 (Panthéon-Sorbonne), and as a research fellow has published several articles on legal history and ancient Greek law.

Vern L. Bullough was a distinguished professor of the State University of New York and the author, coauthor, or editor of numerous books, including *Cross-Dressing, Sex and Gender* (1993, with Bonnie Bullough) and *Handbook of Medieval Sexuality* (1996, coedited with James A. Brundage). He served as the president of the Society for the Scientific Study of Sex. Vern Bullough died in 2006.

William E. Burns is a historian and teacher in Washington, D.C. His books include *An Age of Wonders: Prodigies, Politics and Providence in England, 1657–1727* (2002), *Witch Hunts in Europe and America* (2003) and *Science and Technology in Colonial America* (2005). He is currently working on a study of science in world history.

Sara M. Butler is assistant professor of medieval history at Loyola University New Orleans. She has written a number of articles on women, marriage, and the law, and has a forthcoming book titled *The Language of Abuse: Marital Violence in Later Medieval England*.

ABOUT THE EDITOR AND CONTRIBUTORS

Susannah Mary Chewning teaches British literature, women's studies, and writing at Union County College in Cranford, New Jersey. She has published widely on Chaucer, medieval spirituality, and gender studies. She is the editor of the collection *Intersections of Sexuality and the Divine in Medieval Culture: The Word Made Flesh* (2005) and is currently working on a monograph on medieval mysticism and dream vision poetry.

Clark Chilson is assistant professor of Japanese religions at the University of Pittsburgh. He coedited the *Nanzan Guide to Japanese Religions* (2006, with Paul Swanson) and has published on secretive Pure Land Buddhists in Japan.

Elvio Ciferri is permanent professor of Italian literature and history at Leopoldo and Alice Franchetti Institute, Città di Castello (Italy). He has written extensively on the history of the papal states and hagiography, and is the author of *Tifernati illustri* (2000–2003, 3 volumes) and numerous other books on the history of central Italy and church history. He has contributed to many encyclopedias. In 2002 he won the Atheste Award for distinguished writing in historical research.

Jennifer Della'Zanna is a graduate of Albright College in Reading, Pennsylvania, where she received a bachelor's degree with a triple major in history, German, and classical Greek. She studied medieval history at Temple University in Philadelphia and currently works as a freelance writer in Columbia, Maryland.

Lindsay Diggelmann is a lecturer in the Department of History at the University of Auckland, New Zealand. He completed his PhD thesis, on the topic of political marriages in twelfth-century England and France, in 2004. He has had several articles on related themes published in leading academic journals.

Susanne Enderwitz received a PhD in 1990 with a study of classical Arab love-poetry of al-'Abbas ben al-Ahnaf. From 1991 to 1999 she was assistant professor at the Free University of Berlin. Her 2001 "Habilitation" was a study of modern Palestinian autobiography. She has made several visits abroad to Egypt, France, and Israel. Since 2002 she has been professor of Islamic and Arabic studies at the University of Heidelberg.

Robert M. Frakes is professor of history at Clarion University, Pennsylvania. He is the author of *Contra Potentium Iniurias: The Defensor Civitatis and Late Roman Justice* (2001) and *Writing for College History* (2004).

Silvana A. Gaeta, a scholar of Roman culture, lives in Buenos Aires, Argentina. She has done research on the poet Ennius and Roman Hellenism.

Antonella Ghersetti has a PhD in Semitic linguistics and is a researcher in Arabic language and literature at Università Ca' Foscari, Venezia. Her fields of research are Arabic classical literature, especially the narrative tradition and *adab* literature; the classical Arabic linguistic tradition; and Arabic physiognomics. She is the editor of the Arabic translation of pseudo-Aristotle's *Physiognomics* (*Il Kitab Aristatalis al-faylasuf fi l-firasa nella traduzione di Hunayn b. Ishaq*, 1999). She also translated into Italian, with introduction and notes, the famous physician Ibn Butlan's treatise on the purchasing of slaves (*Il trattato onnicomprensivo sull'acquisto e l'esame degli schiavi*, 2001) and the book on spongers by the historian al-Khatib al-Baghdadi (*L'arte dello scrocco*, 2005).

Jamie A. Gianoutsos is a student in the Baylor University Honors College, Texas, specializing in political science and great texts of the Western tradition. In 2005, she was recognized as outstanding student in both these disciplines. Her current research examines the early writings of John Locke and, in particular, the portrayal of the "Lockian gentleman."

Jeanne L. Gillespie is associate professor of Spanish and director of women's studies at the University of Southern Mississippi.

Mark D. Gossiaux is assistant professor of philosophy at Loyola University New Orleans. He specializes in the history of medieval philosophy and classical metaphysics, with a special emphasis on thirteenth- and fourteenth-century Latin philosophical thought.

David B. Gray is assistant professor of religious studies at Santa Clara University, in Santa Clara, California. He received his PhD in the history of religions from Columbia University, specializing in Buddhist studies. David's interests focus upon the development of the Buddhist Yogini Tantras in India and their dissemination to Tibet and China. He has completed a study and translation of the *Cakrasamvara Tantra*, an important Indian Buddhist scripture focusing on yoga and ritual, one that borrowed heavily from Shaiva Hindu sources, and that later became very popular in Tibet. He is currently completing a translation of the important Cakrasamvara commentary by Tsongkhapa, "The Illumination of the Hidden Meaning." He is also working on the dissemination of Cakrasamvara ritual texts in China from the Yuan dynasty through the contemporary period.

Edward Green is a professor at the Manhattan School of Music. His published scholarly writings range from medieval studies to the music of Haydn, Elgar, Mendelssohn, and the contemporary Chinese composer Zhou Long. In 2006 he won the Isabelle Cazeaux Prize from the Lyrica Society for Word-Music Relations for his essay "Marcabru: An Early Exemplar of Western Song." Currently he is at work on a book about Duke Ellington for Cambridge University Press. An active composer, his music is available on several labels. Among these are Albany Records, for his *Trumpet Concerto*; Arizona University Recordings, for his *Concerto for Saxophone and Strings*; and Traditional Crossroads, for his *Zhou*, which is scored for pi'pa and erhu. In 1995 Edward Green was awarded first place in the prestigious International Kodaly Composers Competition, and in 2004 he received a *Music Alive!* award from the American Symphony Orchestra League. He also holds the position of composer-in- residence at both Imagery Films Ltd. and the Aesthetic Realism Theater Company.

Anne Hardgrove teaches in the Department of History at the University of Texas at San Antonio. She is the author of *Community and Public Culture: The Marwaris in Calcutta, c. 1897–1997* (2002) and is currently working on a history of the *Kama Sutra* and its translations.

Muhammed Hassanali's interests include the philosophical and civilizational aspects of Islam. He has written curricula for high school students that teach Islam from a sociological perspective and has also developed training modules for those teaching Islam.

Dawn Marie Hayes received her PhD in medieval European history from New York University in 1998. Having taught at Iona College and the City University of New York's Borough of Manhattan Community College, she joined the history faculty at Montclair State University in the fall of 2003, where she now teaches the history of medieval Europe. Dr. Hayes has been a speaker in the humanities for the New York Council for the Humanities and a participant in National Endowment for the Humanities Summer Seminars on Gothic Architecture in the Ile-de-France (1998) and Anglo-Saxon England (2004). She is the author of *Body and Sacred Place in Medieval Europe, 1100–1389* (2003), which explores the symbiotic relationship between human bodies and churches in the later Middle Ages. Her current project is *Medieval Maternity*, a book on pregnancy and childbirth in medieval Europe.

Lisa R. Holliday is a graduate student at the University of Kentucky, where she is completing her dissertation. Her research interests are early Christian history, the Roman Empire, and Roman culture.

Alison Jeppesen is working toward her doctorate in Roman social history in the Department of Greek and Roman Studies at the University of Calgary, Alberta, Canada. Her dissertation examines developments in spousal identity in Latin literature and epitaphs from Augustus to Augustine.

Mia Korpiola is doctor of laws and researcher of legal history at the University of Helsinki, Finland. The subject of her doctoral thesis was marriage formation in medieval and early modern Sweden. She has also written many articles on matrimonial and family law and sexual crime in the Middle Ages and the sixteenth century.

Hiram Kümper is assistant for the Didactics of History at the Ruhr-University Bochum's history department. He has published editions, studies, and articles mainly on medieval European law and the history of eighteenth-century jurisprudence.

Tonya Marie Lambert is a PhD student at the University of Alberta in Edmonton, Canada. She studies the history of sexual violence in the medieval and early modern periods, focusing on Tudor-Stuart England.

Jason Lewallen received his BA in 2005 from Baylor University, where he was a member of the prestigious University Scholars Program. His research interests include medieval literature and literary modernism. Jason's honors thesis examined the artist figure in Virginia Woolf's novel *To the Lighthouse*. Jason was selected by the French government to serve as a teaching assistant in Créteil, France, during 2004–2005.

Sergey Lobachev, PhD, is an associate at the Center for European, Russian and Eurasian Studies at the University of Toronto. He has published extensively on the history of seventeenth-century Russia, especially on the relations of church and state.

Deborah Thalheimer Long, who earned her PhD from Princeton University in 2000, is currently pursuing a master's in theology at St. Mary's Seminary and University in Baltimore, Maryland. She has taught at Notre Dame of Maryland, and worked, spoke, and published on the *Charrette Project*.

Mark David Luce is a PhD student at the University of Chicago. He has written a number of articles on women in Afghanistan, the Arab conquests, and Persian literature. He is a medievalist with particular interests in the development of a Persian-Turkish Islamic identity in Khurasan and central Asia from the eighth through the eleventh centuries.

Elizabeth Maxey is a PhD candidate at Cornell University, New York, and is currently working on her dissertation as a Five College Associate. Her work focuses on medieval treatments of Ovid's *Metamorphoses*, particularly the *Ovide Moralisé*.

Claudia M. Mejía is a lecturer at Tufts University, Massachusetts. She has an MA in Latin American literature and culture with a minor in Spanish medieval literature at Boston College.

Patit Paban Mishra is professor of history in Sambalpur University, Orissa, India. He is the author of several books, and his articles have been published in various reputed journals. Dr. Mishra regularly attends national and international conferences and has presented seminar papers and chaired sessions in Amsterdam, Bangkok, Berlin, Dekalb, Edinburgh, Hanoi, Moscow, Singapore, Vientiane, and Warsaw. He is connected with different academic organizations and international projects and has contributed many articles to encyclopedias published in the United States. He was the president, Indian History Congress, Countries other than India, 2004.

Nicole Mitchell is a graduate student at the University of Alabama, pursuing a master's degree in library and information sciences. She previously was the assistant archivist for a public liberal arts university in Georgia. Her research interests include southern history and the Georgia penitentiary.

K. Sarah-Jane Murray received her PhD in 2003 from Princeton University, where she was awarded the Porter Ogden Jacobus Prize for outstanding academic achievement and promise. She is currently assistant professor of medieval literature and French at the Baylor University Honors College. She is also codirector of the award-winning manuscript archive, *The Charrette Project*. Murray's research focuses on the fusion of Celtic and classical traditions in twelfth-century storytelling.

She has published articles on topics ranging from Chrétien de Troyes, Marie de France, Plato's *Timaeus*, and the *Song of Roland*, to humanities, computing, and foreign language pedagogy.

Kathryn O'Keeffe graduated from Princeton University in 2005 with a BA in public and international affairs and certificates in French and Spanish. In 2005–2006, she was selected to participate in the French Embassy exchange, and taught English in Paris. Her major research interests include cultural policy in northern Ireland as well as French and Spanish literature.

T. Brice Pearce is a graduate student in ancient history at the University of New Hampshire. His research focuses on class, race, gender, sexuality, and religion in the ancient Mediterranean world. As an undergraduate at Indiana University of Pennsylvania, he was a founder and the inaugural editor-in-chief of *The Endnote: Student Journal of the Department of History*, and received the Senior Seminar Research Award.

Kim M. Phillips is senior lecturer in history at the University of Auckland, New Zealand, where she has been teaching since 1997. She received her DPhil in medieval studies from the University of York in 1998. Her publications include *Medieval Maidens: Young Women and Gender in England, 1270–1540* (2003) and *Young Medieval Women* (1999). She also coedited *Sexualities in History: A Reader* (2002). Her research covers a wide range of topics relating to medieval gender, sexualities, and the body, and she is working on a new project, *Before Orientalism: Medieval Representations of the Far East*.

Gillian Polack received her MA from the Centre of Medieval Studies, University of Toronto, and her PhD from the University of Sydney. She currently teaches at the Australian National University.

Edward J. Rielly is professor of English at Saint Joseph's College of Maine. His teaching interests include medieval literature, eighteenth-century British literature, popular culture, and writing courses. He has published ten books of poetry, most recently, *Ways of Looking* (2005), as well as *Approaches to Teaching Swift's Gulliver's Travels* (1988), *Baseball: An Encyclopedia of Popular Culture* (2005), *Baseball and American Culture: Across the Diamond* (2003), *The 1960s* (2003), and *F. Scott Fitzgerald: A Biography* (2005).

Margaret Sankey is associate professor of history at Minnesota State University Moorhead, researching early–eighteenth-century Britain. Her book, *Jacobite Prisoners of the 1715 Rebellion: Preventing and Punishing Insurrection in Early Hanoverian Britain*, was published in 2005.

John T. Sebastian is assistant professor of medieval literature at Loyola University New Orleans. He specializes in Middle English writing, especially dramatic and mystical works, and his current projects include an article on processional dramaturgy in the York Cycle. His research spans the literatures of several European vernacular languages and has been supported by two separate Mellon Foundation fellowships.

Katherine Allen Smith is assistant professor of history at the University of Puget Sound in Tacoma, Washington. Her research focuses on monastic communities, devotional culture, and gender in high medieval Europe.

Georgia Tres is currently visiting assistant professor at Oakland University in Rochester, Michigan. She has a PhD from Wayne State University, for which she wrote a dissertation titled *The Discreet Charm of Spanish Patriarchy: The Representation of Masculinities in the Films of Fernando Rey*. She has also contributed to *Women and War: An Historical Encyclopedia* (2006) and *The Age of Imperialism: 1800–1914* (forthcoming).

Jitendra Uttam is assistant professor at Jawaharlal Nehru University in New Delhi, India. She has a deep interest in esthetics and culture.

Sinda K. Vanderpool earned her doctorate in French literature from Princeton University in

2005. She has written on women's writing in the Middle Ages and Renaissance, foreign language learning, and female expressions of religious belief. She is currently the director of Baylor University's College of Arts and Sciences advisement program.

Lavanya Vemsani is assistant professor of Asian history at Shawnee State University, Ohio. She has previously taught Asian religions at McMaster University and St. Thomas University in Canada. Prior to her PhD in religious studies from McMaster University, Canada, she obtained a PhD in history from University of Hyderabad, India.

Susan W. Wade, MA, MPhil, ABD, is a graduate student in medieval history at New York University. She is in the final stages of her PhD dissertation, "Miraculous Seeing and Monastic Identity: Miracles of the Visual from the Monasteries of Lobbes and Nivelles," which examines the influence of medieval discourses of visuality on the formulation and gendering of monastic identity.

Andrew J. Waskey is associate professor of philosophy and government at Dalton State College, Dalton, Georgia, where he teaches courses in government, philosophy, logic, and world religions. He received his PhD from the University of Southern Mississippi in 1978 with a dissertation on John Calvin's doctrine of civil disobedience. His major works include "Federalism" for multiple editions of *People and Politics: An Introduction to American Government*, edited by Mary Kate Hiatt; and *Political Perspectives: A Reader*, which he coedited. He has published over 200 articles in encyclopedias and journals on anthropology, geography, history, law, management, military history, philosophy, politics, political theory, public administration, and religion and has edited a book of philosophy readings. Since the September 11, 2001, terrorist attacks in America, he has published a glossary of Islamic terrorist terms for training law enforcement personnel, and has lectured on Islamic terrorism for the Federal Bureau of Investigation (FBI) and other groups. He is an ordained Presbyterian minister and has been serving a small country church part time since 1990.

Brannon Wheeler is associate professor of history and politics at the United States Naval Academy in Annapolis, where he is director of the Center for Middle East and Islamic Studies. He has published widely in the areas of Islamic studies and the history of religions, and has had visiting appointments and fellowships throughout Europe and the Middle East.

Ping Yao is associate professor of Chinese history at the California State University, Los Angeles. She has written extensively on gender in Chinese history and is the author of *Women's Lives in Tang China* (2004).

Vanessa Yosten is currently pursuing her BA in sociology at Baylor University with a focus on gender studies. Her academic interests include social justice, women's rights and women's history, and foreign cultures. Vanessa's current research includes studying in depth the history, practice, and social implications of all kinds of female genital mutilation, and exploring the Eugenics movements and forced sterilization in the United States.

Hannah Zdansky graduated from the Baylor University Honors College with distinction in 2006, specializing in English. She has received a Fulbright Scholarship to study in Ireland. Her research interests include medieval literature and the Celtic tradition. Hannah's current research focuses on the concept of *caritas* as portrayed in medieval religious and secular writings.